Praise for *The Low-FODMAP Diet Step by Step*

"Low FODMAP eating is a proven remedy for many suffering with chronic digestive problems, but it can be a daunting road to navigate without the right help. Enter the dream-team, Kate and Dédé, top notch professionals who guide you through, step-by-step, with a clear, doable plan and excellent recipes, so you can heal and stay healthy while enjoying delicious food all along the way."

—ELLIE KRIEGER MS RD

"I believe all foods should be celebrated and enjoyed by everyone but for those who suffer with food intolerance this can pose a challenge. I ask you to put your trust in Kate Scarlata and Dédé Wilson, for these two experts have spun fresh, whole ingredients into culinary gold, with their all low FODMAP recipes designed specifically for those who suffer with a sensitive gut. Let the love affair begin with Yogurt Marinated Grilled Lamb Kebobs or Pan Seared Salmon & Greens with Balsamic Soy Glaze to homemade soups, fresh and wholesome salads and delectable baked goods. Sink your teeth into amazing food while you enjoy the freedom from your IBS symptoms in this groundbreaking book, *The Low-FODMAP Diet Step by Step*."

—SUVIR SARAN, EXECUTIVE CHEF, COOKBOOK
AUTHOR, AND FARMER

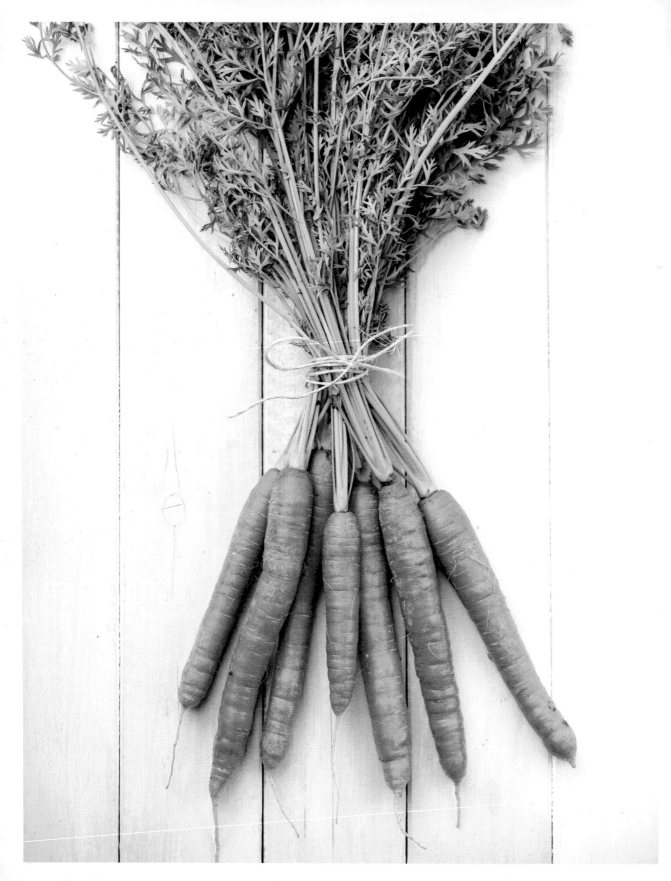

THE
LOW-FODMAP
DIET *Step by Step*

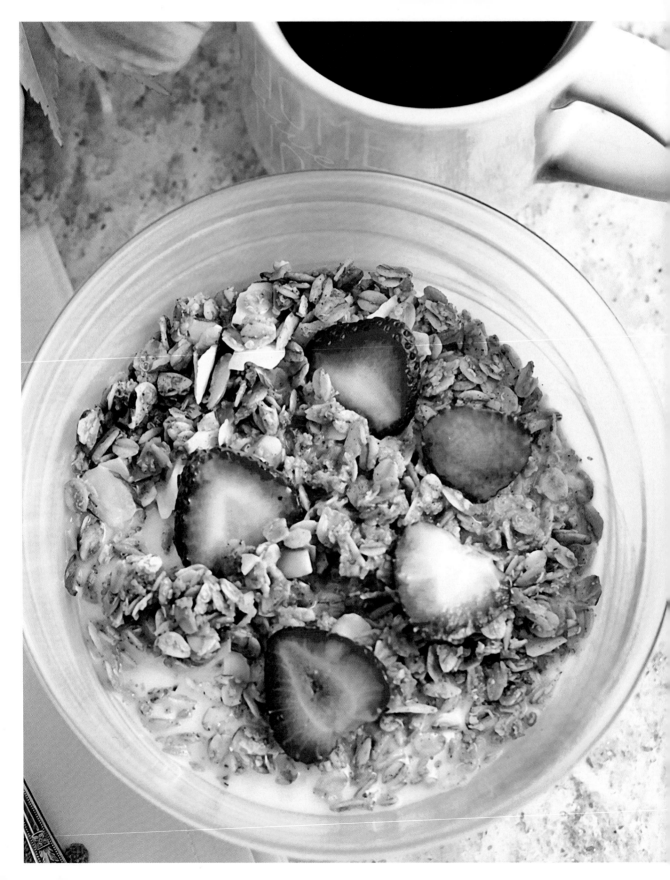

THE
LOW-FODMAP
DIET *Step by Step*

A Personalized Plan to Relieve the Symptoms of IBS
and Other Digestive Disorders—with more than

130 DELICIOUSLY SATISFYING RECIPES

Kate Scarlata RDN, LDN
and Dédé Wilson

Da Capo

LIFE
LONG

PERSEUS BOOKS | HACHETTE BOOK GROUP

Food photography copyright © 2017 by Dédé Wilson. Pages iv, 36, 58, 88, 98, 109, 114, 123, 132, 143, 151, 154, 162, 177, 179, 185, 186, 204, 208, 217, 223, 231, 234, 238, 245, 250, 253, 264, 274, 281, 290, 295, 289, 301, 306, 313, 325, 331, 325, 339, 341

Additional food photography © istockphoto.com. Pages 195, 259; All other photos © 123rf.com.

Da Capo Press
Hachette Book Group
1290 Avenue of the Americas, New York, NY 10104
DaCapoPress.com
@DaCapoPress
Printed in the United States of America

First Edition: January 2018

Published by Da Capo Press, an imprint of Perseus Books, LLC, a subsidiary of Hachette Book Group, Inc.

The Hachette Speakers Bureau provides a wide range of authors for speaking events. To find out more, go to www.hachettespeakersbureau.com or call (866) 376-6591.

The publisher is not responsible for websites (or their content) that are not owned by the publisher.

Print book interior design by Tabitha Lahr.

Library of Congress Cataloging-in-Publication Data has been applied for.

ISBNs: 978-0-7382-1934-9 (paperback), 978-0-7382-1965-6 (e-book)

LSC-C

10 9 8 7 6 5 4 3 2

"As a registered dietitian specializing in digestive health and nutrition for thirty years, I can honestly say the most rewarding work to date has been with IBS patients implementing the low FODMAP-diet approach. Like waving a magic wand, the low FODMAP diet can literally make their debilitating pain disappear in days! I am grateful for the innovative research in the area of diet and gut health and for my wonderful patients that have allowed me to share in their journey back to great health."

–KATE SCARLATA

"I had been suffering with IBS for over twenty-five years until one day, Dr. Joseph P. Tassoni Jr. scribbled the word 'FODMAP' on a piece of paper and handed it to me while I lay in my hospital bed. I had been admitted with extreme abdominal pain related to my gastrointestinal issues. He told me to look up the Monash University smart phone app and give this diet a try. It was quite literally a turning point in my life. This book is dedicated to him and to all the others, like me, who have suffered unnecessarily."

–DÉDÉ WILSON

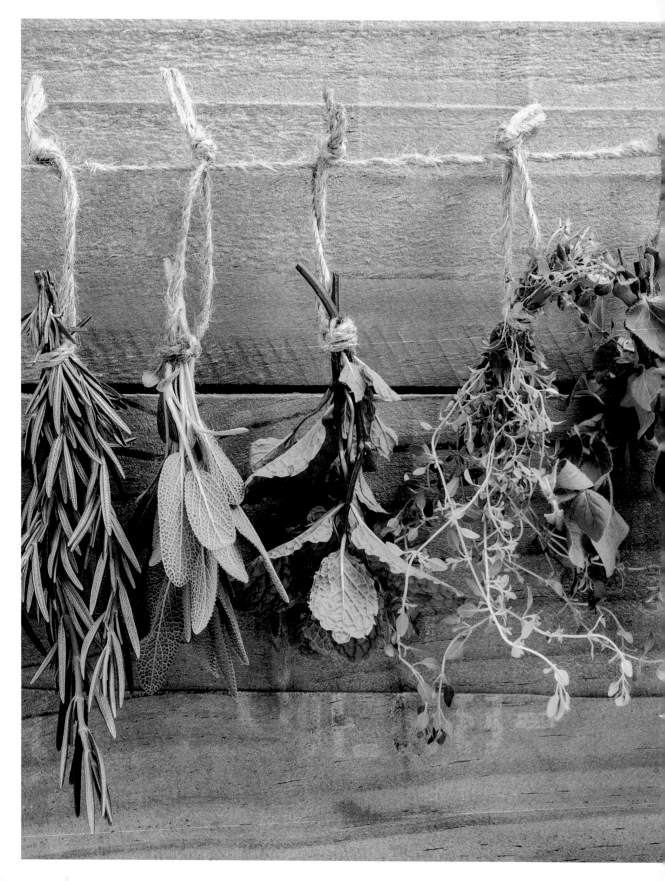

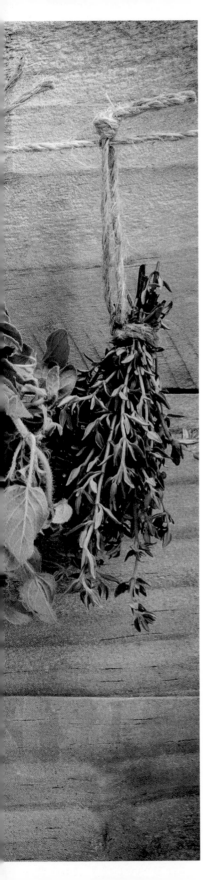

CONTENTS

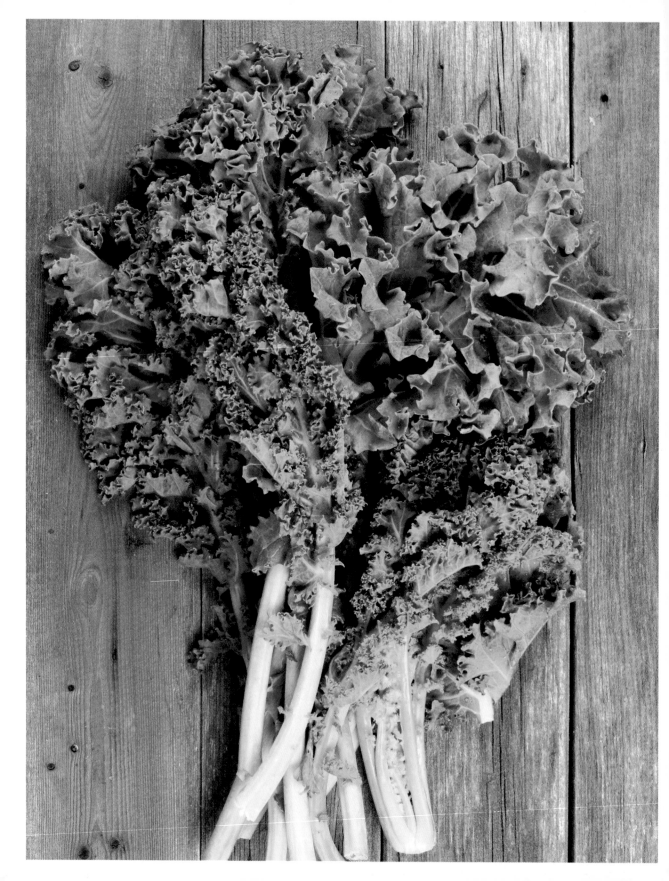

INTRODUCTION

SUFFERING WITH A SENSITIVE TUMMY? We get it. Digestive distress is on the rise globally and can interrupt the quality of life you deserve.

Clinical trials have proven that **up to 70 to 75 percent of those with IBS can attain relief by following a low FODMAP diet.** And modifying FODMAP carbohydrates has been shown to offer symptom benefit in those with GERD, IBD, celiac disease, and intestinal resections, too. Kate Scarlata, RDN, is a pioneer in the low FODMAP field and a research collaborator with Monash University, and Dédé Wilson, a former *Bon Appétit* magazine contributing editor, brings thirty years of proven recipe development for the home cook.

Kate and Dédé both have had up close and personal experience of suffering with IBS symptoms for years. Dédé was diagnosed with IBS in 1990 and Kate suffered a major intestinal resection nearly twenty-three years ago, resulting in debilitating digestive symptoms. Both of us turned our lives around using the innovative low FODMAP diet to manage our unending and painful digestive symptoms.

As FODMAPers ourselves, we understand the pain, fear, and confusion of living with digestive symptoms while also experiencing firsthand what a dramatic difference eating a low FODMAP diet can make. With our insider and expertise knowledge, we have done the heavy lifting for the millions of IBS sufferers like you who really need this resource to adapt to low FODMAP living with ease.

The low FODMAP nutritional approach was created by Australian researchers at Monash University in Melbourne, Australia, and it is time that more sufferers worldwide were aware of its power. For years, gastroenterologists and dietitians had little to offer to help their IBS patients, until now. This book shares the most current research and also provides accurate low FODMAP recipes without sacrificing good taste and good living.

The key is knowing what foods are okay to eat and which ones must be avoided—and then incorporating that knowledge into your everyday life. When you minimize FODMAPs in your diet, you can relieve an enormous amount of physical agony and emotional distress—for some, literally overnight! For up to 20 percent of Americans, the low FODMAP diet is their ticket to a new life. The low FODMAP diet is an empowering solution for an everyday problem. We provide nutritionally sound advice with delicious and approachable recipes to help those with IBS not only feel better—but to thrive.

This book covers everything you need to know, such as what FODMAPs are, why eating a low FODMAP diet might make a difference for IBS symptoms, and, the best part: 125 recipes covering the basics, breakfast, easy-to-pack lunches, snacks, dinners, soups, salads, sides, desserts, and baked goods. As the FODMAPing dietitian, Kate provides the nutritional science and research, while Dédé developed the recipes and both offer lifestyle tips—a powerhouse combo providing you with a book of sound, up-to-date medical advice and delectable recipes for the everyday life of the FODMAPer. These are recipes that will satisfy everyone in your family, whether they are following the diet or not. This book offers real-life solutions to a worldwide problem.

—KATE & DÉDÉ

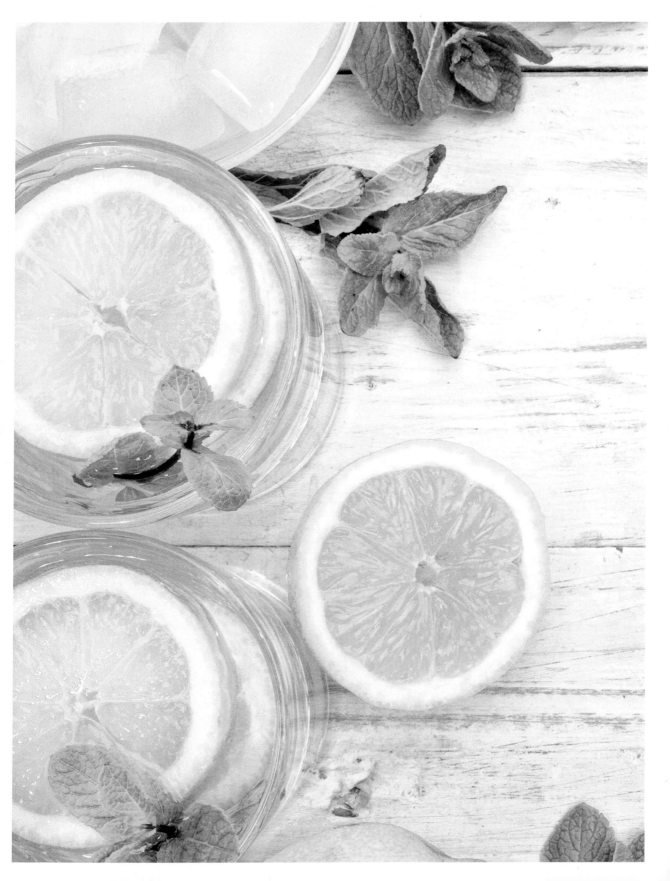

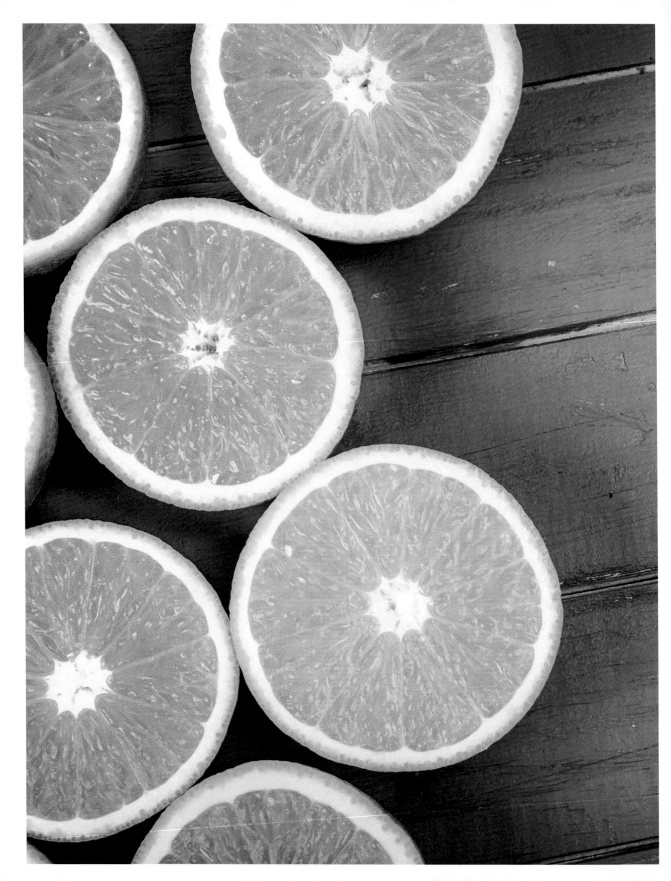

Chapter 1

GUT ISSUES? THE ROLE OF FODMAPS IN DIGESTIVE DISTRESS

DISTRESSED BY DIGESTIVE SYMPTOMS? You are not alone. One in four people in the United States suffers regularly with a faulty gastrointestinal (GI) tract leading to uncomfortable symptoms. Irritable bowel syndrome (IBS), an unrelenting and often debilitating GI motility disorder, strikes one in seven Americans, resulting in gas, bloating, cramping, pain, and alteration in bowel habits.[1] Celiac disease, inflammatory bowel disease, heartburn, and gastro-esophageal reflux (GERD) are just a few of the digestive diseases on the rise, globally. Increasingly, many are stopped in their tracks due to digestive discord. Because GI symptoms can't be seen, just felt, and topics about digestive distress are often taboo, many simply suffer in silence. Here's the good news: We have an effective, holistic nutrition solution for you and your troubled gut!

By simply modifying certain sugars and fibers in your diet, collectively known as FODMAP carbohydrates, you may find your tummy troubles are completely gone, literally in one day! Don't be put off by the big, somewhat intimidating acronym FODMAP. We will break everything down for you in real English. As a brief introduction, FODMAP carbohydrates include lactose, fructose (in excess of glucose in a food), fructans, galacto-oligosaccharides, and polyols, types of sugars and fibers found in everyday foods, such as apple, pear, watermelon, wheat, onion, and garlic, to name a few. When FODMAP carbohydrates are malabsorbed in the intestine, they drag water into the gut, stretching it. Furthermore, the residential gut microbes feast off the poorly digested FODMAPs, creating gas. If you have a sensitive tummy, these malabsorbed carbohydrates can cause a cascade of GI symptoms. Although you may think a diet to calm your digestive woes will be bland, tasteless, and full of deprivation, we have the most delicious solution right here for you, using fresh whole foods that you can easily find in any supermarket. This book will help you customize your own low FODMAP plan; you'll quell your upset belly with easy-to-prepare recipes that will soon be your new family favorites, for the low FODMAP diet followers and their family members alike. Before we get to the plan and recipes, let's talk a bit more about digestive problems and how changing your diet just might turn your life around in only a few days.

Gut Problems? Common GI Disorders

As mentioned, **irritable bowel syndrome (IBS)** is a digestive health condition that presents with abdominal bloating, gas, pain, alteration in bowel habits, urgency, or a feeling of incomplete emptying. It is the most common intestinal disorder diagnosed by gastroenterologists and occurrs in 7 to 20 percent of the US population, impacting the quality of life of 25 to 45 million Americans![2] In addition to experiencing digestive distress, individuals with IBS often suffer anxiety and depression. IBS can develop at any age and is more common in women than men.[3]

The symptoms of IBS appear due to a malfunction in the way your intestine, brain, and nervous system talk and/or work with one another. People with IBS may have other coexisting digestive disorders, such as inflammatory bowel disease (IBD), GERD, celiac disease, lactose intolerance, or nonceliac gluten or wheat sensitivity; IBS can also appear on its own.

For years, patients with IBS have connected food as a symptom trigger. Yet only very recently has the medical community offered an effective nutritional approach that works to keep symptoms at bay. Researchers at Melbourne, Australia's Monash University proved through numerous studies that a specific group of commonly malabsorbed carbohydrates are the culprit for symptom exacerbation in many with IBS. In fact, studies worldwide have shown that about 3 in 4 IBS patients will experience symptom relief from following a diet modified in foods rich in FODMAP carbohydrates.[4]

Gastro-esophageal reflux (GERD) occurs commonly with a sensation of burning in the throat, often referred to as heartburn, a sour or bitter taste in the mouth, difficulty with swallowing, or a dry cough. The changing diet landscape, obesity epidemic, and stress are likely all contributing factors to the rise in this condition. It is estimated that GERD occurs in 18 to 28 percent of North Americans.[5] The low FODMAP diet might help mitigate GERD symptoms, as some indigestible carbohydrates can lower the pressure of the lower esophageal sphincter, the door between the stomach and esophagus. The lower pressure allows the sphincter to open more readily, releasing the acidic stomach contents into the esophagus, causing GERD symptoms. Fructans, a fiber and source of FODMAPs, have been linked with reflux.[6] More on these frustrating fructans later in this chapter.

Inflammatory bowel disease (IBD) is not the same as IBS. It primarily includes **Crohn's disease and ulcerative colitis**, which are chronic autoimmune disorders that present with inflammation in the intestine. They differ slightly: Crohn's disease can occur anywhere in the digestive tract, but most often in the lowest section of the small intestine, whereas ulcerative colitis is limited to the large intestine only. The low FODMAP diet has been shown to help manage ongoing IBS-like symptoms in those with IBD.[7]

Does the Modern Diet Fuel Gut Inflammation?

Gut microbes feast on the foods we don't digest adequately, mostly fibers and carbs, but also some protein and fats. It has been proposed that the Western (modern-day) diet is partly responsible for the rise in digestive diseases and unhealthy changes in our gut microbiome. For instance, animal studies have shown an increase in inflammation in the gut and a shift of bacteria into the small intestine resulting from use of emulsifiers in our food supply.[8] Eating processed fats, refined grains, and sugar has been shown to also alter the microbes in our gut, leading to potential harmful and inflammatory bacterial-derived metabolites. Human-made high-fructose corn syrup (HFCS) intake, a potential source of excess fructose, has skyrocketed in our food supply over the years, and is associated with fatty liver and inflammatory bacterial endotoxins. The connection between diet, gut microbes, and digestive disorders is under vigorous study at this time, and truth be told, researchers have really only scratched the surface of this important area of study. There is no doubt that what we choose to put in our mouth is important for our gut health.

Celiac disease is an autoimmune condition in which gluten is toxic to the small intestine. Celiac disease is on the rise, occurring in at least 3 million, or in about 1 in 133 Americans. Untreated, celiac disease can present with IBS-like symptoms; left untreated, it can also put a person at risk for intestinal cancer, infertility, osteoporosis, anemia, and other autoimmune conditions. Unfortunately, most people with celiac disease don't know they have it. According to the University of Chicago's renowned celiac center, only about 17 percent of individuals with celiac disease have been diagnosed. On average, it takes eleven years for a person with symptoms to be diagnosed. Despite strict vigilance to a gluten-free diet, 20 to 23 percent of treated celiac patients fulfill the diagnostic criteria for IBS.[9] For these individuals, a low FODMAP gluten-free diet may offer improved symptom management.

Small intestinal bacterial overgrowth (SIBO) occurs when abnormal amounts of gut microbes seed the small intestine and overgrow in great numbers. Normally, the small intestine has limited bacteria. When bacteria populate the narrow tube of the small intestine, they will consume and ferment any small carbohydrates that escape digestion. The resultant fermentation can lead to pain, cramping, distention, and bloating; some sufferers may experience constipation; others may have diarrhea. Symptoms of SIBO mimic those seen in IBS. Although not adequately studied in the research setting, many SIBO sufferers find symptom relief on a low FODMAP diet, as FODMAPs are fast food for small intestinal microbes.

Digestion 101

Understanding the science of digestion can be helpful when sorting out your personal digestive challenges. Digestion is individual. What works for you might not work for your best friend. This is due to important factors, such as the genes we inherited from our parents and what microbes reside in our gut. The colon is one of the most diverse ecosystems on Earth! And we all have our very own "fingerprint" of microbes that reside there. Microbes play a big part in the digestive process. They produce digestive enzymes we don't have. In fact, the human body has twenty genes relating to carbohydrate digestion and some microbes have over two hundred! Some microbes, called vigorous fermenters, are capable of creating copious amounts of gas from our undigested food. When microbes ferment carbs, they produce carbon dioxide, hydrogen, and/or methane gas, which can impact intestinal movement. Too much methane gas in the intestine is associated with constipation, whereas elevation in hydrogen gas is associated with diarrhea. Our gut microbes not only help us digest foods but they regulate our immune system and synthesize vitamins for us, too.

The digestive tract comprises the mouth, esophagus, stomach, and small and large intestine. Digestion starts in your mouth. Your pearly whites are meant to break up food, increasing its surface area, which allows the digestive enzymes in your saliva to start the process of digestion. Most of what we eat should be broken down partially in the stomach and in the small intestine, where nutrients are actively transported into the bloodstream to nourish and energize our body. Wolfing down food and rushing while eating incorporates more air into your digestive tract, setting yourself up for faulty digestion and intestinal distress. Try your best to set aside time to eat in a relaxed setting.

Residual undigested food matter, mostly fiber, but also some poorly absorbed protein, carbs, and fats will move from your small intestine into the colon. The primary role of the colon is to absorb water, provide residence to important gut microbes that further break down foods, create important vitamins, and eliminate the end products of digestion. When too much undigested food substrates arrive in the colon, the residential microbes feast and create the all too well-known and felt plentiful amounts of gas.

The human intestine is made up of a complex of nerves and muscles that help move food along the GI tract. Two major modes of operation occur in the intestine: the eating mode and the cleaning mode. When you eat, your intestine is secreting digestive enzymes and sloshing the food around to break down the nutrients into their digestible form. When you are not eating, your intestine will initiate a repetitive and important housecleaning wave, called the migrating motor complex, to clean up the small bowel and to get it prepared for the next meal. It is important to leave three to four hours between eating, to allow this cleansing wave to take place; otherwise, your small intestine can become a petri dish as microbes, food, and debris can accumulate. For this reason, we recommend eating three meals and one snack per day rather than several small meals or a grazing-style eating pattern. Yes, you and your sensitive gut need a little downtime between meals!

Understanding the Gut Microbiome

The gut microbiome is the collection of microbes and all of their genes residing in our gastrointestinal tract and includes bacteria, viruses, and fungi. The combination of microbes that live within us is individual. Which microbes reside in our gut depend on numerous factors, including where we live, what we eat, and what antibiotics we have taken during our lifetime, to name a few. The microbes in our intestine weigh collectively 2.5 to 3 pounds! They help keep our immune system functioning, make vitamins, and aid digestion. Microbes can cohabitate in harmony or can get out of balance, in a condition called dysbiosis. Because what we eat plays a role in the delicate balance of microbes, and the low FODMAP diet is a new therapy, we are unsure of the effects of following the diet strictly for the long term. Research has shown that the low FODMAP diet increases diversity of bacteria in the gut (a good thing), but also reduces some probiotic bacteria, too. This is one of the key reasons that we walk you through the three phases of the low FODMAP diet in this book. We want to help you reintroduce FODMAPs to your personal tolerance level rather than unnecessarily restricting your diet, for your good health and that of your microbes, too!

What You Need to Know Prior to Changing Your Diet

First off, do not self-diagnose yourself with any GI disorder. Visit with your primary care doctor and/ or a gastroenterologist to rule out serious conditions for your GI distress, such as untreated celiac disease, inflammatory bowel disease, small intestinal bacterial overgrowth, GERD, parasitic infections, or even in the rare instance, cancer. Understand that in some instances, diet may be only part of your treatment plan along with other traditional medical therapies.

A special note about celiac disease: It is advised that you be screened for celiac disease before embarking on the low FODMAP diet. Treatment for celiac disease is a lifelong gluten-free diet. Although the low FODMAP diet is not a gluten-free diet, it does reduce gluten intake. Testing for celiac disease requires adequate gluten intake, so the test may not be accurate if it occurs while following the low FODMAP diet.

Gluten and IBS Symptoms

Some people who do not have celiac disease do note symptom improvement on a gluten-free diet. Gluten sensitivity, otherwise known as nonceliac gluten sensitivity (NCGS), presents with a cascade of symptoms associated with eating gluten, including brain fog, depression, hyperactivity, joint pain, and IBS-like symptoms. although these symptoms may occur in people with celiac disease, those with NCGS do not have the genes or antibodies present for celiac disease to occur. The symptoms, however, dissipate when gluten is removed from the diet and reoccur when gluten intake is resumed.

Research has shown that in people with NCGS who have digestive symptoms, the elimination of gluten (which simultaneously restricts FODMAP-containing grains: wheat, barley, and rye) from the diet might lessen gastrointestinal symptoms, but this effect is likely due to the reduction in FODMAPs rather than the elimination of gluten.[10] If you are unsure whether you are gluten sensitive, we recommend you work with a registered dietitian to guide you. If you have irritable bowel syndrome, the research suggests that FODMAPs (not gluten) in your diet are the most likely contributor to your digestive complaints.

Let's Talk FODMAPs

As previously mentioned, FODMAPs are a group of small carbohydrates found in many everyday foods. This collection of small sugars and fibers are commonly malabsorbed in the intestine and can contribute to GI distress in someone with a sensitive gut. "FODMAP" is an acronym for fermentable oligosaccharides, disaccharides, monosaccharides, and polyols. Whew! That's a mouthful.

Unfortunately, you don't often see the terms *oligosaccharide* or *disaccharide* on a food label. Deciphering what foods have these FODMAPs can be tricky. No need to worry; we've got you covered! The following chart offers a closer look at the FODMAP acronym and FODMAP subtypes (lactose, excess fructose, fructans, galacto-oligosaccharides, sorbitol, and mannitol).

Why Are FODMAPs Malabsorbed?

Lactose, the sugar in cow's, sheep's, and goat's milk, is commonly maldigested. For lactose to be adequately absorbed in the intestine, the enzyme lactase needs to be present. Unfortunately, lactase enzyme production reduces as we age, and genetically some ethnicities, such as Asians and African Americans, make less lactase. Small amounts of lactose (0 to 2 grams) as found in hard cheese and butter should not trigger typical lactose malabsorption symptoms, such as gas and bloating, and can be enjoyed while on the low FODMAP diet. Foods with larger amounts of lactose, such as the 12 grams found in 1 cup (240 ml) of milk, however, may trigger IBS symptoms and are not allowed on the low FODMAP diet.

Fructose, a one-chain sugar that is slowly absorbed throughout the small intestine, is best absorbed when glucose is present at the same time. When the fructose content of a food exceeds the glucose content, we call that a source of "excess fructose." Transporters in our intestine help move fructose from our intestine into our blood for absorption and some rely on glucose to guide the process. Some people lack some of the fructose transporters, making fructose malabsorption (FM) more likely. Previous surgical resection of the small intestine or a fast-moving small intestine can also contribute to the malabsorption of fructose. FM is quite common, occurring in 1 in 3 people; however, not everyone experiences symptoms from malabsorbing fructose. For those who

FODMAP: The Acronym	
F: Fermentable	Creates gas by being broken down by gut microbes
O: Oligosaccharides	Oligosaccharides are water-soluble fibers; namely, **fructans and galacto-oligosaccharides (GOS).**
D: Disaccharides	Disaccharide is the two-chain sugar **lactose.**
M: Monosaccharides	Monosaccharide is the one-chain sugar **fructose** (when in excess of glucose in a food).
A: and	
P: Polyols	Polyols, also known as sugar alcohols, include **mannitol** and **sorbitol, isomalt, xylitol,** and **maltitol.**

Note: *Saccharide* is another name for sugar.

develop symptoms with excess fructose ingestion, the low FODMAP approach certainly can help! Foods with equal amounts of fructose and glucose, or those that contain more glucose than fructose, are absorbed more efficiently and considered suitable choices for the low FODMAP diet. It appears that the intestine has a limited capacity to handle too much fructose (even when glucose is present) all at once; therefore, we recommend you limit yourself to one serving of fruit per meal or snack time. The goal is to absorb fructose adequately to ward off any potential GI distress caused by its malabsorption. We will remind you throughout the book how we would like you to modify your fruit servings. Fruit is delicious and nourishing, but like most things in the low FODMAP realm, it is all about moderation and balance.

Lastly, let's talk about fructans, galacto-oligosaccharide (GOS), and polyols. Oligosaccharides (fructans and GOS) are malabsorbed by all humans, as we lack the enzymes to break them apart. GOS are found in all beans, such as kidney beans and black beans. Although we know a big bowl of chili will give rise to intestinal gas in just about everyone, if you have IBS, the gas can lead to debilitating pain. Polyols, also known as sugar alcohols, are poorly absorbed, too, especially when consumed in large quantities. Sorbitol and mannitol are the most prevalent polyols found naturally in foods, but they may also be used as sweeteners in sugar-free gum and mints, along with other manufactured polyols, such as xylitol, maltitol, and isomalt. Note the *-ol* ending when reading labels. Sorbitol and mannitol are absorbed slowly and insufficiently via pores in the small intestine. Some polyols may be absorbed, but all too often, they are too big or move too quickly through the intestine and can contribute to diarrhea, especially when consumed in larger quantities. Inflammation in the intestine may reduce pore size, making polyol malabsorption even more likely. For example, in an individual with newly diagnosed celiac disease or inflammatory bowel disease where inflammation plays a big role, polyol absorption likely will be impaired.

Malabsorbing FODMAPs does not cause IBS or contribute to symptoms for everyone. For individuals with a highly sensitive intestine, however, the malabsorbed FODMAPs can lead to major digestive distress.

How Do FODMAPs Contribute to IBS Symptoms?

Short-chain, in other words, small FODMAP, carbohydrates pull water into the small intestine, stretching the intestinal wall, which can contribute to pain, cramping, and bloating. The extra water travels to the colon, where it can lead to diarrhea in people with a fast-moving intestine. Those with a sluggish intestine might feel cramps and pain from the water stretching the intestine, like a water balloon inside their gut! Moreover, these poorly digested FODMAPs arrive in the colon intact and become a hearty food supply for the millions of microbes that reside there. When the microbes feed off the FODMAPs, the act of fermentation creates copious amounts of gas.

An additional side effect of fermentation is the production of short-chain fatty acids (SCFA). SCFAs can typically be a healthy side effect of fermentation in the intestine, as they can act as nourishing fuel for the cells of the colon. SCFAs, however, can speed the motility of the large intestine, too, and can cause injury to the colon wall if there is an overproduction of these acids. It's all about balance.

The distention caused by the gas and water driven by malabsorbed FODMAPs is one way these poorly absorbed carbohydrates can contribute to GI distress, but additional factors may play a role also. When residential microbes feast on undigested sugars and fibers, they may produce toxic or inflammatory metabolites. The stretching of the intestine may cause the release of even more inflammatory chemicals via mast cells that line the intestine. Mast cells are filled with inflamatory compounds. As previously mentioned, people with IBS often experience anxiety and depressive symptoms. Interestingly, the low FODMAP diet has been shown in emerging research to minimize these symptoms; it appears the low FODMAP diet impacts the immune system of the gut and the brain, too, contributing to a reduction in these mental health conditions.[11] Nutritional science can be complex and the full beneficial effect of a low FODMAP diet for individuals with IBS is still being determined through further research.

Intolerance to FODMAPs Is Not a Food Allergy

When you are **allergic** to a food, your immune system identifies the food as harmful, targets it, and attacks it. Food allergies can lead to anaphylactic reactions (an allergic response that presents with swelling, lowered blood pressure, and dilated blood vessels) and in severe cases, death. The eight most common food allergens are wheat, eggs, tree nuts, peanuts, milk, soy, shellfish, and fish. FODMAP sensitivity is not an allergy; it is a form of food **intolerance**. Symptoms of food intolerance may include gas, bloating, hives, or diarrhea, but there are no anaphylactic reactions or life-threatening events. Let's be clear though, although not life threatening, food intolerance can be life debilitating.

The Low FODMAP Diet Overview: Eliminate-Challenge-Integrate

The low FODMAP diet is a three-phase approach, which we refer to it as Eliminate-Challenge-Integrate. During the first phase, **eliminate**, often referred to as the elimination diet, you will restrict high-FODMAP foods in an attempt to calm your digestive tract. The second phase, **challenge**, involves a methodical reintroduction of FODMAPs back into your diet to help you identify your individual triggers; you will go through "challenges" to see what your body can tolerate. The last phase, **integrate**, allows you to personalize your diet and integrate foods back into your diet that work just for you and your sensitive intestine. This might sound complicated, but it truly isn't. It does take time, but you are in control. You'll do the challenges yourself to learn more about your own body and what it can or cannot tolerate. This isn't something a doctor can simply tell you. Our three-phase process requires your full involvement—and it allows you to really take charge of your health.

The elimination phase of the low FODMAP diet is not a long-term diet. Rather, it is a two- to six-week dietary approach to guide you in identifying your IBS trigger foods, helping you minimize painful, sometimes embarrassing and life-disrupting IBS symptoms. The length of time on the elimination can vary person to person, but typically, by four weeks most people will be able to start the challenge phase. The diet can be tailored to your personal taste, but should include a wide range of healthy foods. It is essentially a learning diet. You will remove all FODMAP-rich foods from your diet to calm your digestive symptoms. Once your symptoms have abated, the challenge phase begins.

You will learn that some FODMAP-containing foods are definite culprits, causing your GI distress, and which others may safely and comfortably be added back to your nutritional repertoire. Once you determine what FODMAPs are *not* your triggers, you will then be able to integrate the nontrigger foods back into your diet, thus expanding your diet into a more personalized and liberal eating plan going forward.

Most people are able to add some FODMAP-containing foods back into their diet. The goal is to eventually eat as varied a diet as possible, adding back the FODMAP-rich foods that your body can tolerate comfortably. Many FODMAP-containing foods are innately healthy and should only be avoided if they cause intestinal distress. Eating a well-balanced and nourishing diet is essential for good health.

As you now know, the low FODMAP diet is not a FODMAP-free diet but one that focuses on **reducing the total amount** of FODMAPs you consume at one meal and over the course of the day. Everyone has an individual tolerance to how many and what types of FODMAPs he or she can handle at one time. That is, the more you have of them at one meal, the more likely you will feel symptoms. Likewise, individual foods that contain multiple FODMAPs may be more likely to trigger symptoms. Watermelon, for instance, has three different sources of FODMAPs—excess fructose, fructans, and mannitol!—so, it might be a tricky food to add back to your diet without symptoms. Additionally, your tolerance to FODMAPs can change over time.

Low- and High-FODMAP Foods

You'll have the most success with the diet if you try to focus on allowable foods rather than grieve the loss of your favorites. And don't *really* grieve the loss of FODMAP-rich foods because it is very possible you will be able to add some FODMAP-containing foods back into your diet after the elimination phase. Even during the elimination phase, you will be able to enjoy foods, such as our Garlic Mashed Potatoes (page 175) or the Slow-Roasted Pork Tacos with Citrus Slaw and Chipotle Mayo (page 235) with optional avocado.

Trust us; you won't go hungry! There are so many delicious and nutritious options, and all of the recipes in this book are suitable for the elimination phase. The following chart provides an overview of foods that are low, moderate, or high FODMAP. Please note that some foods on the low FODMAP list have quantities beside them, such as fruit portions. These are foods that are considered low FODMAP but only in the designated portion; if you eat too much of these particular foods at one sitting, you may get your tummy in a bunch. Our goal is to make you aware and knowledgeable! We want to ensure that you understand the ground rules so you can have the best chance of success with the low FODMAP diet. Lastly, we suggest you place great attention to the Low FODMAP Grocery List on page 45, which tell you all the wonderful foods you can eat while on the low FODMAP diet, including suitable fruits and veggies; low-lactose dairy foods; oils (which are innately FODMAP-free); and protein-rich foods, such as shellfish, eggs, chicken, and meats (most are FODMAP-free, too); along with suitable condiments, flour blends, and more. When you are ready to prepare your grocery shopping and menu plan, our Low FODMAP Grocery List and Pantry Picks will be your new best friends.

Forget about eating the high-FODMAP foods *for now*. Just remember, you likely will be able to add some back and should do so to your personal tolerance after the challenge phase of the diet.

If you are staring at this chart feeling a little nervous, we get it. We've been there personally. We are going to help you through the entire process and we promise you that you are going to be able to eat well and feel great doing it. You might want to flip through the book to take a nice gander at the yummy recipes that will make you feel better. You are about to embark on your new life, eating delicious and nutritious foods, all while eliminating the debilitating pain that has been haunting you, seemingly with no abatement. Our three-phase low FODMAP protocol is ready to take your hand and guide you.

You're in the Driver's Seat

It doesn't take long to learn that the low FODMAP diet has many nuances and can be a tricky diet to follow without guidance. There is a lot of confusion and inconsistent information online, which is partly due to the facts that this dietary approach is fairly new, food composition is variable, and FODMAP food analysis involves a complex testing process, taking up to three weeks to test just one food! FODMAP content in foods can vary depending on where a food has been grown, how ripe the food is, and what food processing has occurred. In fact, drying fruit (as when grapes become raisins) changes their FODMAP content all together.

If you are a rule follower and like things in black and white . . . well, you might just need to give yourself some wiggle room. Remember, the low FODMAP diet is not a FODMAP-free diet. Reducing your total FODMAP intake is generally good enough for most folks to feel symptom improvement. Do your best not to get too frustrated or hung up with discrepancies between our chart and the various food lists online. Although the acceptable low FODMAP foods have been modified over the years, the low FODMAP diet has been successfully helping IBS patients for the past ten years, despite the slight changes on the food lists!

If you have a smartphone or tablet, you may want to look at the Monash University low-FODMAP diet app as a great resource to complement this book. The app is updated regularly with the latest FODMAP food analysis straight from the leaders in the world of FODMAPs. Recommended portion sizes are also provided to help guide you with FODMAP cutoff levels and mealtime limits. Some need to be more diligent than others when following the low FODMAP diet as the degree of their gut sensitivity and microbes differ from one person's to another's. If you have previously tried the low FODMAP diet with only marginal results, perhaps try following our low FODMAP meal plan on page 50 to better guide you. And remember, not all IBS patients will experience 100 percent symptom relief on the low FODMAP diet, though many do. See "When Diet Isn't Enough," page 33, for other potential issues.

7 Days to a New You

In seven days or less you will likely know whether the low FODMAP diet is working.

That's right. A bold statement to be sure, but in Kate's practice and in a Monash University study, most patients notice substantial GI symptom improvement almost immediately. Certainly after a week, you will know if the diet is having a positive effect.[12] In fact, Dédé could "feel" how great the diet felt within 24 hours! Think about the pain and suffering that you have been experiencing, and give the low FODMAP diet a try for a week. That's it. *Seven days*. Promise yourself that you will eat a strict low FODMAP diet for one week. For you. For a new lease on life. It truly has been life changing for both Kate and Dédé and for the thousands of patients Kate has worked with. From people who couldn't travel due to an unreliable digestive tract, to those who feared dating, and many that held off on having a child due to their constant agony; today their lives are forever changed. Now, folks are jet-setting far and wide, enjoying time with new companions, and expanding their family circle. It's time for you to feel joy when you eat real foods that are delicious, nutritious, and leave you pain free with no sense of withdrawal or deprivation! So, turn the page. Let's get started!

FRUIT

Select one serving per meal. For example: ½ banana, 1 medium orange, ½ cup chopped fruit.

Low FODMAP

banana • dried banana chip • blueberries • breadfruit • cantaloupe • clementine • fresh coconut • dragon fruit • durian melon • grapes • ripe guava • honeydew • kiwifruit • lemons • limes • mandarin • orange • papayas • passion fruit • pineapple • plantains • prickly pears • raspberries • rhubarb • star fruit (carambola) • strawberries • tamarind

Moderate FODMAP (Use as accent to meal (~1 tablespoon) vs. consuming large servings as it is easy to exceed FODMAP threshold.)

avocados • dried coconut • dried cranberries • pomegranate • dried raisins

High FODMAP

apples • apricots • blackberries • boysenberries • cherries • currants • dates • figs • grapefruit • mangoes • nectarines • peaches • pears • persimmons • plums • prunes, tamarillo • watermelon

VEGETABLES AND LEGUMES

Low FODMAP

arugula • bamboo shoots • bok choy • bean sprouts • bell peppers • carrots • celery root (a.k.a. celeriac) • chives • collard greens • green or red cabbage (not savoy) • chiles • cucumber • eggplant • endive • fennel (bulb and stalk) • ginger (fresh or ground) • green beans • kabocha squash • kale • leeks (green part only) • lettuce • nori seaweed • okra • olives • parsnips • pattypan squash • potatoes (white) • radishes • rutabaga • scallions (green part only) • spaghetti squash • spinach • summer squash • Swiss chard • tomatoes (canned or fresh) • turnips • watercress • water chestnuts • zucchini

Moderate FODMAP

beet • broccoli • Brussels sprouts • butternut squash • celery • corn on the cob • canned pure pumpkin • sweet potato • taro • yucca; **Legumes:** drained and rinsed canned chickpeas • drained and rinsed canned lentils

High FODMAP

artichokes • asparagus • cauliflower • garlic • leeks • mushrooms • onion and garlic powder • shallots • Most beans (kidney, black, fava) • peas • savory cabbage • sugar snap peas • snow peas • soybeans

GRAINS, CEREALS, FLOURS, BAKED GOODS

Low FODMAP

gluten-free bread • brown rice tortillas • buckwheat • cornmeal • corn tortillas • millet • gluten-free pasta • oats • polenta • quinoa • quinoa flakes • rice (brown, white, basmati) • rice cakes • starch (corn, potato) • sorghum • sourdough spelt or sourdough wheat bread • tapioca • teff; **Note:** Avoid products with inulin or chicory root additives or other FODMAP ingredients.

Moderate FODMAP

amaranth • corn flakes

High FODMAP

rye, wheat, barley, or products made with these ingredients • **Bean-based flours:** chickpea, fava, or soy flour, coconut flour

PROTEIN

Low FODMAP

bacon • beef • eggs • fish • ham (check for FODMAP ingredients) • lamb • pork • poultry shellfish; **Bean-based:** tempeh • firm tofu

High FODMAP

meat products made with honey garlic, onion, or other FODMAP ingredients; **Bean-based:** silken tofu

FAT

Low FODMAP

Pure oils are free of FODMAPs . Avoid consuming particles of onion or garlic in flavored blends.

DAIRY AND DAIRY ALTERNATIVES

Low FODMAP

Beverages: almond milk • canned pure coconut milk (full-fat or light) • lactose-free cow's milk (whole, 2%, 1%, or fat-free) • hemp milk • rice milk; **Cheese:** Brie • Camembert • Colby • Cheddar • feta, goat cheese • Havarti • mozzarella • Parmesan and Parmigiano-Reggiano • pecorino and Pecorino Romano • Swiss • lactose-free cottage cheese • lactose-free cream cheese; **Other:** lactose-free ice cream (without FODMAP ingredients) • sorbet from acceptable fruits • goat's milk yogurt • lactose-free yogurt • coconut yogurt • lactose-free sour cream • whipped cream

▶

Moderate FODMAP (Limit to just a spoonful if lactose intolerant.)
Greek yogurt • cream cheese • sour cream

High FODMAP
cow's, sheep's, or goat's milk • buttermilk • cottage cheese • condensed milk • custard • evaporated milk • ice cream • pudding • ricotta cheese • traditional yogurt

NUTS AND SEEDS

Low FODMAP (Limit to a handful of nuts and seeds per meal.)
Brazil nuts • chestnuts • macadamia nuts • peanuts • pecans • pine nuts • walnuts;
Seeds: chia seeds • poppy seeds • pumpkin seeds • sesame seeds • sunflower seeds

Moderate FODMAP (Limit to 1–2 tablespoons.)
almonds • hazelnuts

High FODMAP
cashews • pistachios

SWEETENERS & CHOCOLATE

Low FODMAP
pure maple syrup • rice malt syrup • stevia • granulated sugar • light brown sugar • palm sugar • raw sugar • dark chocolate

Moderate FODMAP
golden syrup

High FODMAP
agave syrup • fructose • honey • isomalt • maltitol • mannitol • sorbitol • xylitol • carob, milk, or white chocolate

OTHER: FIBER ADDITIVES, TEAS & COFFEE, ALCOHOL

Low FODMAP
Fiber: chia seeds • flax seeds • oat bran • rice bran; **Tea:** black • green • peppermint • white; Coffee; **Alcohol:** most wine and beer • gin • vodka • whiskey

High FODMAP
Fiber: chicory root extract • FOS (fructo-oligosaccharides) • inulin; **Tea:** chamomile • fennel • oolong; **Alcohol:** rum

FAQs

What Does FODMAP Stand For?

FODMAPs are a certain group of sugars and fibers that are commonly malabsorbed and can trigger irritable bowel syndrome (IBS) symptoms. The term "FODMAP" is an acronym that stands for: F—fermentable (creates gas); O—oligosaccharides (fructans and galacto-oligosaccharides, water-soluble fibers); D—disaccharide (lactose); M—monosaccharide (fructose); A— and; P—polyols (sugar alcohols).

How Do FODMAPs Trigger IBS Symptoms?

FODMAPs contribute to IBS symptoms due to their ability to be rapidly fermented by gut microbes, contributing to intestinal gas. As small carbohydrates, they have been shown to pull water into the small intestine, too. The combination of excess water and gas stretches the intestine and can lead to pain and cramping, frequent bathroom trips, and/or bloating.

What Is a Low FODMAP Diet?

This nutritional approach to help manage symptoms of IBS is a learning diet. High-FODMAP foods are removed from the diet for two to six weeks, then FODMAP food sources are reintroduced one at a time to test individual tolerance to specific FODMAPs. Well-tolerated foods are then added back, to allow the diet to be as liberal as possible while still maintaining good symptom control. Research has shown that the low FODMAP diet manages IBS symptoms in 75 percent of those who suffer with this condition.

Will I Have to Eat Low FODMAP Forever?

No! Typically, you follow the initial phase of the diet for two to six weeks, followed by the challenge phase, during which you will determine which foods trigger symptoms and which do not. Once you establish which foods do *not* trigger your IBS symptoms, those will slowly be added back to your diet. There may be some high-FODMAP foods that you will eliminate for the long term, but the goal is to have a more moderate FODMAP intake when possible.

How Common Are FODMAPs in Our Diet?

Onion and garlic, sources of FODMAPs, are in hidden in most savory foods; FODMAPs also lurk in wheat products (see next FAQ). Many fruits and vegetables contain FODMAPs though, thankfully, many are low FODMAP, allowing for healthful options. Dairy items that are rich in lactose are restricted on the low FODMAP diet; however, hard cheeses, butter, and lactose-free milks and lactose-free yogurt are allowed as they provide little to no lactose to the diet.

▶

Is the Low FODMAP Diet a Gluten-Free Diet?

No. The low FODMAP diet modifies small-chain carbohydrates; gluten is a protein. Wheat, barley, and rye contain fructans, a source of FODMAP carbohydrates as well as gluten. As the low FODMAP diet minimizes these foods, gluten intake will likely be minimized as well; however, this diet is not entirely gluten-free.

Is Soy a Source of FODMAPs?

Different forms of soy may or may not contain FODMAPs. Soy lecithin, soybean oils, edamame, and firm tofu are low FODMAP sources; however, whole mature soybeans, soy milk made with the whole soybean, silken tofu, and soy flour do contain FODMAPs and would not be suitable for this diet.

Can I Eat Sweets and/or Chocolate on the Low FODMAP Diet?

Yes, you can eat sweets, within reason, on the low FODMAP diet. Selecting one serving of one of the many delectable dessert recipes in this book is a great way to get your sweet fix. More than a tablespoon of milk and white chocolate contains lactose, so should be limited (to up to 15 g per serving) on the low FODMAP diet; however, dark chocolate (semisweet, bittersweet) is allowed. Granulated, or table, sugar is not a source of FODMAPs; still, we recommend that sugar intake be enjoyed in moderation for good health.

How Do I Know Whether the Low FODMAP Diet Is Right for Me?

The low FODMAP diet is a science-based approach to help manage symptoms for those with IBS. Do not self-diagnose! If you are struggling with GI distress, see your primary care doctor and/or a gastroenterologist to help determine whether the low FODMAP diet is appropriate for you.

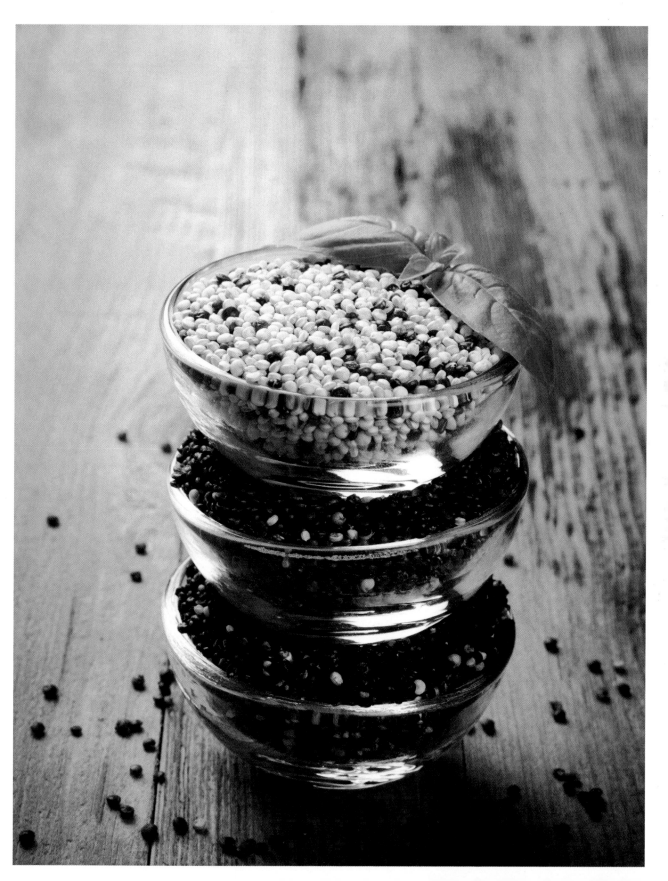

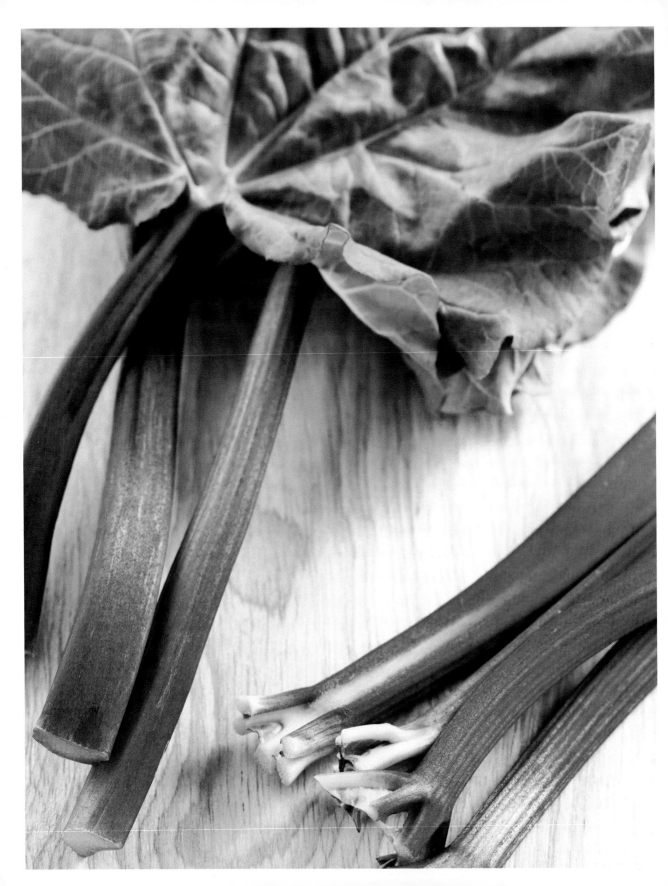

Chapter 2

THE WELL-BALANCED LOW FODMAP DIET: ELIMINATE, CHALLENGE, INTEGRATE!

IF YOU'RE FEELING A BIT OVERWHELMED, keep in mind that the low FODMAP elimination phase of the diet is not a forever diet, but rather a short-term nutrition experiment. The goal of this unique and personalized approach is to help you identify your individual FODMAP food triggers, quell your disruptive GI symptoms, and allow you to get on with your life! Let's start by detailing the three phases of the low FODMAP diet: eliminate, challenge, and integrate, followed by some basic helpful details on nutrition and digestion.

The 3 Low FODMAP Diet Phases

Phase 1: Eliminate

This initial phase typically lasts two to six weeks, depending on how quickly you respond to the diet. In this phase, you eliminate FODMAP-rich foods from your diet. Remember, the low FODMAP diet is not a FODMAP-free diet, but you will be reducing your FODMAP intake substantially at this time. The more organized and FODMAP knowledgeable you are, the easier and more effective the elimination phase will be! We suggest you create a weekly menu plan (we have included a sample for you, on page 50) with your favorite low FODMAP foods. Scan through our Low FODMAP Grocery

List on page 45 before you make your first market run as an official FODMAPer. In addition to stocking your pantry, be sure to select a few recipes from this book so you can dive right into the very delicious side of low FODMAP eating.

In working with patients, Kate has found the most common slip-ups on the elimination phase are consuming commercial food items with hidden FODMAP ingredients (especially cereals or granola bars with fructan additives called chicory root or inulin); overconsuming low FODMAP fruit portions (especially in fruit smoothies); and missing a meal and then overeating at the next meal, exceeding recommended portion limits of FODMAP-containing foods. If you find you are particularly hungry during this phase, add an extra scoop of rice or a big baked potato to your dinner (they are virtually FODMAP-free), increase your portion of fish or chicken (again FODMAP-free), or add an extra snack to your meal plan. We have many suggestions for snacks and menu-planning tips in Chapter 3.

Phase 2: Challenge

Once your symptoms are adequately controlled during the low FODMAP elimination diet, the next step is to add high-FODMAP foods methodically back onto your plate during the FODMAP challenge. This phase will help you identify your personal trigger foods and enable you to create your personal FODMAP barometer, highlighting what foods you can comfortably add back to your diet. FODMAPs are reintroduced one at a time by each FODMAP subtype: lactose, excess fructose, fructans, GOS, and polyols (mannitol and sorbitol). The challenge phase should be done in a systematic manner to best identify which FODMAP subtypes are contributing to your symptoms. Take your time with this challenge phase. It isn't hard, but it does require that you pay close attention to what you eat and how your body responds. Each and every person will have different responses. You might find out that excess fructose is an issue for you, whereas family members or friends might realize that polyols are their biggest trigger. Or you might determine that certain FODMAPs are very portion sensitive for you: perhaps small amounts of lactose are fine, but larger quantities are not. This challenge phase is what allows you to come away with your unique and personalized food road map that will keep you symptom-free. Undergoing the challenge phase will take six to eight weeks, depending on how you react to the various challenges. We do encourage that if you experience undesirable symptoms during a FODMAP challenge, you return to the low FODMAP elimination diet and wait until you are symptom-free for three days before embarking on the next challenge.

When you select a food to add back to your diet, it should only contain the FODMAP subtype you are challenging. To simplify the process for you, we have included a list of foods to choose, their amounts, and sample challenge day templates to guide you when you are reintroducing a specific FODMAP back into your diet. Let's review the challenge FODMAP phase in a bit more detail.

During this phase, you will stay on your low FODMAP elimination diet and select which FODMAP subtype you would like to challenge. Try to begin the challenges with a FODMAP

What Constitutes a Failed Challenge?

A failed FODMAP challenge would be one in which you experience uncomfortable or undesirable symptoms consisting of diarrhea, cramping, bloating, constipation, or those symptoms experienced typically with an IBS flare. If adding back the FODMAP triggers undesirable IBS symptoms, stop the challenge. Let your body rest on the low FODMAP elimination diet and initiate the next FODMAP food challenge when you have been symptom-free for three days.

subtype that you don't think is a major trigger for you. For example, if you know you are highly sensitive to lactose, you can hold off on challenging lactose and skip to the next FODMAP subtype, excess fructose. It's normal to be a little tentative in getting started with adding back FODMAPs when without them you feel great, but it is important to not overrestrict your diet unnecessarily. Passing your first FODMAP challenge will certainly be a positive reinforcement for you! When selecting a food within a FODMAP subtype to challenge, use the following guide. We have carefully selected the challenge foods, ensuring they only contain the FODMAP subtype you are challenging. For example, you might think an apple would be a good food to test to learn whether you are sensitive to excess fructose; however, in addition to excess fructose, apples also contain sorbitol. If eating an apple results in symptoms for you, it might be from the sorbitol, the excess fructose, or the combination of both of them! In other words, you would not know which FODMAP subtype triggered your symptoms. Thus, it is vital to isolate each subtype in your choice of challenge foods.

After you have challenged all the initial FODMAP subtypes you can assess your tolerance to multiple FODMAPs in one food. For instance, if you pass both sorbitol and excess fructose, then testing your tolerance to apples is a good next step. You might be feeling that you need a PhD in nutritional science to undertake the challenge phase, but we promise, it really is a whole lot easier than it sounds; just make sure to keep detailed notes. The challenge phase is an important step, as eating a more restrictive diet than you need to can impair your quality of life and in the long term may not be ideal for your gut health. Besides, it is more enjoyable to know how broadly you can eat!

Here are some general challenge phase tips:
- Test one FODMAP subtype (lactose, excess fructose, etc.) at a time.
- Be sure to follow the guidelines for the challenge food choices and amounts we have outlined for you. They will ensure that you are selecting challenge foods that only have the FODMAP subtype you are challenging.
- There is no need to overeat the challenge food; try to keep the portion in line with the quantity you would normally consume.
- Try to incorporate the test food three times in the test week (only once per day).

- Note challenge foods are listed as raw food measurements, but you can serve them cooked. For instance, start with ½ cup (37 g) of raw button mushrooms for the mannitol challenge. If cooked they will reduce in volume, but eat only the cooked amount that began as ½ cup raw.
- If you do not experience any symptoms at all, you can move directly onto the next challenge. If your symptoms flare during a food challenge, be sure to allow your symptoms to abate for at least three days before undergoing your next challenge.
- Track your diet and symptoms during the challenge days to help define your reactions to your food challenges.

If you pass a food challenge, good for you! But don't add any new foods back into your everyday diet yet! All challenges must be done while you otherwise remain on the low FODMAP elimination diet. Because FODMAPs effects are additive, if you are consuming other FODMAP-containing foods, even those that don't appear to cause symptoms while you are doing a FODMAP food challenge, it might skew the results of the other FODMAP challenge tests. In other words, if you pass the sorbitol challenge, make note of it for the integration phase, but do not eat any sorbitol-rich foods during the other challenges.

FODMAP CHALLENGE FOODS AND AMOUNTS

Lactose
½ cup (120 ml) cow's milk
¾ cup (171 g) plain cow's milk yogurt (without high-fructose corn syrup or other FODMAP ingredients)

Excess Fructose
½ (104 g) mango
2 teaspoons (10 ml) honey
¼ cup (30 g) raw sugar snap peas

Polyols
Mannitol
½ cup (37 g) raw chopped or sliced button mushrooms
¼ cup (33 g) raw chopped cauliflower
½ medium-size (19 g) raw celery stalk
1 cup (140 g) raw diced sweet potato
Sorbitol
5 (25 g) blackberries
½ medium (73 g) yellow peach
½ (80 g) avocado

Fructans

We recommend three separate challenges for fructans: a wheat, a garlic, and an onion challenge. We encourage various fructan challenges for a couple of reasons. First, fructans can vary in size in different foods and this may impact how they elicit symptoms. Second, wheat bread has other components, such as gluten, that may trigger symptoms.

Onion: 1 tablespoon (cooked versus raw is often better tolerated, so we suggest trying onion in cooked form first)

Garlic: ½ to 1 garlic clove (1–3 g)

Wheat: 1 to 2 slices of traditional whole wheat sandwich bread (60 g); if you have not tested slow-leavened sourdough wheat bread during the elimination phase, we suggest you trial 2 slices of slow leavened sourdough wheat bread first as it typically has less fructans and gluten than traditionally prepared wheat bread and may be tolerated better. Of course, if you are gluten intolerant or have been advised to avoid wheat for other conditions, skip this challenge.

Note: What is slow-leavened sourdough bread? It is bread made with live active sourdough culture (contains yeast and bacteria) that leavens the bread for 24 hours. No baker's yeast is added to speed the rising process. The microbes in the active culture contain ferment (consume), the FODMAPs (fructans), and protein (gluten) in the bread, reducing them, thus making the bread more tolerable for some.

GOS

½ cup (85 to 105 g) cooked beans (black beans, red kidney beans, soybeans)

GENERAL TIPS AND TEMPLATES FOR FODMAP CHALLENGES DAY BY DAY

The following tips will provide general guidance for undergoing the FODMAP challenges. We have also included detailed challenge phase templates to direct you through each FODMAP subtype challenge. These templates can be found on page 25.

FODMAP CHALLENGE, DAY 1

- Add the first serving of the FODMAP food you are challenging. For example, for lactose, you may add ½ cup (120 ml) of lactose-containing cow's milk to your diet at one of your meals.
- We encourage you to test the food or beverage you are challenging as part of a meal as it may be tolerated better with other food than by itself.
- Note any symptoms you may feel adding in the new high FODMAP food. If you experience minor but not painful symptoms (e.g., you feel a gas bubble traveling through

your intestine), this may be noted, but should not be considered a failed FODMAP challenge. See the sidebar on page 21 about what constitutes a failed challenge.

FODMAP CHALLENGE, DAY 2

- Double the portion of the FODMAP challenge food. In the event that you would *never* eat a double portion of the food you are testing, then stick with the same portion you tested on Day 1.
- Note any symptoms you may experience on your symptom log. Stop the challenge if you are experiencing an IBS flare or undesirable symptoms, and again, wait it out until you are symptom-free for three days before trying another challenge.

FODMAP CHALLENGE, DAY 3

- You may triple the food portion of the initial FODMAP challenge food amount if this would be an amount you would normally consume. If not, stick with the portion you used on Day 1 or 2, as appropriate to your normal eating habits and preference.
- Note any undesirable symptoms on your symptom log. If you experience undesirable symptoms during the challenge phase, we suggest you avoid foods that contain the FODMAP subtype you challenged. If you like, you could wait until you are symptom-free for three days and retry that FODMAP subtype with a *half*-portion of the test food or another food within that FODMAP subtype. You could also consider repeating that challenge in a month or two, as tolerance to FODMAPs can change over time. Why would your tolerance to FODMAP change over time? A number of factors may alter the way we process FODMAPs: the types of microbes in our intestine can change; or constipation can slow the movement of our small intestine, possibly allowing some microbes to creep farther up into our small intestine, where they may interact with our food and ferment it in the small bowel, which is smaller and less adaptable to gas production.

Now that you've completed one challenge cycle, move on to the next FODMAP challenge, using the challenge templates on page 25 to guide you.

CHALLENGING MULTIPLE FODMAPS SUBTYPES

When you have completed all the initial FODMAP subtype challenges, you might consider trying to add back foods with multiple FODMAPs. Again, it is recommended that you do this somewhat systematically, to get a good sense of what FODMAP subtypes trigger your symptoms. A favorite among the foods with multiple FODMAPs is an apple! Kate has learned that she can eat half of an apple without any digestive distress. Instead of avoiding this fruit, adding a few apple slices to a salad or snacking on apple slices are perfect ways to add smaller servings of apple to the diet.

If you found that you were able to incorporate some fructose and sorbitol during your challenge trials, you can try to challenge your digestive tract with an apple, too.

To walk you through a multiple challenge phase, we have constructed a template to guide you through this phase of the diet, also found on page 29.

Here is a list of a few combo FODMAP subtype challenges:

Sorbitol plus excess fructose:

½ (83 g) Pink Lady apple

Fructans and sorbitol:

1 (66 g) plum, 4 (32 g) prunes, or 4 (28 g) dried apricots

GOS and mannitol:

1 cup (120 g) raw diced butternut squash

Fructans and fructose:

2 slices raisin toast (wheat based) (75 g), or ½ medium-size (25 g) Jerusalem artichoke

LACTOSE CHALLENGE		
DAY 1	**DAY 2**	**DAY 3**
Add ½ cup (120 ml) cow's milk or ¾ cup (171 g) suitable yogurt to one of your meals.	Add 1 cup (240 ml) cow's milk or 1½ cups (342 g) suitable yogurt to one of your meals.	Add 1½ cups (360 ml) cow's milk or 2¾ cups (513 g) suitable yogurt to one of your meals. **Note:** You could maintain the amounts outlined in Day 2 if the amounts in Day 3 exceed what you would normally consume.
Use your food and symptom log to document food and symptoms.	Use your food and symptom log to document food and symptoms.	Use your food and symptom log to document food and symptoms.
If your IBS symptoms are triggered after reintroducing the FODMAP, stop the challenge.	If your IBS symptoms are triggered after reintroducing the FODMAP, stop the challenge.	If your IBS symptoms are triggered after reintroducing the FODMAP, stop the challenge.

FRUCTOSE CHALLENGE		
DAY 1	**DAY 2**	**DAY 3**
½ (104 g) mango or 2 teaspoons honey	1 (208 g) mango or 1 tablespoon plus 1 teaspoon honey	1½ (312 g) mangoes or 2 tablespoons honey **Note:** You could maintain the amounts outlined in Day 2 if the amounts in Day 3 exceed what you would normally consume.
Use your food and symptom log to document food and symptoms.	Use your food and symptom log to document food and symptoms.	Use your food and symptom log to document food and symptoms.
If your IBS symptoms are triggered after reintroducing the FODMAP, stop the challenge.	If your IBS symptoms are triggered after reintroducing the FODMAP, stop the challenge.	If your IBS symptoms are triggered after reintroducing the FODMAP, stop the challenge.

POLYOL CHALLENGES Sorbital		
DAY 1	**DAY 2**	**DAY 3**
5 (25 g) blackberries, ½ (73 g) medium yellow peach, or ½ (80 g) avocado	10 (50 g) blackberries, 1 (145 g) medium yellow peach, or 1 (160 g) avocado	15 (75 g) blackberries, 1½ (218 g) medium yellow peaches, or 1½ (240 g) avocados **Note:** You could maintain the amounts outlined in Day 2 if the amounts in Day 3 exceed what you would normally consume.
Use your food and symptom log to document food and symptoms.	Use your food and symptom log to document food and symptoms.	Use your food and symptom log to document food and symptoms.
If your IBS symptoms are triggered after reintroducing the FODMAP, stop the challenge.	If your IBS symptoms are triggered after reintroducing the FODMAP, stop the challenge.	If your IBS symptoms are triggered after reintroducing the FODMAP, stop the challenge.

POLYOL CHALLENGES		
Mannitol		
DAY 1	DAY 2	DAY 3
½ cup (37 g) raw chopped or sliced raw button mushrooms, or ¼ cup (33 g) chopped cauliflower	1 cup (74 g) raw chopped or sliced raw button mushrooms, or ½ cup (66 g) chopped cauliflower	1½ cups (111 g) chopped or sliced raw button mushrooms, or ¾ cup (99 g) chopped cauliflower **Note:** You could maintain the amounts outlined in Day 2 if the amounts in Day 3 exceed what you would normally consume.
Use your food and symptom log to document food and symptoms.	Use your food and symptom log to document food and symptoms.	Use your food and symptom log to document food and symptoms.
If your IBS symptoms are triggered after reintroducing the FODMAP, stop the challenge.	If your IBS symptoms are triggered after reintroducing the FODMAP, stop the challenge.	If your IBS symptoms are triggered after reintroducing the FODMAP, stop the challenge.

FRUCTAN CHALLENGES		
Wheat		
DAY 1	DAY 2	DAY 3
2 slices wheat bread	4 slices wheat bread Note: You can maintain the amounts in Day 1 if the amounts in Day 2 exceed what you normally would consume.	6 slices wheat bread **Note:** You could maintain the amounts outlined in Day 1 or 2 if the amounts in Day 3 exceed what you would normally consume.
Use your food and symptom log to document food and symptoms.	Use your food and symptom log to document food and symptoms.	Use your food and symptom log to document food and symptoms.
If your IBS symptoms are triggered after reintroducing the FODMAP, stop the challenge.	If your IBS symptoms are triggered after reintroducing the FODMAP, stop the challenge.	If your IBS symptoms are triggered after reintroducing the FODMAP, stop the challenge.

Garlic		
DAY 1	**DAY 2**	**DAY 3**
½ garlic clove (1.5 g)	1 garlic clove (3 g)	1½ garlic cloves (4.5 g) **Note:** You could maintain the amounts outlined in Day 2 if the amounts in Day 3 exceed what you would normally consume.
Use your food and symptom log to document food and symptoms.	Use your food and symptom log to document food and symptoms.	Use your food and symptom log to document food and symptoms.
If adding back the FODMAP triggers your IBS symptoms, stop the challenge.	If adding back the FODMAP triggers your IBS symptoms, stop the challenge.	If adding back the FODMAP triggers your IBS symptoms, stop the challenge.

Onion		
DAY 1	**DAY 2**	**DAY 3**
1 tablespoon (15 g) chopped white or yellow onion Note: Most tolerate best when cooked.	2 tablespoons (30 g) chopped white or yellow onion	3 tablespoons (45 g) chopped white or yellow onion **Note:** You could maintain the amounts outlined in Day 2 if the amounts in Day 3 exceed what you would normally consume.
Use your food and symptom log to document food and symptoms.	Use your food and symptom log to document food and symptoms.	Use your food and symptom log to document food and symptoms.
If your IBS symptoms are triggered after reintroducing the FODMAP, stop the challenge.	If your IBS symptoms are triggered after reintroducing the FODMAP, stop the challenge.	If your IBS symptoms are triggered after reintroducing the FODMAP, stop the challenge.

GALACTO-OLIGOSACCHARIDE CHALLENGES		
DAY 1	**DAY 2**	**DAY 3**
½ cup (85 to 105 g) cooked black beans, soybeans, or kidney beans	1 cup (170 to 210 g) cooked black beans, soybeans, or kidney beans	1½ cups (255 to 417 g) cooked black beans, soybeans, or kidney beans **Note:** You could maintain the amounts outlined in Day 2 if the amounts in Day 3 exceed what you would normally consume.
Use your food and symptom log to document food and symptoms.	Use your food and symptom log to document food and symptoms.	Use your food and symptom log to document food and symptoms.
If your IBS symptoms are triggered after reintroducing the FODMAP, stop the challenge.	If your IBS symptoms are triggered after reintroducing the FODMAP, stop the challenge.	If your IBS symptoms are triggered after reintroducing the FODMAP, stop the challenge.

EXAMPLE OF A MULTIPLE FODMAP CHALLENGE Sorbitol and Excess Fructose Challenge		
DAY 1	**DAY 2**	**DAY 3**
½ (83 g) medium apple	1 (165 g) medium apple	1½ (248 g) medium apples **Note:** You could maintain the amounts outlined in Day 2 if the amounts in Day 3 exceed what you would normally consume.
Use your food and symptom log to document food and symptoms.	Use your food and symptom log to document food and symptoms.	Use your food and symptom log to document food and symptoms.
If your IBS symptoms are triggered after reintroducing the FODMAP, stop the challenge.	If your IBS symptoms are triggered after reintroducing the FODMAP, stop the challenge.	If your IBS symptoms are triggered after reintroducing the FODMAP, stop the challenge.

Phase 3: Integrate

Once you determine what FODMAPs you can tolerate (as identified by the challenge phase), those foods may be integrated back *slowly* to your baseline diet. The integrate phase will help you create your very own personalized moderate-FODMAP diet plan.

Although you very likely will be able to eat more than you have been lately, it is possible that you may not be able to consume every FODMAP-rich food you passed during the challenge phase, *all at one meal*. You may find spreading them out throughout the day or perhaps throughout the week will allow for your best tolerance. As you experiment, it will become quite intuitive what works and what doesn't work for your body. Don't be afraid to advance to this phase of the diet; go gently and remind yourself this is an important part of the plan! If your IBS symptoms seem to flare, a day or two of the low FODMAP elimination diet should bring you back to good symptom control. You will have a much better understanding of how your diet impacts the way your tummy feels. Whereas your intestines might have had a mind of their own before you started the low FODMAP diet, you will now feel that you are in full control. It can be very empowering!

HOW TO INTEGRATE FODMAPS ONTO YOUR PLATE

To illustrate how the integration phase of the diet might look, here is an example of an integrated meal plan for a person that passed both the lactose and sorbitol challenges.

Breakfast:
Greek yogurt, 10 blueberries, 1 tablespoon chia seeds
Suitable low FODMAP toast and peanut butter

Lunch:
Mixed salad greens with cottage cheese and balsamic and olive oil dressing
5 to 10 blackberries and 10 almonds

Dinner:
Grilled salmon
Baked potato
Tomato, mozzarella, and avocado salad with fresh lemon juice and garlic-infused oil

Note: Greek yogurt and cottage cheese have been added back to the diet. These lactose-containing foods should not pose any symptoms. Adding back into the diet sorbitol-rich foods, such as 5–10 blackberries and the larger avocado serving, should be well tolerated.

General Menu Planning Tips

- Make food from scratch when possible. This allows full control over the ingredients you add to your diet.
- Choose foods in their natural state when possible. Snack on 10 strawberries and a handful of almonds rather than choosing a handful of packaged low FODMAP cookies.
- Plan your meals *and* snacks in advance. Having a general idea of what you plan on eating for the day will keep you on track with the low FODMAP diet and ensure you are good to go when you get hungry.
- If eating away from home, at a friend's home or at a restaurant, be sure you get a heads-up on the menu items available. Bring along some snacks; offer to bring an appetizer or a salad, or perhaps your whole meal.
- Bring along your own gluten-free roll vs. eating a bunless burger when dining out.
- All the recipes in this book are suitable for the elimination phase, so dive in and start adding them to your weekly meal plans!

WELL-BALANCED LOW FODMAP LIVING

Eating a low FODMAP diet may be the start of symptom relief for you, but of course, we want to keep you and your gut healthy for the long haul. This means eating more *whole foods first* and a mixture of nutrient-dense foods. Whole plant foods are nourishing for your gut as they contribute to a more diverse and healthy gut microbiome. We trust that Mother Nature had it right and encourage you to choose more plant-based whole foods versus packaged foods made in a plant.

No need to be perfect; just try your best to choose more nourishing real food. For starters, just take a look at our colorful and nourishing Rainbow Chopped Salad (page 163). All the recipes in this book were developed to soothe your GI tract, nourish your body, and keep you delightfully satiated. But, of course, we did throw some rich comfort foods (like Baked Mac 'n' Cheese, page 204) and sweet dessert recipes in to the book, too, because everyone deserves a treat now and again! Just use the decadent recipes in moderation.

BALANCED-PLATE NUTRITION

It's all about balance. Just like life itself, digestion works when the food on your plate is balanced. Too much fiber or fat can delay stomach emptying, making you feel too full and/or bloated. And as you have just learned, too many FODMAPs consumed together often trigger IBS symptoms. We find that most people do best with well-balanced meals containing a mixture of low FODMAP carbs and produce, lean protein, and healthy fats. When creating your menus for the week, use these general rules of thumb: fill one quarter of your plate with protein-rich meats, poultry, shellfish, fish, or firm tofu; one quarter of your plate with carb-rich grains or starches, such as gluten-free pasta or bread, rice, quinoa, baked potato, ½ cup (30 g) of cooked, mashed sweet potato; and on the remaining half of your plate, 1 cup (240 ml) of a variety of cooked low FODMAP veggies; plus a smattering of healthy fats: drizzle of olive oil, or allowable nuts, nut butters, and/or seeds.

What does a balanced plate look like?

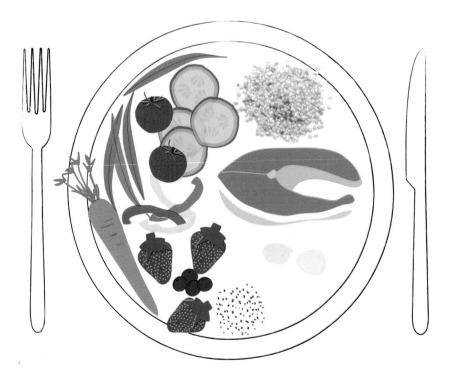

PORTION SIZE COUNTS!

Because FODMAPs in food have cumulative effects in the intestine, portion size matters. Pay attention to what you are eating as well as the amounts. You might not be able to eat a whole avocado at one sitting; however, eating the equivalent of an eighth of an avocado, as in our Maki Roll Bowl (page 127), might agree better with your digestive tract. It is all about finding out what works for you! We hope you will use this book for the amazing low FODMAP recipes, but also for creating a low FODMAP lifestyle that works for you, personally.

Some portion-planning tricks to incorporate into your eating style include:
- Limit to one fruit serving per meal or snack time; forgo a smoothie with 4 bananas and a cup of strawberries! A low FODMAP serving size would equate to approximately ½ banana, 1 medium orange, ½ cup chopped fruit.

- Balance your meals with a mix of nutrient-rich foods; this will help you automatically keep your portions in check while nourishing your body. Don't eat just vegetables for lunch. Be sure to include a starch, fruit, vegetable, protein, and healthy fat. When your plate is balanced, you will feel balanced, too! Plus, eating a wide variety of foods often helps moderate your mealtime FODMAP intake. For more specifics on how to balance your plate, see page 30 for tips.

When Diet Isn't Enough

Diet is a controllable variable in treating your digestive distress, but sometimes nutritional change only offers partial relief . . . and in some, no relief at all. IBS is a complicated disorder and a symptom-based diagnosis. This means that many people with IBS may have arrived at the diagnosis via different paths. Some might have been born with very slow intestinal transit (i.e., a slow-moving intestine); others may have developed food-borne illness and landed with an IBS diagnosis. Working closely with a forward-thinking gastroenterologist and a dietitian specializing in digestive disorders is a good way to uncover a bit more about the underpinnings of your particular IBS case. Perhaps simply trying a probiotic might help soothe your digestive woes. Or maybe you have developed a treatable condition, such as small intestinal bacterial overgrowth (SIBO). As previously mentioned, symptoms of SIBO mimic those seen in IBS, such as chronic diarrhea, postmeal fullness, bloating, abdominal distention, and gas. These symptoms may occur due to increased gas production, toxic by-products of bacterial metabolism, or bile salts that have been rendered inactive by the microbes. Current treatment of SIBO is specialized antibiotics.

Dyssynergic defecation, or pelvic floor dyssynergia, occurs when the muscles and nerves of the pelvic floor do not work in coordinated fashion to allow for a normal bowel movement. Associated commonly with constipation-predominant IBS, the muscles contract versus relax in the rectum during a bowel movement. Treatment with physical therapy and biofeedback can be very effective for this condition.

Most people with IBS have been screened for other conditions, such as celiac disease, inflammatory bowel disease, and gastroparesis (delayed stomach emptying), but if you have not, meet with your gastroenterologist to discuss the need for additional testing based on your medical history. The more you understand about digestive health and your body, the best you can advocate for yourself.

Picking a Probiotic

The World Health Organization defines *probiotics* as "live microorganisms which when administered in adequate amounts confer a health benefit on the host."[2] To be labeled a probiotic, scientific evidence for the health benefit would have to be acknowledged. Select a probiotic that has research to support its use for the condition you are trying to improve. A great guide to use is the Clinical Guide to Probiotic Products; this is available in an app form or online at http://usprobioticguide.com.

When selecting a probiotic during the low FODMAP diet, select one that does not contain prebiotic FODMAP-containing ingredients, such as chicory root extract, fructooligosaccharides (FOS), or inulin. In practice, Kate uses Align, Culturelle (without inulin), and VSL#3, Florastor probiotics with her IBS patients most frequently. If you are just starting the elimination phase and are not currently on a probiotic, we encourage you to wait before starting one. It's best to change one part of your treatment plan at a time to better assess what is helping you. If you add a probiotic and change the diet at the same time, it will be less clear which is helping or hindering your symptoms.

Low FODMAP Forever?

Finally, you may ask, "If I feel so much better on a diet lower in FODMAPs, can't I just follow it for a lifetime?" If you have reached the integration phase, then you have added some FODMAP-rich foods back in, while still lowering your FODMAP intake from where you were initially. It is our goal with this book to get you to that point. On the other hand, remaining on the full low FODMAP elimination phase of the diet over the long term may have a potential downside. Research has shown that some beneficial intestinal probiotic bacteria populations decline when individuals follow the low FODMAP elimination phase over the long term. Some of these beneficial microbes produce butyrate, one of the short-chain fatty acids produced by our gut bacteria as a result of fermentation, which offers positive health effects, such as reducing the risk of colon cancer. The acidity of the colonic contents may reduce a bit, especially during the low FODMAP diet elimination phase, and this may increase the risk of pathogenic bacteria getting a foothold in your colon. This is why it is so important to take yourself through the challenge phase of the diet, so that you will know which foods that do contain FODMAPs are tolerated by you and can be reintroduced into your diet.

On the other hand, the low FODMAP elimination diet has been shown to increase the diversity of microbes in the intestine, which is viewed as a positive side effect. More recent research has revealed that lowering the intake of FODMAPs lowers inflammatory chemicals in urine.[1] What we eat impacts what gut microbes grow in our gut and what they produce.

In the next chapter, we show you how to navigate the supermarket aisles and get into the kitchen, where we help you create incredibly delicious low FODMAP meals.

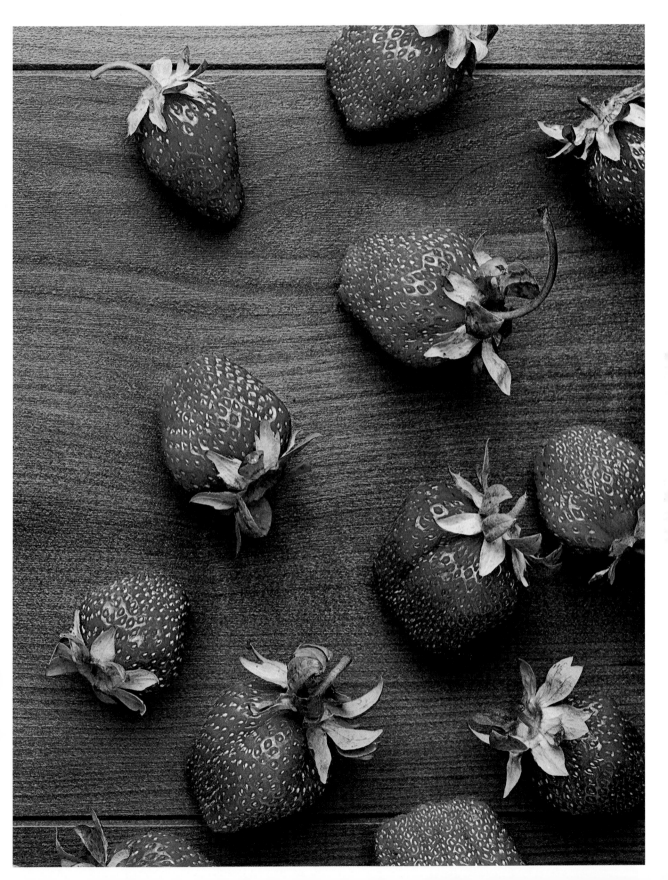

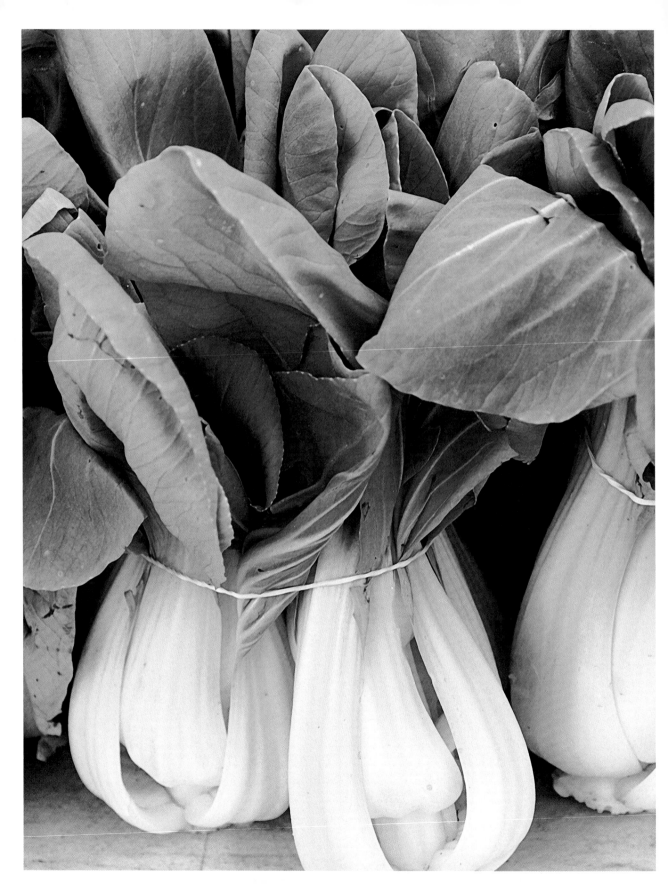

Chapter 3

PUTTING THE LOW FODMAP DIET INTO PRACTICE

IT IS EMPOWERING TO BE AWARE of the foods you can safely eat and to know how happy and healthy you will feel when you follow our personalized FODMAP diet. The recipes that follow are all low FODMAP according to the latest research and will leave you feeling satisfied. It's time you felt less deprivation, desperation, pain, or bloating. To help you do this, we offer our best tips and practices in this chapter. We'll start with the most important:

Stock Your Home with Low FODMAP Foods and You Will Never Go Hungry!

This might sound obvious, but one of the easiest ways to slip up is to become hungry and reach for something that you end up paying for later. Hey, we have all been there. With good planning, however, this can easily be prevented. And since the ingredients in this book, and low FODMAP foods in general, are all easily found at a typical supermarket, shopping is easy.

We think it's important that if you are truly going to test your FODMAP sensitivity, do the testing right. Don't try to "sort of" do the low FODMAP diet. Go in prepared, educated, and ready to roll. In this chapter, we will provide you with meal and snack inspirations. As a general guide, we have provided seven days of low FODMAP menu plans. You can mix and match the various menus or create your own adaptions if you feel confident in your ability to do so. By the end of seven days, you will know whether you are FODMAP sensitive or not. You may still experience symptom benefit after the initial seven days, but if you do not feel an ounce better by day seven, you can keep at it for another week. However, it is possible that you fall in the 25 percent of those with IBS where FODMAPs are not the cause of symptom exacerbation. Some may only experience partial benefit from the low FODMAP diet. In this case, the other condition(s), which we discussed in Chapter 2, may be impairing your ability to feel symptom-free.

If you like to follow directions, then having a set meal plan to start your low FODMAP dietary experiment might be the way to go. Just take a look at the seven days of menus later in this chapter. If you are a nutrition guru or foodie and want to create your own low FODMAP menu framework, by all means go for it!

Keep Low FODMAP Snacks Handy

Most of us are pretty good about planning what we will eat for our meals, but less organized when it comes to our snacks. We all get hungry between meals, and this can be a crucial time for FODMAPers. Why? Because if you don't have the right food around, you may veer into dangerous territory. If you find yourself aimlessly staring into a vending machine or gazing around a convenience store, you are going to have to be very careful—and most likely, will not find anything low FODMAP that you can eat. Always have an emergency snack on hand to prevent a slip-up. Keep our Fruit & Nut Protein Kinder Bars (page 134) handy!

If you pack lunch every day and find that you need more than your main offerings, add something else, such as a ½-cup (120 ml) container of Cucumber, Tomato & Feta Salad (page 158) or Quinoa Tabouleh (page 184). A snack doesn't always have to be a starchy carb, such as a granola bar. Mix it up. *Be prepared. Don't let yourself get overly hungry.* Some of our favorite snack suggestions can be found on page 133.

To Graze or Not to Graze

We are all about eating the occasional snack to keep your energy up, but eating all day long may have a downside. In case you missed this info in Chapter 1 (Digestion 101), the human intestine is made up of a complex of nerves and muscles that help move food along the GI tract. Two major modes of operation occur in the intestine: the eating mode and the cleaning mode. When you eat, your intestine secretes digestive enzymes and sloshes food around to break down the nutrients into their digestible form. When you are not eating, your intestine will initiate a repetitive and important housecleaning wave to clean up the small bowel and get it ready to digest again. It is important to allow three to four hours between eating to allow this cleansing wave to take place; otherwise, your small intestine can become a petri dish where microbes, food, and debris will accumulate. For this reason, we recommend eating three meals and one snack per day, rather than several small meals or following a grazing-style eating pattern. Yes, you and your sensitive gut need a little downtime between meals!

Keeping Up Your Fiber Intake

It's possible that as you remove the vast majority of wheat from your diet, your fiber intake may plummet. Fiber is important for gut health, from keeping us regular to feeding healthy gut microbes. Fiber is the indigestible component of plant-based carbohydrates. Fiber, or roughage, found in plant foods, will add bulk to your intestinal contents and keep things moving along the digestive tract. Fiber travels down to the end of the small intestine and into the colon, intact. *Fiber is an umbrella term*, meaning fiber comes in many sizes and shapes. Some fiber, such as most skins of fruits and veggies, is not fermented by microbes in the colon, whereas others, such as FODMAP fibers found in wheat, beans, onion, and garlic, are rapidly fermented—often resulting in copious amounts of gas. To ensure that you consume a variety of different types of fiber during your low FODMAP diet, we suggest you try a few of our favorite low FODMAP fiber sources: chia seeds, pumpkin seeds, whole white potato with skin, navel oranges, kiwifruit, strawberries, oats, quinoa, and green beans.

How much fiber do you need? The National Academy of Sciences Institute of Medicine recommends that adults consume 20 to 35 grams of dietary fiber per day, but most of us are falling short on fiber with the average American's daily intake of dietary fiber being only 12 to 18 g![1]

To guide fiber through your intestine, adequate fluid intake is key. Your body signals thirst when it's in need of fluids; be sure to listen! As a general rule of thumb, we suggest you include a 12-ounce (360 ml) glass of water with each meal and sip water whenever your body signals thirst or the color of your urine appears a darker yellow.

What Would 20 to 35 Grams of Fiber Look Like?

Breakfast: ½ cup (115 g) cooked oats (2 grams fiber), 1 tablespoon chia seeds (5 grams fiber), 10 medium-size (140 g) strawberries (2 grams fiber). Total breakfast fiber: 9 grams fiber.

Lunch: 1 cup (38 g) raw baby spinach (1 gram fiber), 1 cup (185 g) cooked quinoa (5 grams fiber), 3 ounces grilled chicken (0 grams fiber), 1 medium-size (130 g) orange (3 grams fiber). Total lunch fiber: 9 grams fiber.

Dinner: Salmon steak (0 grams fiber), 1 medium-size (122 g) white potato, baked (3 grams fiber), 1 cup (180 g) cooked zucchini (2 grams fiber), 2 small kiwi fruit (150 g) (4 grams fiber). Total dinner fiber: 9 grams fiber.

Full Menu Plan Fiber: 27 grams fiber

A Word About Magnesium

Magnesium is a vital mineral that your body relies on to perform hundreds of biochemical reactions, and one you may fall short of getting in sufficient amounts. Adequate magnesium is essential to support your immune function, heart, bone, and gut health. Recommended amounts of magnesium vary per gender and age. For men aged 19 to 30, 400 milligrams is the recommended daily intake, and increases to 420 milligrams for those aged 31 and over. For women, the amounts are 310 milligrams for those aged 19 to 30, and ups to 320 milligrams for those aged 31 and over. Research suggests that magnesium plays a role in fighting inflammation in your body; many chronic diseases, including many in the GI tract, including IBS, involve inflammation. Our favorite magnesium-rich boosters include pepitas (shelled pumpkin seeds), almonds, quinoa, peanuts and peanut butter, and small amounts of acceptable legumes, such as ¼ cup (42 g) of canned, drained and rinsed chickpeas.

Bone Up with Calcium

Your calcium intake can take a hit on the low FODMAP diet. Calcium is an essential mineral required for blood vessel contraction and dilation, proper function of your muscles and nerves, and bone and teeth health. In fact, 99 percent of your body's calcium is safely stored in your bones and teeth. Dairy foods are the most abundant source of dietary calcium. It is difficult to meet your calcium needs on a dairy-free low FODMAP diet. Fortunately, our low FODMAP diet is not dairy-free! With careful planning, you can easily meet your calcium needs by incorporating lactose-free cow's milk, lactose-free yogurt, and hard cheeses; even kale has some calcium, and chia seeds do, too! The recommended dietary allowance for calcium for men and women aged 19 to 50 years old is 1,000 milligrams per day. For women over age 50, the recommended amount is 1,200 milligrams per day. For those who cannot tolerate dairy foods, be sure to speak with your health professional about whether you need a calcium supplement or creative ways to boost your intake.

Time to Get Grocery Shopping Ready and Label Reading Savvy

Creating a list of your weekly menus will make grocery shopping less stressful and more efficient, and might even save you a few bucks. Grocery shopping is best done after you have come up with some menu items for the week ahead. Review the recipes in this book and write out your menus for the week or review those we have provided as a guide to help create your market list. Don't forget to add to your list breakfast, snacks, desserts, and foods for on the go! Having the right foods at your fingertips will help you navigate the diet much more easily. If you don't have the low FODMAP foods within reach, it's easy to fall off the diet and feel poorly again.

We recommend you choose as many foods as possible in their whole food (unprocessed) form versus choosing mostly packaged, manufactured foods. Why? Because they tend to be healthier that way! Of course, we also realize that you will need to stock some prepared food products for your pantry. To guide you, following are two lists of common label ingredients: the first list contains acceptable low FODMAP ingredients and the second list details the ingredients to avoid. Commercially prepared product labels with multiple ingredients can be a bit challenging to decipher, but our lists will help you.

These lists are not exhaustive as many ingredients have yet to be tested, but they will provide a good framework for you when reading a label. Remember, the low FODMAP diet is *not* a FODMAP-free diet; the goal is to reduce your intake, not eliminate every little FODMAP. Yes, you need to read labels, but remember the bulk of your diet should come from the low FODMAP recipes in this book. And remember, too, that when you stick with whole foods, such as a fresh orange or ripe and delicious strawberries, over a box of low FODMAP cookies—at least most of the time—you will probably feel better and have a better sense of your FODMAP intake. We get it, cookies taste good and we all deserve a treat, however, by choosing more whole foods versus packaged products, you remove the hassle of label reading. Our low- and high-FODMAP ingredient lists will help you when you do pick up those few convenience products at the grocer's.

Here are a few main points to remember:
- Be sure to focus your attention on the order of the ingredients on labels; they are listed, greatest quantity first, according to how much of the ingredient is in that prepared food. This will be important information for you to have as you assess your tolerance to different food products.
- Avoid onion and garlic that is added to any food in any form.
- Some FODMAP-containing foods, such as honey or wheat, might be tolerated if they are one of the last ingredients listed in a manufactured food.
- Note the term *natural flavors*: In goods regulated by the United States Department of Agriculture (animal-based products), such as chicken or beef broth, this can denote garlic or onion has been added to the product. In other food products regulated by the Food and Drug Administration, however, onion and garlic ingredients would be listed, such as in a vegetarian broth.

Low FODMAP Ingredients

Note: We have not called out in the following list those items that may have gluten, as the low FODMAP diet by nature is not gluten-free. If you are following a gluten-free diet be sure to select gluten-free as well as low FODMAP ingredients. For example, select a gluten-free soy sauce or gluten-free oats.

Condiments and dried spices:	allspice, asafetida, Asian fish sauce, cardamom, cayenne pepper, chili powder (without onion and garlic), cinnamon, citrus juice and zest, cloves, coriander, cumin, curry powder (without onion and garlic), fennel seeds, ginger, malt extract, miso paste, mustard, mustard seeds, nutmeg, oyster sauce, paprika, pepper (whole peppercorns or ground), red pepper flakes, saffron, salt, soy sauce, star anise, tamari, turmeric, vanilla extract, vinegar
Fresh and dried herbs:	basil, bay leaves, cilantro, coriander, curry leaves, dill, fenugreek leaves, lemongrass, mint, oregano, parsley, rosemary, sage, tarragon, thyme
Sweeteners and other derivatives of sugar:	aspartame, bar sugar, beet sugar, berry sugar, cane juice crystals, cane sugar, castor sugar, corn syrup (not high-fructose corn syrup), dextrose, evaporated cane sugar, glucose, granulated sugar, high-maltose corn syrup, invert sugar, light brown sugar, maltose, maltodextrin, pure maple syrup, palm sugar, raw sugar, refined sugar, rice malt syrup, stevia, sucrose, superfine sugar
Leavening agents:	active yeast, baking soda, baking powder
Flours and grains:	almond meal up to ¼ cup (25 g) per serving, brown rice flour, buckwheat flour, buckwheat groats, corn flour, cornmeal, cornstarch, millet and millet flour, oat bran, oats, polenta, potato starch, quinoa, quinoa flour or flakes, rice (brown, basmati, white), rice bran, rice flour or flakes, sorghum flour, tapioca starch, teff flour, wheat starch, yam flour
Thickeners:	cornstarch, guar gum, modified food starch, pectin, potato starch, tapioca starch, wheat starch (despite the "wheat" name, this is allowed as it contains a longer-chain carbohydrate and is not a FODMAP), xanthan gum

Nuts and seeds:	almonds, Brazil nuts, chestnuts, chia seeds, hazelnuts, macadamia nuts, peanuts, pecans, pepitas (hulled pumpkin seeds), pine nuts, poppy seeds, sesame seeds, sunflower seeds, walnuts
Oils:	all oils; garlic-, shallot-, and onion-infused oils used for flavor (do not eat any flesh of onion or garlic added to seasoned oil mixtures)
Milks:	almond milk, canned coconut milk, hemp milk, lactose-free cow's milk, rice milk
Other:	cocoa powder, semisweet or bittersweet chocolate, soy lecithin, whey protein isolate

High-FODMAP Ingredients

Sweeteners:	agave syrup, crystalline fructose, fructose, fruit juice concentrate, high-fructose corn syrup, honey, isomalt, lactitol, maltitol, mannitol, molasses, polydextrose, sorbitol, xylitol
Flours and grains:	amaranth flour, almond meal greater than ¼ cup (25 g) per serving, barley and barley flour, bean flours, bulgur wheat, einkorn flour, emmer flour, freekeh, kamut, lupin flour, rye flour, soy flour, spelt flour (allowed in sourdough spelt bread only), wheat flour and derivatives (all-purpose, pastry flour, white wheat flour, whole wheat flour; allowed in sourdough wheat bread)
Fiber additives:	chicory root extract, fructo-oligosaccharides (FOS), inulin
Flavorings:	garlic, onion; note that the term *natural flavor* (in products regulated by USDA [products made with meat, e.g., chicken or beef broth], could denote onion or garlic)
Milk:	Cow's milk, cream, dry milk solids, goat's milk, sheep's milk
Other:	rum

Soy and the Low FODMAP Diet

Soy is a tricky ingredient to tease out in the low FODMAP diet. Let us explain. Whole soybeans contains fiber, which contains the FODMAP subtype GOS and fructans, therefore they are a high-FODMAP food. Soy protein without the fiber is low FODMAP. Firm tofu is made by separating the protein from the water-soluble-containing GOS and fructan FODMAP fibers, making it an acceptable low FODMAP food. Silken tofu is made with a different process, whereby the soybeans are curdled and combined without any draining of the GOS and fructan fibers. For this reason, silken tofu is a high-FODMAP food. Soy flour contains the whole bean; consequently, it is high FODMAP. Soy sauce and the emulsifier soy lecithin, found in many commercial products, do not contain the fiber from soy; thus they are low FODMAP, too. Edamame, an immature soybean, has less GOS and fructans than the mature soybean and is low FODMAP in small servings.

What follows is our **Low FODMAP Grocery List** to guide you. Copy or scan these lists to help assist you during your weekly menu planning and shopping trip. Or simply snap a pic with your smartphone! Having the right foods around—and eliminating the ones that could sabotage you—sets you up for success.

(**Note:** Many of these specific products have not yet been tested for FODMAP content, but appear suitable based on the ingredients listed on their food label. Food companies developing low FODMAP-certified foods currently include FODY Food Co. and Casa de Santé, so be on the lookout for these low FODMAP-certified products on the shelves of your grocer's or online shops.)

Breads, Cereals, Crackers, Pasta, Grains, and Snacks

☐ **Bread:** Udi's white sandwich bread, Berlin Natural Bakery sourdough spelt bread, Iggy's sourdough (specifically Iggy's country or Francese bread selections that have been slow leavened), Foods by George gluten-free plain English muffins

☐ Gluten-free pizza crust (Udi's thin and crusty pizza crust comes in a two-pack)

☐ Plain corn tortillas

☐ **Boxed breakfast cereals:** Environkidz Gorilla Munch and Panda Puffs

☐ Brown rice crackers, such as Ka-Me plain rice crunch or sesame rice crunch crackers, or Blue Diamond Almond Nut Thins (not smokehouse flavor); choose regular almond nut thins with a hint of sea salt or pecan-flavor nut thins

☐ Gluten-free pasta

☐ Rice cakes, plain or lightly salted

☐ Popcorn

☐ Popchips, salted flavor

☐ Plain old-fashioned oats

☐ Gluten-free pretzels (such as Snyder's of Hanover gluten-free pretzels)

☐ **Rice:** brown, white, basmati, jasmine (raw or prepared, such as Trader Joe's frozen plain, microwavable jasmine rice)

☐ Quinoa (such as Ancient Harvest red quinoa and Trader Joe's frozen precooked, plain microwavable white quinoa) and quinoa flakes

The Dairy Case (Dairy, Egg, Butter Section)

☐ Lactose-free yogurt, vanilla or plain (such as Green Valley Organics)

☐ Greek yogurt, plain (such as Fage brand). Greek yogurt is often tolerated as it is lower in lactose than traditional yogurt, but if you are very sensitive to lactose or unsure, select lactose-free yogurt.

☐ Lactose-free milk (such as Organic Valley lactose-free milk)

☐ Eggs

☐ Butter

☐ Margarine (individuals following a dairy-free or vegan diet should choose a margarine made with oil as the first ingredient. Choose tub style [e.g., Earth Balance original or soy-free] versus stick as tub styles typically have less trans fat and/or saturated fat)

☐ Dairy-free milk alternatives: We suggest unsweetened milk alternatives when possible, but those made with sugar or sugar derivatives, such as evaporated cane juice in small quantities, used in coffee or a small bowl of cereal are suitable, too.

☐ Almond milk (Silk or Almond Breeze brand)

☐ Canned coconut milk (such as Trader Joe's or Thai Kitchen canned light coconut milk)

☐ Hemp milk

☐ Rice milk

Cheese

- ☐ (**Note:** Most cheeses are low FODMAP, except "wet," cheeses, such as ricotta and cottage cheese.)
- ☐ Brie cheese
- ☐ Cheddar cheese
- ☐ Lactose-free cottage cheese (such as Lactaid brand)
- ☐ Feta cheese
- ☐ Muenster cheese
- ☐ Parmigiano-Reggiano cheese
- ☐ Provolone cheese
- ☐ Shredded part-skim mozzarella cheese
- ☐ Swiss cheese

Produce

Fruit

- ☐ Avocados
- ☐ Bananas (best to select unripe)
- ☐ Blueberries
- ☐ Cantaloupe
- ☐ Dragon fruit
- ☐ Clementines
- ☐ Kumquats
- ☐ Grapes
- ☐ Guavas (ripe)
- ☐ Kiwifruit
- ☐ Lemons
- ☐ Limes
- ☐ Mandarins
- ☐ Honeydew melon
- ☐ Navel oranges
- ☐ Passion fruit
- ☐ Papayas
- ☐ Pineapple
- ☐ Plantains
- ☐ Raspberries
- ☐ Rhubarb
- ☐ Star fruit (carambola)
- ☐ Strawberries

(**Note:** You may substitute frozen unsweetened low FODMAP fruit as listed above)

Vegetables

- ☐ Arugula
- ☐ Bean sprouts
- ☐ Green beans
- ☐ Bamboo shoots
- ☐ Beets
- ☐ Bell peppers (red, green)
- ☐ Bok choy
- ☐ Broccoli
- ☐ Brussels sprouts
- ☐ Carrots
- ☐ Celeriac
- ☐ Chile peppers
- ☐ Collard greens
- ☐ Cucumbers
- ☐ Eggplant
- ☐ Endive
- ☐ Fennel bulbs and leaves
- ☐ Ginger
- ☐ Green or red cabbage
- ☐ Kale
- ☐ Leeks (use green parts only)
- ☐ Lettuce greens
- ☐ Spring onion and scallions (use green parts only)
- ☐ Okra
- ☐ Parsnips
- ☐ Potatoes, sweet
- ☐ Potatoes, white
- ☐ Radishes
- ☐ Spinach
- ☐ Summer squash
- ☐ Swiss chard

- ☐ Taro
- ☐ Tomatoes (canned, cherry, grape, common beefsteak, plum)
- ☐ Turnip
- ☐ Water chestnuts
- ☐ Yam
- ☐ Zucchini

Fresh and Dried Herbs

- ☐ Basil
- ☐ Bay leaves
- ☐ Chives
- ☐ Cilantro
- ☐ Curry leaves
- ☐ Dill
- ☐ Fenugreek leaves
- ☐ Lemongrass
- ☐ Mint
- ☐ Oregano
- ☐ Parsley
- ☐ Rosemary
- ☐ Sage
- ☐ Tarragon
- ☐ Thyme

Canned or Jarred Vegetables

- ☐ Butterbeans, drained, without onion and garlic
- ☐ Capers
- ☐ Chickpeas, drained, without onion and garlic
- ☐ Lentils, drained, without onion and garlic
- ☐ Olives (black, green)
- ☐ Pure pumpkin puree (not pumpkin pie mix)
- ☐ Tomatoes, diced or fire-roasted, without onion or garlic

Meats, Poultry, Seafood

- ☐ Fresh meats, poultry, and fish, unseasoned
- ☐ Rotisserie chicken, unseasoned
- ☐ Sliced deli turkey breast (such as Applegate brand organic roasted turkey slices without onion or garlic)
- ☐ Canned tuna
- ☐ Shellfish (clams, scallops, quahogs, etc.)

Meat Alternatives

- ☐ Firm and extra-firm tofu
- ☐ Quorn grounds
- ☐ Tempeh (without FODMAP ingredients, such as wheat, barley, onion, or garlic)

Condiments and Baking/Cooking Supplies

☐ Peanut butter, all-natural or other styles without honey or high-fructose corn syrup

☐ Low FODMAP flour blend (such as Bob's Red Mill Gluten Free 1 to 1 Baking Flour or King Arthur Gluten Free All Purpose Flour)

☐ Cocoa powder, unsweetened, natural, or Dutch-processed

☐ Coconut oil

☐ Ghee

☐ Grapeseed oil

☐ Olive oil

☐ Rice bran oil

☐ Sesame oil

☐ Garlic-infused oil (such as Garlic Oil by Boyajian)

☐ Vinegar: cider, balsamic, or rice vinegar

☐ Mayonnaise (avoid those with high-fructose corn syrup, onion, or garlic)

☐ Mustard (such as Maille or Grey Poupon Dijon, or Trader Joe's yellow mustard)

☐ Asian fish sauce

☐ Miso paste

☐ Oyster sauce (such as Kikkoman brand)

☐ Soy sauce or tamari (such as San-J brand)

☐ Nori seaweed

☐ Pure maple syrup (not pancake syrup)

☐ Marinara sauce, without onion and garlic (such as

Rao's Sensitive Formula Marinara or FODY certified low FODMAP marinara or tomato basil sauce)

☐ Orange marmalade, made without high-fructose corn syrup or chicory root

☐ Strawberry jam, made without high-fructose corn syrup or chicory root

☐ Pepper

☐ Salt

☐ Semisweet chocolate chips and bulk semisweet or bittersweet chocolate

☐ Sugar (granulated, light brown, confectioners')

☐ Pure almond extract

☐ Pure vanilla extract

Spices

☐ Allspice

☐ Bell's seasoning

☐ Cardamom

☐ Cayenne pepper

☐ Chili powder (such as McCormick Chipotle Chile Pepper, made without added onion and garlic)

☐ Chinese five-spice powder

☐ Cinnamon

☐ Cloves

☐ Coriander

☐ Cumin

☐ Curry powder (without added onion and salt)

☐ Fennel seeds

☐ Ginger

☐ Mustard seeds

☐ Nutmeg

☐ Old Bay Seasoning

☐ Oregano

☐ Paprika

☐ Red pepper flakes

☐ Saffron

☐ Star anise

☐ Turmeric

☐ Casa de Santé certified FODMAP-friendly spice blends

☐ FODY Food Co. certified low FODMAP spice blends

Nuts and Seeds

Nuts

- ☐ Almonds
- ☐ Brazil nuts
- ☐ Chestnuts

- ☐ Hazelnuts
- ☐ Macadamia nuts
- ☐ Peanuts
- ☐ Pecans

- ☐ Pine nuts
- ☐ Walnuts

Seeds

- ☐ Chia seeds
- ☐ Pepitas (hulled pumpkin seeds)

- ☐ Poppy seeds
- ☐ Sesame seeds
- ☐ Sunflower seeds

Reference: Adapted from the Monash University Low FODMAP App; Brand name ingredient labels, USDA Nutrient Composition Databases

---

Although having digestive woes can feel as if you picked the short straw at times, you might feel a stroke of luck has come your way when you bite into our tasty dishes with a new sense of relief and digestive calm.

You are now ready to embark on the elimination phase of the low FODMAP diet. As promised, we have provided seven days' worth of low FODMAP menus to help get you started. Bear in mind you may need to tweak the portions depending on your nutrient needs, which may vary depending on your height, weight, sex, and activity level. If you find you are still hungry while following the menu plans, simply add an extra snack or up the protein, rice, or potato portion to increase your satiety level. You don't need to follow these plans exactly; they serve as a basic framework and inspiration to create menus for the week. If you have additional dietary restrictions, such as following a gluten-free, dairy-free, or vegan or vegetarian diet, we have provided a sample menu for each of these special diets along with the low FODMAP diet modifications to guide you as well.

7 DAYS OF DELICIOUS LOW FODMAP MENU PLANS

| DAY 1 | DAY 2 | DAY 3 |

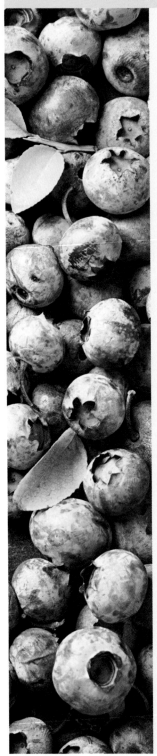

BREAKFAST: ¼ cup (25 g) old-fashioned oats cooked according to the package directions, sprinkled with a pinch of ground cinnamon and topped with 20 blueberries (28 g) and 1 tablespoon chopped walnuts. Enjoy with 8 ounces (227 g) of vanilla lactose-free yogurt.

LUNCH: 2 cups (150 g) salad greens topped with sliced chicken (from Whole Roast Chicken with Lemon and Herbs, page 276), or sliced turkey (from Citrus Sage Turkey Breast, page 282) or roast beef (without onion or garlic), 1 ounce (¼ cup [62 g]) of feta cheese (if desired), a handful of baby carrots, 5 slices of cucumber, and 5 cherry tomatoes. Dress with red wine vinegar and olive oil, salt, and pepper. Enjoy with an orange and a handful of rice crackers.

DINNER: Roast Chicken Thighs with Smoked Paprika, Lemon & Herbs, Carrots & Potatoes (page 278)

SNACK: Lactose-free cottage cheese with salt, pepper, ¼ cup (36 g) of chopped black olives, and a sprinkle of chopped fresh chives. Use as a flavorful dip with suitable crackers, bell pepper slices, and/or baby carrots.

BREAKFAST: Portable Breakfast Sandwich (page 95) and 2 small (150 g) kiwifruit

LUNCH: Tarragon Chicken Salad with Grapes & Pecans (page 118) served on low FODMAP bread with a handful of baby carrots or red pepper slices and 8 ounces (227 g) of lactose-free yogurt

DINNER: Lasagne the low FODMAP Way (page 196). Enjoy with a side garden salad prepared with romaine lettuce, 5 cherry tomatoes, and sliced green pepper, drizzled with olive oil and vinegar, and an orange.

SNACK: Rice cake spread with peanut butter and topped with 1 tablespoon of semisweet chocolate chips and 1 tablespoon of pepitas (hulled pumpkin seeds), served with 1 cup (240 ml) of lactose-free milk

BREAKFAST: ¼ cup (30 g) of Quinoa Oat Granola with Coconut (page 90) sprinkled over 8 ounces (227 g) of lactose-free yogurt and topped with 10 strawberries (140 g), sliced

LUNCH: Rice tortilla rollup filled with 1 cup (38 g) of raw baby spinach or kale, sliced chicken, 1 slice of provolone cheese, a few thin slices of cucumber and tomato, and mustard or mayonnaise. Serve with a side of tortilla chips and 1 cup (150 g) of grapes.

DINNER: Slow-Roasted Shredded Pork (page 297) served with Garlic Mashed Potatoes (page 173) and steamed carrots

SNACK: Peanut butter banana chocolate sorbet: Blend 1 medium-size just ripe banana with 1 teaspoon of natural or Dutch-processed cocoa powder and 1 tablespoon of all-natural peanut butter (add water to thin to desired consistency).

DAY 4

BREAKFAST: Blueberry Muffin (page 300), coffee or suitable tea with lactose-free milk, 8 ounces (227 g) lactose-free vanilla yogurt

LUNCH: 2 slices low FODMAP bread spread with 2 tablespoons of peanut butter and 1 tablespoon of strawberry jam (without high-fructose corn syrup), served with 1 cup (240 ml) of lactose-free milk or 8 ounces (227 g) vanilla or plain lactose-free yogurt, 2 cups (16 g) of salted popcorn, and baby carrots

DINNER: Baked half chicken breast, ½ small cooked sweet potato (about ½ cup raw [70 g]) topped with a pat of butter and pinch of ground cinnamon, and green beans sautéed in olive oil and topped with 1 tablespoon of sliced almonds. Enjoy with 2 small (150 mg) kiwifruits.

SNACK: 1 string cheese snack (28 g), 10 rice cracker rounds, and 1 cup (150 g) of grapes

DAY 5

BREAKFAST: 2 slices low FODMAP bread, toasted and lightly buttered, plus scrambled eggs cooked with a handful of baby spinach, and an orange

LUNCH: Simple green salad topped with 5 grape tomatoes, 5 slices of cucumber, and grilled chicken, dressed with a 1-tablespoon mixture of oil and vinegar or Balsamic Dijon Vinaigrette (page 73). Enjoy with a Fruit & Nut Protein Kinder Bar (page 134).

DINNER: Pan-Seared Salmon & Greens with Balsamic Glaze (page 244), a baked potato topped with shredded Cheddar cheese and dollop of butter, and a side of carrot rounds sautéed in garlic-infused oil

DESSERT: Chocolate Walnut Brownie (page 323) and 1 cup (240 ml) of lactose-free milk

SNACK: 8 ounces (227 g) of vanilla or plain lactose-free yogurt topped with 10 medium-size (140 g) strawberries and 10 (20 to 30 g) pecans or walnuts, chopped

DAY 6

BREAKFAST: Lemon Ginger Scone (page 308) and 8 ounces (227 g) of vanilla lactose-free yogurt topped with 1 tablespoon of chopped walnuts

LUNCH: Asian Chicken Salad (page 168)

DINNER: Margherita pizza for one: starting with a low FODMAP pizza crust for one (such as Udi's gluten-free pizza crust), coat the circumference of the crust with 1 tablespoon of garlic-infused olive oil; arrange ½ small (59 g) common beefsteak tomato, sliced, and ½ cup (57 g) part-skim shredded mozzarella cheese on top of the crust, sprinkle with ¼ teaspoon of dried oregano, and bake as directed on the package. Scatter 2 tablespoons of fresh basil leaves, torn into strips, on top of the cooked pizza. Serve immediately with a salad of lettuce, 5 slices of cucumber, and shredded carrot dressed with about a 1-tablespoon mix of oil and vinegar or Balsamic Dijon Vinaigrette (page 73).

SNACK: 10 rice cracker rounds, a slice (1½ ounces) of Brie cheese, and 1 cup (150 g) grapes

DAY 7

BREAKFAST: 8 ounces (227 g) of vanilla or plain lactose-free yogurt topped with ¼ cup (30 g) of Quinoa Oat Granola with Coconut (page 90) and 20 (28 g) blueberries

LUNCH: Egg Drop Soup (page 265) with 10 rice cracker rounds. Enjoy with 1 cup (140 g) of chopped pineapple.

SNACK: 1 Fruit & Nut Protein Kinder Bar (page 134)

DINNER: Grilled pork chop brushed with 1 teaspoon of pure maple syrup mixed with 1 teaspoon of Dijon mustard, with side of a baked Yukon gold potato and grilled baby bok choy (slice in half, then lightly brush with sesame oil and a dash of soy sauce, prior to grilling)

DESSERT: One to two 3-Ingredient, 17-Second Peanut Butter Cookies (page 321) and 1 cup (240 ml) of lactose-free milk

Navigating Special Diets: Vegan, Vegetarian, Gluten-Free, and Dairy-Free

We understand that you may be following additional dietary modifications due to other health conditions, religious, or ethical reasons. We do recommend that you work closely with a registered dietitian to ensure your diet is nutritionally adequate and that you are not unnecessarily restricting food groups, as combining diet strategies can easily lead to nutrient inadequacy, and in some cases, malnutrition. In clinical practice, Kate tends to shorten the low FODMAP elimination phase to two weeks for her clients that have multiple dietary restrictions, to avoid nutritional shortcomings. We also understand that merging more than one dietary restriction can be a challenge for you; therefore, we provided a day's worth of menus to help provide some guidance to those following additional diet modifications.

THE LOW FODMAP VEGAN AND VEGETARIAN

For the low FODMAP vegan and lacto-ovo vegetarian struggling with GI distress, we have provided a few pearls of wisdom for you as you embark on a low FODMAP diet trial. First, for the vegetarian (lacto-ovo), include low-lactose dairy products, such as lactose-free milk, hard or semisoft cheeses, lactose-free yogurt, and eggs to help you meet your protein, calcium, and vitamin D needs. Vegans, however, relying mostly on legumes to fulfill their protein requirement, may have trouble eating enough protein during the FODMAP elimination phase. This is because vegans rely on FODMAP-rich legumes (kidney beans, black beans), soy milk, silken tofu, and the like for their protein needs. While it is possible to do the low FODMAP elimination diet as a vegan, we don't advise you stay on the elimination phase for longer than two weeks, as the combination of a vegan and a low FODMAP diet can easily be nutritionally incomplete without strict attention to detail. We encourage all FODMAPers to meet with a registered dietitian when possible prior to starting the low FODMAP diet approach, but when blending the low FODMAP diet with a vegan diet modification, this recommendation is strongly encouraged. Without careful planning, a vegan diet can fall short on vitamin B12, vitamin D, omega-3 fats, iron, protein, calcium, and zinc. Some suitable low FODMAP vegan protein sources include drained and rinsed canned chickpeas (¼ cup [42 g] limit), and canned lentils (½ cup [46 g] limit), canned butter beans (¼ cup [35 g]), peanuts and peanut butter, edamame (1 cup [50 g]), and firm and extra-firm tofu.

A few additional low FODMAP-suitable selections for the vegan or vegetarian FODMAPer:

Dairy equivalents: Choose unsweetened and unflavored almond, macadamia, quinoa, hemp, rice, canned coconut, or soy milk (made from soy protein only).

Vegetarian diet followers can add lactose-free dairy milk; hard and semisoft cheese; such as feta and goat cheese; and suitable lactose-free yogurt.

Grains and seeds: Choose more of the protein-rich and nutrient-dense grains and seeds: quinoa, buckwheat, millet, sorghum, oats, oat bran, chia, flaxseeds, pumpkin seeds, sesame seeds, walnuts, pecans, or sunflower seeds.

Soy products: Choose firm or extra-firm tofu or tempeh (select products without added FODMAPs), edamame and soy milk made with soy protein isolate, not the whole soybean.

One-Day Sample Low FODMAP Vegan Menu

Breakfast

Quinoa flakes with fortified almond, hemp, macadamia, quinoa, or rice milk, topped with 20 (28 g) of blueberries, 1 tablespoon of pepitas (hulled pumpkin seeds) and 1 tablespoon of chia seeds

Lunch

Vegan Rice bowl: Place a scoop of cooked basmati or brown rice in a dish and top with bell pepper slices, grape tomatoes, sliced radish, kale, and shredded carrot plus ¼ cup (42 g) of drained and rinsed canned chickpeas or ¼ cup (35 g) of canned butter beans. Drizzle with balsamic vinegar and olive oil dressing and 2 tablespoons of toasted walnuts.

Snack

10 (12 g) almonds, 10 rice cracker rounds, and 1 cup (150 g) of grapes

Dinner

Tofu stir-fry: ⅔ cup (160 g) of firm or extra-firm (not silken) tofu sautéed in sesame oil with chopped bok choy, sliced kale, red bell pepper, and carrot, seasoned with soy sauce and served over cooked quinoa. Add 1 tablespoon (11 g) of toasted sesame seeds for flavor and crunch. Enjoy with an orange and 1 cup (240 ml) of fortified rice, almond, macadamia, quinoa, or hemp milk.

One-Day Low FODMAP Vegetarian Menu

Breakfast

¼ cup (25 g) of old-fashioned oats, cooked as directed on the package and served with 1 cup (240 ml) of lactose-free cow's milk or almond, hemp, macadamia, quinoa rice, or canned coconut milk, and topped with 10 medium-size (140 g) sliced strawberries and a tablespoon (12 g) of chia seeds.

Lunch

Grilled cheese and tomato sandwich made with suitable low FODMAP bread (for more info on bread, see page 45; for recipe, see page 121), a side salad of romaine lettuce, carrot, olives, and 2 tablespoons (23 g) of pepitas (hulled pumpkin seeds), drizzled with freshly squeezed lemon juice or 1 tablespoon (21 g) balsamic vinegar and olive oil, sea salt, and pepper.

Snack

1 or 2 rice cakes topped with a smear of peanut butter, a few pepitas, and ⅓ (33 g) ripe banana, sliced.

Dinner

An omelet made with 2 eggs, a handful of spinach, feta cheese, and chives, served with 2 slices of suitable low FODMAP bread, toasted, or breakfast potatoes (cut 1 baked Yukon gold potato into bite-size pieces and brown in a skillet with 2 teaspoons of vegetable oil, sea salt, and pepper). Enjoy with a fresh orange and handful of roasted peanuts (without added FODMAP ingredients).

LOW FODMAP, GLUTEN-FREE

Since wheat, barley, and rye are sources of gluten in the diet and also contain appreciable FOD-MAPs, adapting a low FODMAP diet to be one that is also gluten-free just requires a few extra tweaks. If you have celiac disease, Kate recommends using gluten-free-certified products when choosing crackers, cereals, suitable deli meats, condiments, and other commercially packaged food, whenever possible. A few common food swaps to adjust from a low FODMAP diet to a low FODMAP gluten-free-compliant diet include:

Low FODMAP Diet	Gluten-Free Low FODMAP Swaps
Soy sauce: regular wheat-containing soy sauce is allowed	Gluten-free soy sauce or tamari
Oatmeal, oat bran	Gluten-free oatmeal or gluten-free oat bran, if tolerated
Gluten-free or slow-leavened sourdough wheat bread	Gluten-free bread options made with only low FODMAP ingredients
Baking powder	Gluten-free baking powder
Wheat-based pretzels or crackers	Gluten-free options, such as rice crackers or nut and rice crackers

Sample Low FODMAP Gluten-Free Menu

Breakfast

8 ounces (227 g) of lactose-free yogurt topped with 10 (14 g) blueberries, and ¼ cup (30 g) Quinoa Oat Granola with Coconut (page 90) made with gluten-free oats

Lunch

2 slices suitable gluten-free and low FODMAP bread filled with sliced grilled chicken, a handful of spinach leaves, 1 to 2 slices of tomato, and suitable mayonnaise, with a side of red pepper strips and a fresh medium-size orange

Snack

¼ cup (about 38 g) of Protein-Packed Trail Mix (page 144)

Dinner

Grilled salmon, chicken, or lean steak; a baked potato topped with butter and chives; and sautéed green beans (sautéed in garlic-infused oil) topped with 2 tablespoons (12 g) of sliced almonds. Enjoy with a kiwifruit.

DAIRY-FREE DIET

Eight foods account for 90 percent of all food-allergy reactions, and milk is one of these foods. To be clear, a dairy intolerance is more than just being lactose intolerant. Dairy-free means a diet devoid of cow's milk or ingredient derivatives of milk, even lactose-free options. (Note: Eggs are allowed on a dairy-free diet.) If you have either a dairy intolerance or a dairy allergy, steer clear of the following foods and ingredients: milk, butter, butter fat, buttermilk, casein, casein hydrolysate, caseinates, cheese, cream, curds, custard, diacetyl (found in some butter, margarine, and butter substitutes), ghee, lactose, milk protein hydrolysate, sour cream, whey, whey protein hydrolysate, and cow, sheep, or goat yogurt.

Dairy provides a good source of calcium, protein, riboflavin, and vitamin D, key nutrients for bone health. Low FODMAP and dairy-free alternatives food options for these important nutrients are shown in the following chart. As mentioned, because calcium needs are more difficult to meet on a dairy-free low FODMAP diet, discuss calcium supplement options with your registered dietitian or health-care provider.

Non-dairy sources of key nutrients found in dairy that are acceptable on the low FODMAP diet:

Vitamin D	Sardines, canned tuna, egg yolk, beef liver
Riboflavin	Spinach, beef, pork, liver, shellfish, fish
Calcium	Almonds, broccoli, bok choy, chia seeds
Protein	Meats, fish, poultry, eggs, nut butters, firm tofu

Sample Dairy-Free and Low FODMAP Menu

Breakfast

¼ cup (25 g) old-fashioned oats, cook as directed on the package, and topped with 20 (28 g) of blueberries and 1 tablespoon (12 g) of chia seeds. Enjoy with 1 cup (240 ml) of almond milk (fortified with calcium).

Lunch

Chicken rice veggie bowl: 1 cup cooked jasmine rice topped with baby kale, grated carrot, ½ cup (47 g) of raw broccoli (lightly blanched or microwaved to soften), scallion (green parts only), and 2 tablespoons (28 g) of pepitas (hulled pumpkin seeds), dressed with a 1-tablespoon mix of red wine vinegar and olive oil. Enjoy with 1 medium-size orange.

Dinner

Grilled salmon and grilled summer squash and zucchini wedges (brushed with olive oil, sea salt, and pepper prior to grilling) served with a side of quinoa, plus ½ cup (90 g) of diced cantaloupe

Snack

Fruit & Nut Protein Kinder Bars (page 134) and 1 cup (240 ml) of almond milk (fortified with calcium)

Note: If you are new to a dairy-free diet and could benefit from additional resources, check out our recommended websites in the resource section in the back of the book.

Chapters 5 through 13 provide many mouthwatering, tummy-taming recipes. Most are keyed with icons that flag them as safe for special diets, such as gluten-free or vegetarian, or include ingredient notes that help you make the right choice for special diets. You will note that many of the recipes also include "Post–FODMAP Challenge Options" ingredient add-ins. The purpose of this is to ensure that these recipes can be used for the elimination phase as well as after you have liberalized your diet and reintegrated the FODMAP-rich foods that you can tolerate. We cannot emphasize enough that the purpose of the low FODMAP approach is to manage your symptoms with the least restrictive diet as possible. After the challenge phase, feel free to add small amounts of the Post–FODMAP Challenge Options provided in the recipes as appropriate for you. You will find that we may provide multiple recipe adaptions in these options and we suggest you simply add them to your degree of tolerance: at first, just add one postchallenge ingredient, but as you go along and feel more confident with your body and what it can tolerate, feel free to add more than one. If you find you overdo it with the add-ins and develop symptoms, pull back the next time. Tolerance to FODMAPs can change over time and sometimes people can get overconfident with what they think they can eat and are reminded with a tummyache! We promise, you will soon be very intuitive with what you can eat and what you can't. Ready to dive into the best low FODMAP recipes ever? Then, turn the page!

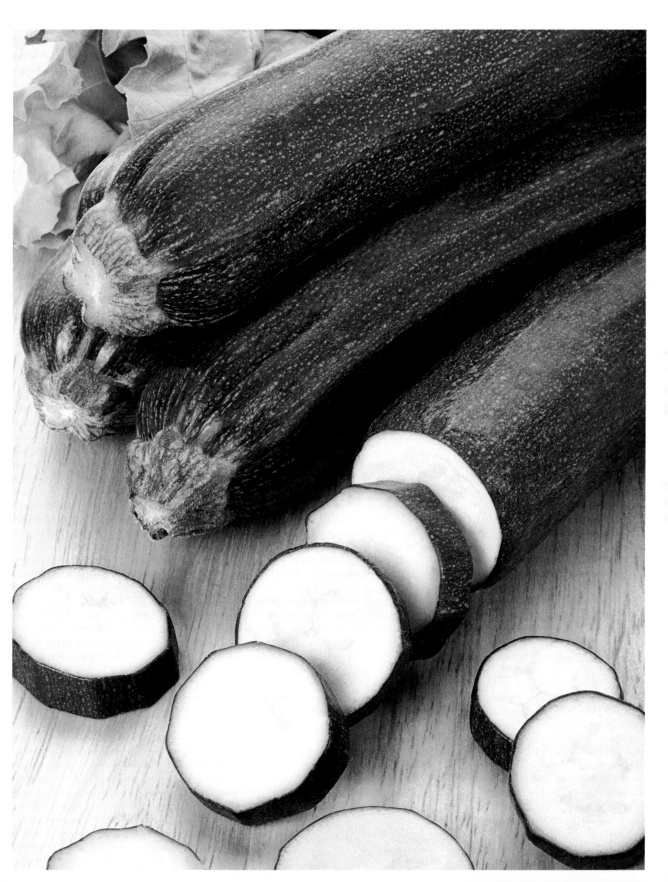

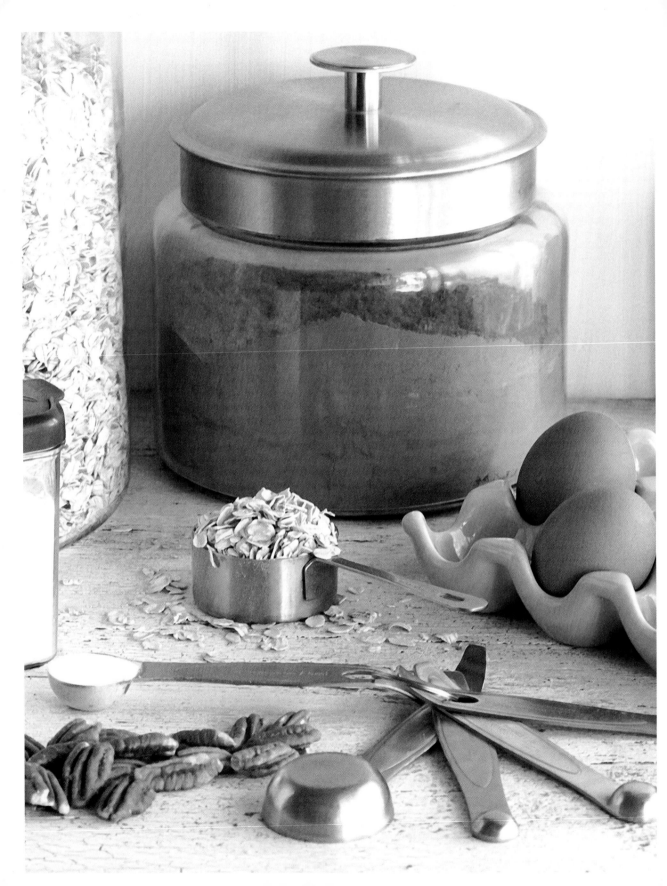

Chapter 4

HOW TO SUCCEED IN THE FODMAP KITCHEN

Making the Best Darned Tasting Low FODMAP Food Ever

NOW THAT YOU KNOW WHAT FODMAPS ARE and you have some strategies for eating low FODMAP, it's time to put it all into practice. These next chapters show you how to make low FODMAP food taste simply fabulous.

There is nothing "diet-y" about these recipes, nor will you find anything beyond standard cooking techniques. These are dishes you'll enjoy eating, made with high-quality ingredients, crafted with attention to detail.

The Importance of Flavor, Texture, Aroma, and Even Visuals

A "diet" can leave you disappointed when it does not satisfy—and then you quit. Our low FOD-MAP approach is about real food, satisfying all of your senses and keeping your digestive symptoms in check. This is the kind of food you want to eat and would even feel good about serving to guests. But while looks are important, taste is always paramount, and since there are a few common flavor-filled ingredients that you won't be using, particularly during the elimination phase—we are looking at you, garlic and onions—you have to learn how to make some key changes.

Salt, Pepper, Herbs, and Spices Are Your Friends

Giving up garlic and onions during the elimination phase might seem near to impossible; the good news is that you can use garlic- or onion-infused oil (homemade or store-bought, page 68; also, see Resources). But beyond that, you'll want to pay attention to your flavorings: plain old iodized salt is not the same as sea salt or kosher salt or large flake Maldon salt; stale ground pepper from a tin cannot provide the bite and complexity that come from freshly ground Tellicherry peppercorns. Freshly juiced lemons and lemon zest are powerhouses compared to bottled lemon juice. To shift the focus away from what you cannot have, make your food as flavorful and inviting as possible by choosing fresh and tasty low FODMAP ingredients. In addition to buying high-quality proteins, grains, dairy, oils, fruits, and vegetables, think about your salt, pepper, herbs, spices, and other flavoring agents. It all makes a difference.

FODMAPing Doesn't Have to Be Hard

We have developed the recipes in this book to please all members of the family so that you are not cooking twice at every meal. The ingredients are easy to find, the recipes are easy to follow, and we are here to support you in any way we can.

READ THE RECIPE—AND FOLLOW IT!

We know this sounds trite, but home cooks notoriously do not follow this simple advice. Do any of the following scenarios sound familiar? The recipe calls for an 8-inch (20 cm) cake pan but you use a 9-inch (23 cm) because it's what you have. Or that stick of salted butter in the fridge gets put to use when unsalted butter is called for. These seemingly small changes that you make on the fly can truly change the outcome of your dish. Follow the recipe to the letter the first time and take notes. Did you like the amount of salt? Was the dish a bit overdone or undercooked for you? Maybe you would like to use pecans instead of walnuts. You can make changes next time and make it yours— just make sure to stick with the low FODMAP guidelines.

Basic Ingredients

Eggs: All eggs used are graded large.

Butter: All butter is unsalted.

Oils: We use coconut oil, olive oil, and vegetable oils; the specific ones will be notated in the ingredient lists where necessary. For frying, we like a vegetable oil with a high heat point, such as grapeseed or rice bran. Buy all oils in amounts you will use quickly, and store in a cool, dark location. When buying nonstick spray, be sure to avoid any that contain flour.

What's a Post-FODMAP Challenge Phase Option?

You will note that we have included alternative recipe ingredients that contain FOD-MAPs for you to experiment with after you have completed the challenge phase of the low FODMAP diet. These ingredient options are under the header "Post-FODMAP Challenge Phase Option(s)" at the end of many recipes. For example, if you learn during the challenge phase that garlic is not a trigger for you, you can search for recipes where we have provided garlic in the Post-FODMAP Challenge Phase Options. Keep in mind, the amount we have included in this section is for the entire recipe, not just your portion. And, yes, you can opt to go a little light on ingredients, such as onion and garlic, if you want to better gauge your tolerance level. However, if you pass the wheat challenge, and note wheat flour as a possible post-challenge option, be sure you adhere to the quantities in the recipe, as using a little less flour could lead to a poorly executed baked good. One caveat: Wheat flour does not weigh the same as most gluten-free blends. If you want to substitute wheat flour, use the weight amount, not the volume.

Salt: In savory cooking, we use kosher salt for its very pure flavor. In baking recipes, we use non-iodized table salt, which has a much finer grain and dissolves readily. If a recipe calls for kosher salt, it will say so. Where it simply says "salt," you should use non-iodized table salt. Kosher salt and table salt measure differently, so please use what is called for.

We tested these recipes with Diamond kosher salt, which is also important to note because it does not measure the same as other brands of kosher salt, some varying by as much as 50 percent, as is the case with Morton's, the other most common brand. Make adjustments based on the salt you use.

Pepper: We recommend freshly ground black Tellicherry peppercorns.

Dried and fresh herbs and spices: We like to buy dried herbs and spices in bulk, for economy. If you do not have a good source near you, try Penzeys.com. Store dried herbs and spices in a cool, dark location, such as a drawer or cabinet away from the stove. Most dried herbs and spices have a shelf life of six months. If you haven't replaced yours in a while, it is time.

If a fresh herb is called for in a recipe, it will specify.

Gluten-free all-purpose flour: We tested these recipes with Bob's Red Mill Gluten Free 1 to 1 Baking Flour, which is Dédé's favorite due to its mild flavor and exceptional performance. The Bob's Red Mill Gluten Free 1 to 1 Baking Flour contains xanthan gum; not all blends do. In addition to the particular flours used in this product, the inclusion of xanthan gum plays an important role in the final texture of our recipes; flour blends without xanthan gum should not be considered a good substitute. You can try other blends, but the end result might not be the same.

Equipment & Techniques

Quality pots and pans do make a difference. Our recipes do not call for anything fancy, but when we suggest using a heavy Dutch oven or a sturdy rimmed baking sheet, know that it is for a good reason. We have used these items during recipe testing and their use can promise the best results.

We assume you have basic kitchen tools, such as a colander, a vegetable peeler, spatulas, a whisk, and the like. Here, we highlight some especially helpful tools.

Oven thermometer: Ovens frequently vary by 25°F (–4°C) or even as much as 50°F (10°C), which can lead to poor results with your baking and roasting. This can be remedied easily by following the oven manufacturer's instructions for calibrating your oven.

Dry measuring cups: We keep a wide array of heavy-duty, well-constructed stainless-steel measuring cups in the test kitchen in the following sizes: ⅛ cup, ¼ cup, ⅓ cup, ½ cup, ⅔ cup, ¾ cup, 1 cup, 1½ cups, and 2 cups. Dented cups will not provide accurate measuring; ditto for cheap sets from the dollar store, or decorative sets. Toss 'em and look for quality cups. We like those from King Arthur Flour and Cuisipro brands.

A Note on Measuring

Most Americans still use volume measurements, by use of dry and liquid measuring cups. Much of the world cooks and bakes by weight and also uses metric. We have provided all of this information in the recipes, but it comes with a caveat. For amounts less than ¼ cup (60 ml), we have chosen to stick with tablespoons, as that is how you will actually measure while cooking—2 tablespoons of vinegar, for instance. The metric amounts of ingredients have been translated from volume and there is not always a precise equivalent. In general, metric amounts have been rounded up, for convenience. We mostly work with volume amounts when measuring and these recipes will yield best results if you follow that approach.

Also we made certain executive decisions about the way we have presented ingredients. In the preceding chapters, where we described the Elimination and Challenge Phases of the diet, attention to detail is paramount. Since the Monash University low FODMAP app lists strawberries as 10 medium-size berries as one serving, so did we. The following chapters are about integrating foods into your life in a very real way. Remember our Eliminate-Challenge-Integrate motto? It's time to integrate all that you have learned through your challenges into actual recipes and cooking and so, for instance, with our 3-Berry Crisp (page 333), we were not going to ask you to count out hundreds of berries; rather, we provide volume as well as weight amounts. Always pay attention to serving size and you will be well on your way to cooking the Low FODMAP Diet Step by Step way.

Technique for measuring dry ingredients: We use a dip-and-sweep method. Aerate whatever dry ingredient is called for, such as gluten-free flour, by whisking until fluffy. Then take the exact-size measuring cup that is called for and dip it into the ingredient, allowing it to overfill. Use the flat edge of a butter knife or icing spatula to sweep off the excess, flush with the cup. You will not get the same results by spooning your ingredients into the cup, tapping the cup on the counter, or any other way. If the recipe calls for a sifted ingredient, sift first, then dip and sweep.

Measuring spoons: Just as with measuring cups, not all spoons are constructed precisely. Follow the previous guidelines for assessing quality construction. We use spoons from King Arthur Flour, Cuisipro, and Williams-Sonoma.

Technique for using measuring spoons: Dip the correct-size spoon into a dry ingredient so that spoon is overfilled. Use the flat edge of a butter knife or icing spatula to sweep off the excess, flush with the spoon. Small amounts of liquids, such as vanilla extract or lemon juice, may be measured with spoons in quantities less than ¼ cup (60 ml). For greater quantities, use a liquid measuring cup.

Liquid measuring cups: Do not use dry measuring cups for liquids or vice versa. Having 1-cup (240 ml), 2-cup (480 ml) and 4-cup (960 ml) sizes on hand will be helpful. As with dry measuring cups, not all cups are created with accuracy. We prefer Pyrex brand.

Technique for measuring liquid ingredients: Place the liquid measuring cup on a flat surface and fill to the correct measurement line. Bring your eye down to its level to assess measurement. Use a measuring cup that is most similar in size to the amount to be measured. In other words, do not measure ½ cup (120 ml) of liquid in a 4-cup (960 ml) measuring cup.

Digital scale: This is the most accurate kind of scale and is useful for certain ingredients, such as bulk chocolate or cheese. Look for a scale that easily toggles between ounces and grams.

Baking sheets: For cookies, pizza, and other recipes, we use commercial-weight aluminum half sheet pans. They do not warp and they conduct heat beautifully. They measure 18 x 13 inches (46 x 33 cm) and are easy to find.

Pots, pans, Dutch ovens, and skillets: In the Test Kitchen we use a variety, from triple-ply stainless steel, to cast iron, nonstick, and enamel-coated cast iron. Equipment can be expensive but can last a lifetime (except for nonstick, which does need timely replacing as the coating can wear unevenly; see next item). A good pot can actually help you be a better cook. Certain foods, such as highly acidic tomato sauces, need a nonreactive pot, which means it is constructed from a material that will not react with the food it comes in contact with. Reactive metals, such as aluminum and copper, can impart a metallic taste and off color to foods when they come in direct contact with acids. Where non-reactive pots are suggested, use stainless steel, triple-ply, or enamel-coated cast iron. Heatproof glass is also nonreactive.

Nonstick pans: Make sure the nonstick surface of your equipment is intact and unblemished (free of nicks, cuts, and scrapes). The coating should be on a heavy base. Ours are PFOA-free and based upon heavy-gauge anodized aluminum for even heating and lasting wear.

Silicone spatulas: These are used to fold and combine ingredients and also to stir hot items while they are cooking on the stove. Most withstand temperatures up to 450°F (230°C) and even higher, depending on the manufacturer.

Food processor: Food processors make grating large amounts of carrots or cheese a breeze. We like the Cuisinart Prep 11 Plus 11-cup food processor; make sure you choose a model with a metal blade as well as slicing and shredding disks.

Stand mixer: We use our 5-quart KitchenAid mixer all the time. The baking recipes in this book are not complicated and can be made with a stand mixer, a handheld electric mixer, and in many cases, by hand.

Microplane rasp-style zester: Box graters come in handy but we find that we use a Microplane rasp-type zester much more often. Microplane zesters are supersharp and offer more control, which makes it easier to leave the bitter, white pith behind when grating citrus. We also use them for grating small amounts of vegetables, cheese, chocolate, and nutmeg and consider these must-have tools. We have versions with small, medium, and larger cutting blades on hand.

Parchment paper: Parchment paper provides easy cleanup, a somewhat nonstick surface, and some insulation.

You'll see some icons by the recipes; here's what they denote. Apart from watching for these icons, read the recipes carefully for additional notes or tips that tell you how to adapt the ingredients to suit a gluten-free, dairy-free, vegan, or vegetarian diet.

Q "Quick" recipes are ready to use or serve in 30 minutes or less.

E "Easy" recipes can be prepped in less than 15 minutes but then might have unattended chilling or standing times or very easy and short cooking methods.

GF totally gluten-free

DF totally dairy-free

VG totally vegetarian (lacto-ovo: eggs, butter, and milk included)

V totally vegan (no animal ingredients)

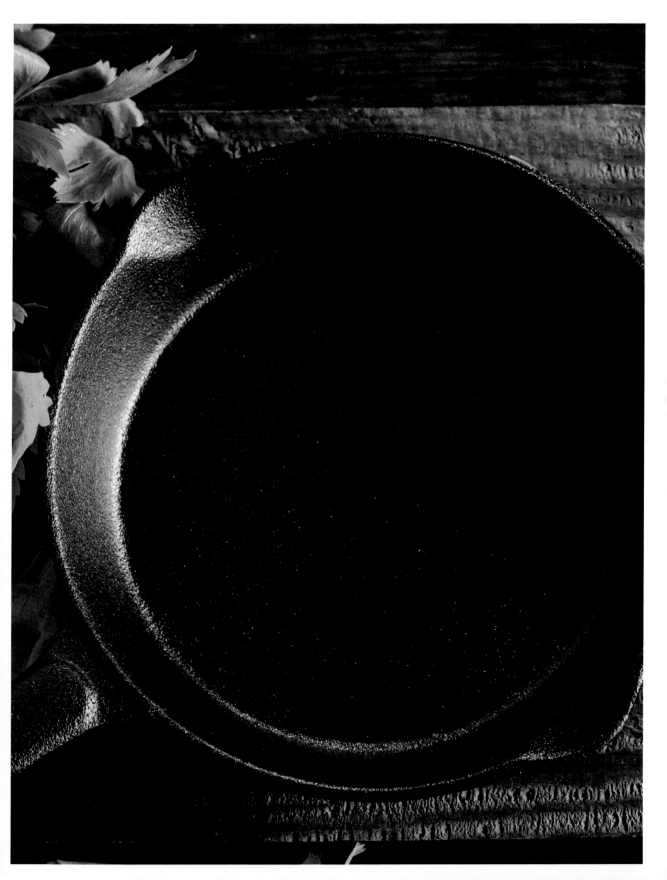

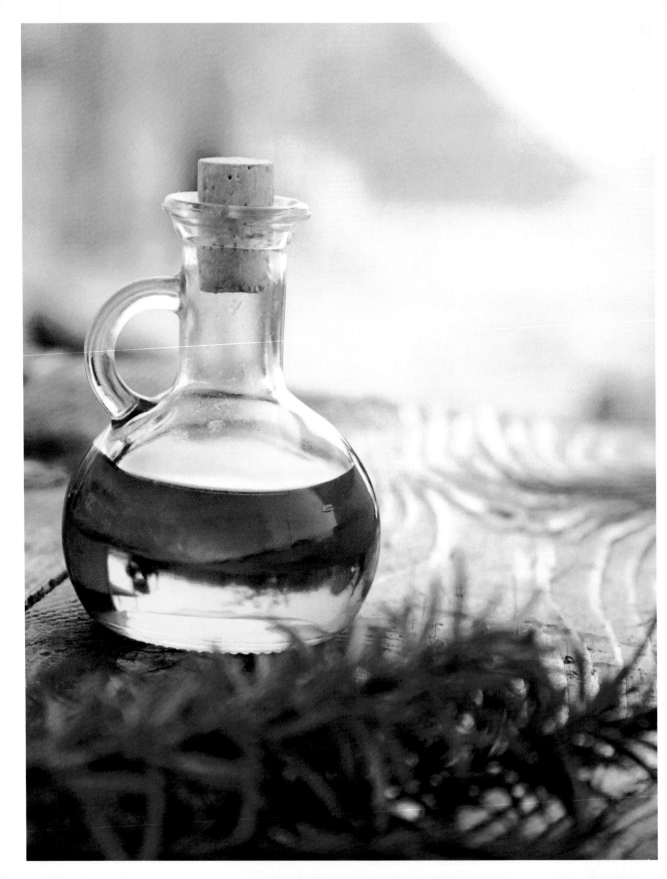

Chapter 5

RECIPE BASICS

AS WITH ANY COOKING APPROACH, you need some basics in your reper-toire for following a low FODMAP diet; these are the recipes that act as building blocks for other recipes, such as a good Chicken Stock (page 70) or Garlic-Infused Oil (page 68), or ones that you will turn to again and again in the course of a week, such as Balsamic Dijon Vinaigrette (page 73) or Salsa Fresca (page 80). Many of these can be made in larger batches, and can keep for a week or more to be on hand as needed. Others freeze well and offer that versatility, such as our vegeta-ble broth (page 69). By the way, being told "you can't have garlic or onions" was one of the most devastating pieces of news for both of us. Dédé, being newer to this low FODMAP world, didn't realize until she met Kate that the offending fructans in garlic were water soluble, but not oil sol-uble. When Kate told Dédé that she could infuse oils with onion and garlic (or buy such products as Boyajian Garlic Oil, which has a pure olive oil base), that was big news! What a relief! So, if you have been agonizing about the lack of garlic in your recipes, fret no more and try the Basil Pine Nut Pesto (page 83) to see what we are talking about.

Garlic-Infused Oil

     MAKES 2 CUPS (480 ML)

These oils mean you can have garlic and onion flavors without fear of intestinal distress. The more garlic or onion you use, the more potent the oil will be. After you make a batch, taste and assess whether you want more or less garlic flavor the next time around.

One important caveat: You should refrigerate the flavored oil to stave off any issues, such as botulism growth, and use it within three days, per FDA recommendations. Simply refrigerate in a clean, airtight glass jar and bring to room temperature before using, or use a measuring spoon to scoop out what you need. See Kate's Notes for purchasing ready-made.

---

2 cups (480 ml) extra-virgin olive oil or vegetable oil, such as canola, grapeseed, or rice bran

6 large garlic cloves, peeled

Have ready a glass storage container, jar, or bottle with an airtight lid. Rinse with boiling water and dry thoroughly; set aside.

Place the oil in a small saucepan and heat over low heat just until just warm to the touch but no hotter, then remove from the heat. Smash the garlic cloves lightly with the broad side of a knife or cleaver. Add the garlic to the oil and allow to sit for about 2 hours. Strain into the clean jar, discarding all the garlic. Cover and refrigerate, and use within 3 days.

VARIATION:

Onion-Infused Oil: Follow the above recipe, replacing the garlic with one medium-size white or yellow onion, peeled and roughly chopped. You can also try red or sweet onion, such as Maui or Walla Walla, for a slightly different flavor profile. Make sure to remove all pieces of onion before using.

KATE'S NOTES

I buy Boyajian Garlic Oil and use it regularly. Boyajian has many infused and flavored oils; the quality is always high and consistent, and they are easily found online or in many brick-and-mortar stores, such as Whole Foods Market.

Vegetable Broth

    MAKES ABOUT 4 QUARTS (3.8 L)

Commercial and homemade vegetable broths typically contain onion and very often garlic as well. Our homemade version is easy to make and freezes well. This is deliberately very mild—we even keep the salt level low—creating a very versatile broth. You can use it to thin and enhance Roasted Tomato Soup (page 258) or as a base for Hearty Vegetable Soup (page 263).

---

2 tablespoons Garlic-Infused Oil (page 68) made with olive oil, or purchased garlic-infused olive oil

1 medium-size white or yellow onion, peeled and quartered

1 large bunch flat-leaf parsley

6 sprigs thyme

1 teaspoon black peppercorns

1 large bay leaf

2 medium-size carrots, unpeeled, scrubbed, and cut into 1-inch (2.5 cm) pieces

2 medium-size leeks, green parts only, washed well and sliced

1 medium-size fennel bulb, root end trimmed, bulb sliced, fronds (the top, feathery leaves) and stems chopped

1 large turnip, scrubbed, ends trimmed, sliced into ½-inch (12 mm) rounds

Place the oil in a 5- to 6-quart (4.7 to 5.7 L) stockpot and heat over medium-low heat. Add the onion and sauté over medium heat, stirring often, for about 5 minutes, or until beginning to soften but not brown. Remove all the onion pieces. This step is very important, to keep the broth low FODMAP approved. Place the parsley, thyme, peppercorns, bay leaf, carrots, leek greens, fennel, and turnip in the pot.

Add water just to cover the solids. Cover the pot and bring to a simmer over medium heat, then lower the heat to a low simmer and cook for 1 hour, skimming off any fat or froth that rises to the top during the first half-hour and adding water if necessary to keep all the solid ingredients just submerged.

When the broth is done, strain into a clean pot or storage container(s) and discard the solids. Allow to cool to room temperature, then refrigerate overnight. Skim all the fat off the surface, then divide the broth into airtight storage containers (we like to make 1-cup [240 ml], 2-cup [480 ml], and 4-cup [960 ml] amounts) and either refrigerate for up to 3 days or freeze for up to 6 months. You can also freeze the broth in ice cube trays, then place the frozen cubes in resealable plastic freezer bags for easy access.

Chicken Stock

   MAKES ABOUT 4 QUARTS (3.8 L)

Most commercially prepared chicken stock is made with onions and/or garlic. Luckily, chicken stock is easy to make—it just takes time, practically unattended on the stove—and when you make it from scratch, you can control the choice and quality of ingredients and the preparation technique. You can use this stock to make Tortilla Soup with Chicken & Lime (page 266) and Egg Drop Soup (page 265). Note that we do call for onion; however, it is only used to infuse the fat with flavor, as a base. For a low FODMAP prepared version, check out Reduced Sodium Chicken Broth Concentrate at Savorychoice.com.

---

6 pounds (2.7 kg) chicken backs, or
  1 (6-pound [2.7 kg]) chicken, cut into pieces

1 medium-size white or yellow onion,
  peeled and quartered

1 large bunch flat-leaf parsley

10 sprigs fresh thyme

6 black peppercorns

1 large bay leaf

2 medium-size carrots, unpeeled, scrubbed,
  and cut into 1-inch (2.5 cm) pieces

Trim the chicken of most of its fat, reserving about 1 cup (240 ml) of fat pieces. Place the reserved fat in the bottom of a 10- to 12-quart (9.5 to 11.4 L) stockpot and cook over medium-low heat to render (melt) the fat. Add the onion and sauté over medium heat, stirring often, for about 5 minutes, or until beginning to soften but not brown. Remove all the onion pieces. This step is very important to keep the stock low FODMAP approved. Place the parsley, thyme, peppercorns, bay leaf, and carrots in the pot, then add the chicken pieces.

Add water just to cover the solids. Cover the pot and bring to a simmer over medium heat, lower the heat to a low simmer, and cook for 3 hours, skimming off any fat or froth that rises to the top during the first half hour and adding water if necessary to keep all the solid ingredients just submerged.

When the stock is done, pour through a fine wire-mesh strainer into a clean pot or container and set the solids aside (see Dédé's Tips). Allow the stock to cool to room temperature, then refrigerate overnight. Skim all the fat off the surface, then divide the stock into airtight storage containers (we like to make 1-cup [240 ml], 2-cup [480 ml], and 4-cup [960 ml] amounts) and either refrigerate for up to 3 days or freeze for up to 6 months. You can also freeze the stock in ice cube trays, then place the frozen cubes in resealable plastic freezer bags for easy access.

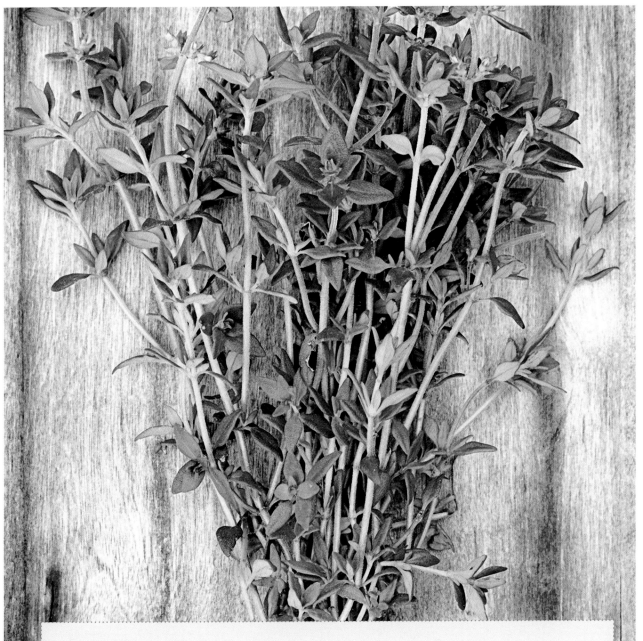

DÉDÉ'S TIPS

You can certainly add salt to taste after you have strained the stock, but remember that most likely it will become part of another dish; salting after the stock is incorporated is our preferred approach.

   After you strain out the solids, the herbs and carrots should be discarded, but there might be some chicken meat, especially if you used a whole chicken to make the stock. We love to use this meat for such recipes as Chicken Tostadas (page 226).

Quick Tomato Sauce

     MAKES ABOUT 12 CUPS (2.8 L)

This tomato sauce is featured as part of our Meatballs for Spaghetti or Subs (page 249) and our Lasagne the Low FODMAP Way (page 196), among other dishes, or use it anytime you need a basic tomato sauce. It's quick, too. If you have the garlic oil on hand, you can make this sauce in less than 15 minutes.

Note: Some tomato products contain added garlic and onion. Be sure to scan the ingredients label on all canned tomatoes—crushed, diced, and so on, to ensure they do not contain these high-FODMAP ingredients.

⅓ cup (75 ml) Garlic-Infused Oil (page 68) made with olive oil, or purchased garlic-infused olive oil

2 teaspoons dried basil

2 teaspoons dried oregano

4 (28-ounce ([794 g]) cans crushed tomatoes (without garlic or onion)

2 teaspoons salt

½ teaspoon sugar

Freshly ground black pepper

Heat the oil in a large saucepan over low heat and add the basil and oregano. Stir to combine for about 1 minute; the heat will release the flavors of the herbs. Add the tomatoes, salt, sugar, and pepper to taste. Bring to a simmer, partially covered, over medium-low heat and cook for about 10 minutes, stirring occasionally. The sauce is ready to use, or allow to cool to room temperature and refrigerate in airtight container for up to 1 week or freeze for up to 3 months.

DÉDÉ'S TIPS

This sauce can be doubled or halved, but why make less? I made a huge batch of this for a pasta potluck and everyone was thrilled–they didn't even know that it was low FODMAP approved. If you want, you can also use half garlic-infused oil and half Onion-Infused Oil (see variation, page 68) for an additional layer of flavor.

Balsamic Dijon Vinaigrette

     MAKES ABOUT 12 CUPS (2.8 L) | SERVING SIZE 2 TABLESPOONS

The classic vinaigrette ratio is 3:1 oil to vinegar, and while that does give us a starting point, it makes for a fairly rich mixture. This vinaigrette is sharper and allows the balsamic vinegar to take center stage. This not only provides loads of flavor but reduces the calorie count as well. Dijon mustard adds flavor and body (the vinaigrette is almost creamy in consistency) and also acts as an emulsifier. Know that old saying of how oil and water (in this case, vinegar) don't mix? An emulsifier brings these two opposing liquids together into a smooth mixture.

⅓ cup (75 ml) balsamic vinegar

2 teaspoons Dijon mustard (use gluten-free if necessary)

¾ cup (180 ml) extra-virgin olive oil or Garlic-Infused Oil (page 68) made with olive oil, or purchased garlic-infused olive oil

Kosher salt (optional)

Freshly ground black pepper (optional)

Whisk the vinegar and mustard together in a small bowl. Slowly whisk in the oil until smooth and combined. You can also shake the mixture together in a covered jar. Season to taste with salt and pepper, if desired. The vinaigrette is ready to use, or may be refrigerated in a covered container for up to a week. Bring to room temperature before using. You may hasten this by warming the jar in a bowl of warm water. Shake well before using.

KATE'S NOTES

Balsamic vinegar should be limited to a 1-tablespoon serving per meal, as larger amounts qualify as a moderate excess fructose source. Our delicious balsamic vinaigrette recipe can be enjoyed as a 2-tablespoon serving on the low FODMAP elimination diet.

POST-FODMAP CHALLENGE PHASE OPTION

Fructan: If you passed the fructan garlic challenge, consider adding one garlic clove, finely chopped, to the salad dressing ingredients. If you do add garlic, use the dressing right away.

Sweet Poppy Seed Dressing

    MAKES ABOUT ¾ CUP (180 ML) | SERVING SIZE 2 TABLESPOONS

If you are used to tangy, savory vinaigrettes, this sweet dressing might surprise you. It is a great option on a simple green salad and really perks up salads with similarly sweet components. Using red wine vinegar creates a pretty pink-tinged dressing with a bit more bite. We have been known to balance out the sweetness with a few grinds of black pepper as well. Toss this together with torn romaine, shredded carrot, and blueberries for a start or try our Kale Cabbage Coleslaw (page 160).

½ cup (120 ml) vegetable oil, such as canola or grapeseed

¼ cup (60 ml) white wine vinegar

2 tablespoons plus 1 teaspoon sugar, or 1 tablespoon pure maple syrup

1½ tablespoons poppy seeds

1 teaspoon Dijon mustard (use gluten-free if necessary)

¼ teaspoon kosher salt

Place all the ingredients in an airtight jar, cover, and shake until well mixed. Use immediately, or refrigerate for up to a week. Shake well before using.

Blue Cheese Dressing

   MAKES ABOUT 1½ CUPS (360 ML) | SERVING SIZE ¼ CUP (60 ML)

Whether you like your blue cheese as a dip for Baked Buffalo Chicken Wings (page 149) or slathered on a wedge of iceberg lettuce, this low FODMAP version satisfies with lots of blue cheese and a tangy edge from the yogurt, lemon juice, and white wine vinegar. Blue cheeses vary in saltiness, so use your taste buds to guide the seasoning. Also, we do like the balance created by both the lemon juice and vinegar, but feel free to use all of one or the other to streamline the recipe or if you have only one on hand.

Best of all, you can make this in five minutes! You will never buy bottled again.

---

6 ounces (170 g) blue cheese (see Kate's Notes)

6 tablespoons (84 g) lactose-free sour cream, such as Green Valley Organics

6 tablespoons (84 g) lactose-free yogurt, such as Green Valley Organics

¼ cup (57 g) mayonnaise

1 tablespoon freshly squeezed lemon juice

1 tablespoon white wine vinegar

Salt

Freshly ground black pepper

2 tablespoons finely chopped fresh chives, for garnish (optional)

Crumble the blue cheese into a mixing bowl, then add the sour cream, yogurt, mayonnaise, lemon juice, and vinegar. Whisk together until combined, leaving some lumps of blue cheese. Season to taste with salt and pepper. We strongly recommend the chive garnish as it adds another layer of flavor. The dressing is ready to serve, or refrigerate in an airtight container for up to 2 days.

KATE'S NOTES

Not everyone considers blue cheese to be gluten-free, hence the lack of that designation. Although gluten testing has shown most blue cheese to have low enough gluten levels to be considered gluten-free, we opted to be careful and not included recipes with blue cheese as suitable for those on a gluten-free diet.

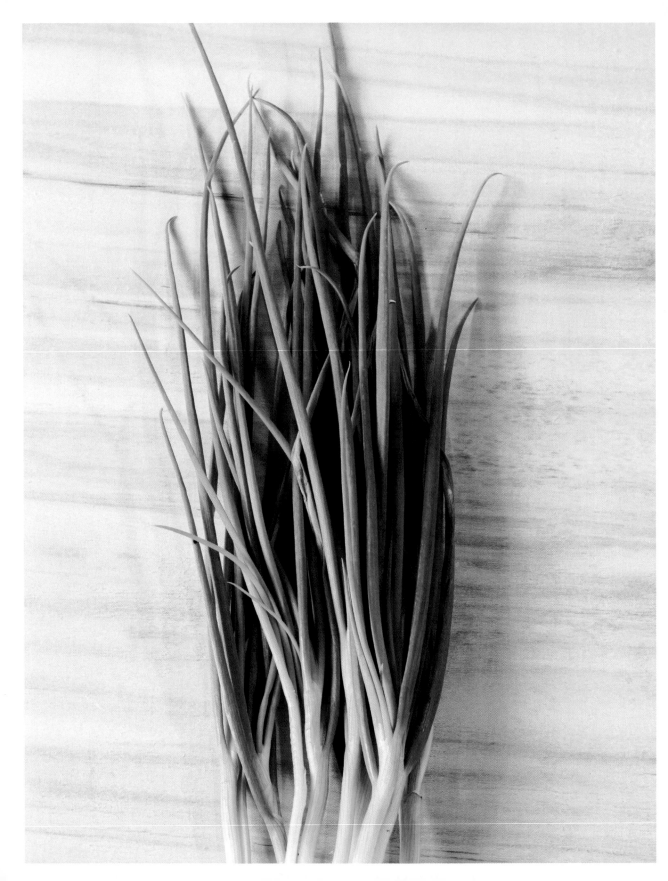

Ranch Dressing

   MAKES ABOUT 1 CUP (240 ML) | SERVING SIZE ¼ CUP (60 ML)

If you have only had bottled ranch dressing, you are in for a treat with homemade. Although you can make this with dried herbs in a pinch, and directions are given for that, we encourage you to use fresh herbs; it makes all the difference. This is great as a dip for Fully Loaded Stuffed Potato Skins (page 222).

½ cup (120 ml) lactose-free milk (whole, 2%, 1%, or fat-free)

2 teaspoons freshly squeezed lemon juice

½ cup (113 g) mayonnaise

1 tablespoon finely chopped scallion, green parts only

2 tablespoons finely chopped fresh chives, or 2 teaspoons dried

1 tablespoon finely chopped fresh dill, or 1 teaspoon dried

1 tablespoon finely chopped fresh flat-leaf parsley, or 1 teaspoon dried

2 teaspoons Garlic-Infused Oil (page 68) made with vegetable oil, or purchased garlic-infused vegetable oil

½ teaspoon Dijon mustard (use gluten-free if necessary)

Kosher salt

Freshly ground black pepper

Combine the milk and lemon juice in a 2-cup (480 ml) lidded jar and allow to sit, uncovered, for 5 minutes, or until slightly thickened. Add the mayonnaise, scallion greens, chives, dill, parsley, oil, and mustard. Cover the jar and shake very well. Season to taste with salt and pepper. The dressing is ready to use, or refrigerate for up to 3 days.

DÉDÉ'S TIPS

For a bit more tang, use ½ cup (114 g) of lactose-free yogurt instead of the milk and lemon juice combo. The dressing will be a bit thicker and can be thinned with lactose-free milk, if desired.

Carrot Ginger Dressing

    MAKES ABOUT ⅔ CUP (165 ML) | SERVING SIZE 2 TABLESPOONS

While a simple oil and vinegar dressing has its place, every now and then we want something with a little more pizzazz. This vivid orange dressing has a kick from fresh ginger and an Asian flavor profile from soy sauce and sesame oil. Try it on greens or get creative; you can use it in one of our Mason Jar Salads (page 124), where it enlivens an array of colorful veggies. You do need a blender and this dressing is best used right after preparing, as it will separate upon sitting. The recipe may be halved or doubled.

2 medium-size carrots, ends trimmed, scrubbed or peeled, and broken into pieces

1 (2-inch [5 cm]) piece fresh ginger, peeled and roughly chopped

¼ cup (60 ml) rice or distilled white vinegar

1 tablespoon plus 1 teaspoon low-sodium soy sauce or tamari (use gluten-free if necessary, such as San-J Organic)

1 tablespoon plus 1 teaspoon toasted sesame oil

2 teaspoons firmly packed light brown sugar

2 teaspoons hot tap water

Place all the ingredients in a blender and blend on high speed until very smooth. Use immediately.

POST-FODMAP CHALLENGE PHASE OPTION

Fructan: If you passed the fructan garlic challenge, consider adding one to two garlic cloves, finely chopped, to the salad dressing ingredients. If you do add garlic, use the dressing right away.

Green Goddess Dressing

    MAKES ABOUT 1 CUP (240 ML) | SERVING SIZE ¼ CUP (60 ML)

Are you a creamy dressing fan? The classic Green Goddess is jam-packed with fresh herbs and garlic, with a flavor punch from anchovies. Garlic, you say? Yes, from our Garlic-Infused Oil (page 68) or, if you have passed your fructan garlic challenge with flying colors, see the Post-FODMAP Challenge Phase Option below. Don't even think about making this with dried herbs; fresh are a must. Try this dressing in one of our Mason Jar Salads (page 124).

½ cup (120 ml) lactose-free whole or 2% milk

1½ tablespoons freshly squeezed lemon juice

½ cup (113 g) mayonnaise

⅓ cup (17 g) roughly chopped fresh flat-leaf parsley

¼ cup (11 g) roughly chopped fresh chives

2 tablespoons roughly chopped fresh tarragon

2 anchovy fillets, packed in oil, drained

1 teaspoon Garlic-Infused Oil (page 68) made with vegetable oil, or purchased garlic-infused vegetable oil

Combine the milk and 1½ teaspoons of the lemon juice in a blender and let sit without blending for 5 minutes, or until thickened. Add the remaining ingredients, including the remaining tablespoon of lemon juice, to the blender and blend on high speed until very smooth. The dressing is ready to use, or refrigerate in an airtight container for up to 3 days. Stir before using.

> **POST-FODMAP CHALLENGE PHASE OPTION**
>
> **Fructan:** If you passed the fructan garlic challenge, consider adding one garlic clove, finely chopped, to the salad dressing ingredients. If you do add garlic, use the dressing right away.

Salsa Fresca

       MAKES ABOUT 2 CUPS (480 ML) | SERVING SIZE ½ CUP (120 ML)

Most commercially prepared salsas contain a good amount of onions and often garlic as well. This homemade salsa is best enjoyed the day of, or maybe the day after it is made, but it is so quick to put together that once you make it, we think you'll be able to whip it up without the recipe. It's all about using good tomatoes and then tasting to get the balance right between the heat (jalapeño), acid (lime juice), and salt. Serve with corn tortilla chips or with our Chicken Tostadas (page 226).

---

1 pound (455 g) ripe plum tomatoes (about 6 medium-size)

¼ cup (16 g) chopped scallion, green parts only

½ medium-size jalapeño pepper, seeded and minced, or more to taste (see Dédé's Tips)

2 tablespoons chopped fresh cilantro leaves

2 teaspoons freshly squeezed lime juice, or more to taste

Salt

Use a sharp paring knife to remove the stem and core of each tomato. Cut the tomatoes in half lengthwise, then into quarters. Chop into roughly ½-inch (12 mm) dice and scrape into a nonreactive mixing bowl along with any juice. Stir in the scallion greens, jalapeño, cilantro, and lime juice. Add salt and taste. Adjust as needed with more jalapeño, lime juice, and/or salt. Serve immediately, or refrigerate in an airtight container for up to 24 hours. Bring to room temperature before serving.

DÉDÉ'S TIPS

Take care when handling the jalapeño—the membranes and seeds are hot and spicy. Either wear gloves or at the very least do not touch your eyes, nose, or mouth while handling and wash your hands well afterward.

If you want more color, add ⅛ orange or yellow bell pepper, seeded and diced, which will also add some sweetness.

POST-FODMAP CHALLENGE PHASE OPTIONS

Fructans: If you passed the fructan garlic challenge, consider adding one garlic clove, finely chopped, to the salsa ingredients. Or, if you passed the fructan onion challenge, add ¼ cup (36 g) of finely chopped red, white, or yellow onion.

Pineapple Salsa

       MAKES ABOUT 1½ CUPS (360 ML) | SERVING SIZE ½ CUP (120 ML)

This gorgeous fresh and fruity alternative to the tomato-based Salsa Fresca (page 80) is a little bit sweet from the ripe pineapple and red bell pepper, and offers a little bit of heat from the jalapeño and a herbaceous kick from cilantro. Set this out with corn tortilla chips, or try it with grilled chicken or fish, such as our Grilled Swordfish with Pineapple Salsa (page 225). This recipe may be doubled.

---

1 cup (140 g) finely diced fresh pineapple

½ red bell pepper, seeded and finely chopped

3 tablespoons finely chopped fresh cilantro

3 tablespoons finely chopped scallion, green parts only

1 tablespoon seeded and finely chopped jalapeño pepper

1 tablespoon freshly squeezed lime juice

Kosher salt

Stir together all the ingredients in a bowl, seasoning to taste with the salt. The salsa is ready to use but tastes even better a few hours later after the flavors have merged. The salsa may be refrigerated overnight in an airtight container, although it does lose a bit of freshness.

POST-FODMAP CHALLENGE PHASE OPTION

Fructose: If you pass the fructose challenge, consider using an equivalent amount of diced mango in place of the pineapple (or try them half and half).

Chipotle Chiles in Adobo Sauce

    MAKES ABOUT 1¼ CUPS (300 ML)

Canned chipotle chiles in adobo sauce provide heat, smoky flavor, and convenience, but they usually contain onion and garlic. This is our low FODMAP homemade version. It's not as easy as opening a can; however, the initial preparation time is less than 30 minutes, including the 20 minutes that it takes to rehydrate the dried chiles. The rest of the time is largely unattended. When done, you can freeze small portions and have this incredibly flavorful seasoning on hand for months (you can even double the recipe so you have more for later). Try these in our Chipotle Mayo (page 233) and our BBQ Sauce (page 84).

---

1 ounce (30 g) dried chipotle peppers (12 to 15 medium-size)

Boiling water

1¼ cups (300 ml) canned tomato puree (without garlic or onion)

⅓ cup (27 g) finely chopped leek, green parts only

⅓ cup (75 ml) distilled white vinegar

1½ teaspoons sugar

½ teaspoon freshly ground black pepper

½ teaspoon kosher salt

Remove any stems from the chipotles (if any are attached) and place the chiles in a heatproof bowl. Cover with boiling water, place a large lid or plate on the bowl to keep the heat in, and allow to sit for about 20 minutes. Check the chiles; they should be pliable. Drain all the chiles, discarding the soaking water.

Place half of the chiles in a blender along with tomato puree, leek greens, vinegar, sugar, pepper, and salt. Blend until smooth.

Scrape the blended mixture into a saucepan. Roughly chop the remaining chiles and add them to the pot, including the seeds, skin, and any juice they exude.

Bring to a boil over medium-high heat, stirring often. Lower the heat, cover, and keep at just a simmer for 45 minutes to 1 hour, stirring occasionally and adding extra water if needed. Cook until the mixture is thick and darkened.

Remove from the heat, allow to cool, then store in small, airtight containers (we like ¼-cup [60 ml] portions). Refrigerate for up to 1 month or freeze for up to 6 months.

Basil Pine Nut Pesto

   MAKES ABOUT 1¼ CUPS (270 ML) | SERVING SIZE ¼ CUP (60 ML)

This is our version of the Italian classic, but instead of fresh garlic, we use a very garlicky olive oil. Use double the garlic when preparing our Garlic-Infused Oil (page 68) for a closer-to-the-traditional end result with this pesto.

3½ cups (50 g) lightly packed fresh basil leaves, washed, dried, and large stems removed

⅔ cup (165 ml) double-strength Garlic-Infused Olive Oil (page 68) (see headnote), made with olive oil

Generous ½ teaspoon kosher salt

¼ cup pine nuts (36 g) or sliced almonds (22 g), very lightly toasted

¾ cup (75 g) finely grated Parmigiano-Reggiano cheese

Combine the basil, oil, salt, and pine nuts in a food processor fitted with a metal blade. Pulse, then process until a paste forms, scraping down the bowl as needed. Add the cheese and process until combined and somewhat smooth. It will retain some texture, which is fine. Scrape into an airtight container and refrigerate for up to a week. (The surface might discolor. To prevent this and possibly extend storage, pour a film of oil directly on top of the pesto).

DÉDÉ'S TIPS

In terms of flavor and texture, you can vary the amount of basil, oil, salt, and cheese to your liking. This recipe makes a fairly firm pesto, which will be thinned with pasta water before tossing with pasta. You can make it more fluid with more oil, if desired.

POST-FODMAP CHALLENGE PHASE OPTION

Fructan: If you passed the fructan garlic challenge, add two garlic cloves, finely chopped, along with the olive oil, rather than using garlic-infused oil.

BBQ Sauce

 MAKES ABOUT 1¼ CUPS (360 ML) | SERVING SIZE ¼ CUP (60 ML)

Barbecue sauces get people talking. Just ask a group of people what makes a great one and you will get as many answers as there are folks in the room. This low FODMAP version of a basic barbecue sauce is a little sweet, a little hot, and there is no onion or garlic in sight. Slather on grilled chicken, pork chops, or ribs or anytime that you like to use barbecue sauce. You will need to make Chipotle Chiles in Adobo Sauce (page 82). If you have passed both the onion and garlic fructan challenges, feel free to substitute canned chipotle in adobo sauce, chopped finely.

---

1 cup (240 ml) canned tomato sauce (without garlic or onion)

¼ cup (60 ml) cider vinegar, distilled white vinegar, or rice vinegar

¼ cup (60 ml) pure maple syrup

2 tablespoons firmly packed light brown sugar

2 to 4 teaspoons Chipotle Chiles in Adobo Sauce (page 82), or to taste

2 teaspoons Worcestershire sauce (use gluten-free if necessary; see Kate's Notes)

1 teaspoon Dijon mustard (use gluten-free if necessary)

Kosher salt

Cayenne pepper (optional)

Whisk the tomato sauce, vinegar, maple syrup, brown sugar, chipotle in adobo, Worcestershire sauce, and mustard together in a medium-size saucepan until combined. Simmer over medium heat for about 5 minutes, whisking occasionally, until the sauce is well blended and slightly thickened.

Add salt to taste. If you would like more spice, add more chipotles in adobo sauce or a bit of cayenne. Cook for 1 minute more to blend the flavors. Remove from the heat, allow to cool to room temperature, then refrigerate in an airtight container for up to 1 week.

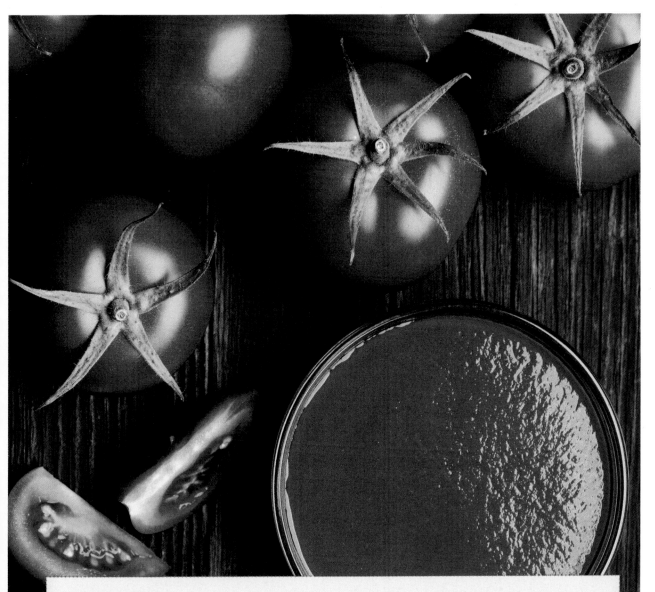

KATE'S NOTES

Monash University has noted that Worcestershire sauce is low FODMAP despite the fact that most varieties contain some garlic and molasses. This is likely due to the small amounts of these ingredients. I find my clients can tolerate Worcestershire sauce in small amounts, such as the 2 teaspoons in this recipe. If you are following a gluten-free diet, please read the ingredients to ensure the product you are using is gluten-free, such as the Lea & Perrins brand.

POST-FODMAP CHALLENGE PHASE OPTIONS

Fructans: If you passed the fructan garlic and onion challenges, feel free to use a commercially prepared tomato sauce that contains them. If you passed the fructan garlic challenge, use canned chipotle in adobo sauce, which contains garlic.

Whipped Cream

    MAKES ABOUT 2 CUPS (480 ML) | SERVING SIZE ½ CUP (120 ML)

Ah, the joys of navigating the low FODMAP diet. Heavy cream, which is what we use to make whipped cream, is not approved as low FODMAP in large quantities. Once whipped, however, an enormous amount of air is incorporated into the cream—and this process creates a finished product where the amounts of lactose (FODMAP) is low enough to allow up to a ½-cup (120 ml) serving size of the finished whipped cream. We FODMAPers can enjoy whipped cream every now and then, in moderation.

1¼ cups (300 ml) heavy cream, whipping cream, or heavy whipping cream, chilled

2 to 3 tablespoons granulated or confectioners' sugar

¼ teaspoon pure vanilla extract (optional)

In a chilled bowl, beat the cream, sugar, and vanilla, if using, on medium-high speed with an electric mixer, until very soft peaks form. (Use a wire whip attachment if using a stand mixer.) Lift the beaters to assess the texture. The cream should come to a peak that softly curves over onto itself. This is "softly whipped" cream perfect for topping desserts. Continue to whip if a stiffer texture is desired. Take care, as it firms up in texture quickly. The whipped cream is best if used immediately.

> ### DÉDÉ'S TIPS
> Pure granulated sugar will lend your whipped cream the purest sweetening flavor; however, if you need the cream to hold up for a while, use the confectioners' sugar.

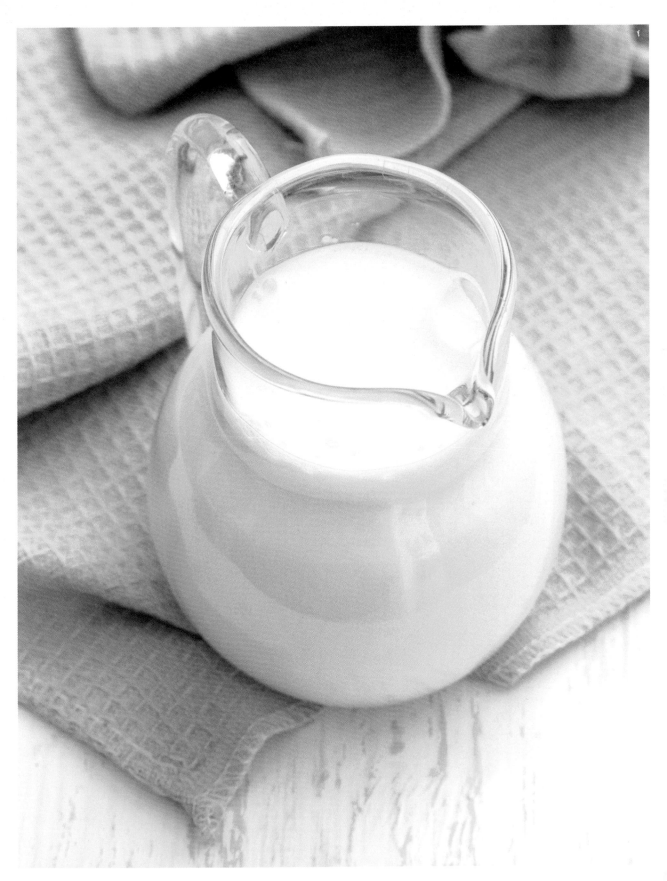

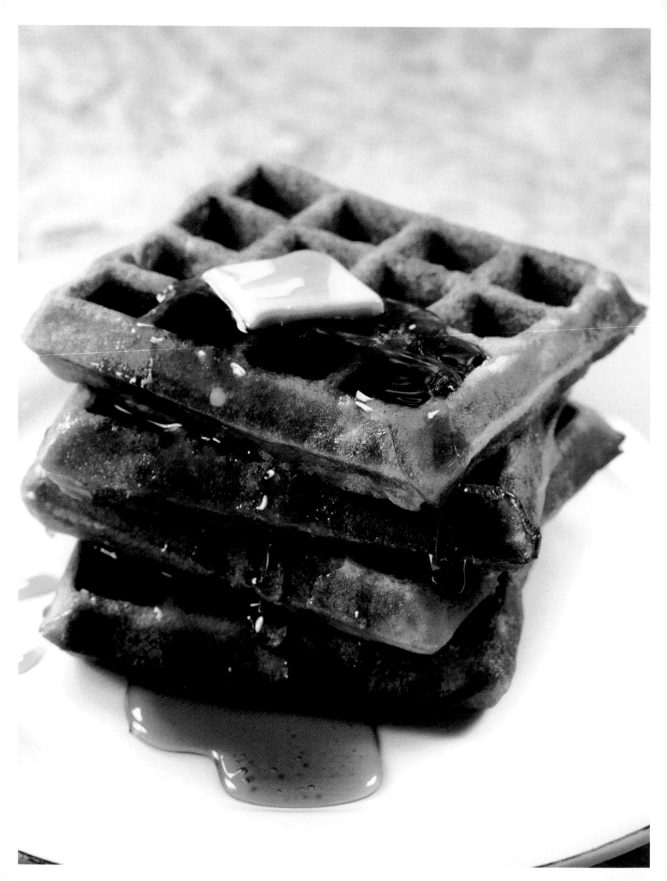

Chapter 6

START THE DAY RIGHT! BREAKFAST AT HOME & ON THE GO

KATE WILL BE THE FIRST ONE to tell any and all of her patients that starting out the day right sets you up for success. Having a good breakfast not only fills your tummy but allows you to focus better at work or school and generally have a better outlook on the day. When you feel good, all things feel possible! But now you have low FODMAP parameters to follow, and during workdays, probably a time crunch as well. This chapter offers variety, from freezable Buckwheat Oat Raisin Breakfast Cookies (page 106) and Mix & Match Fruit Smoothies (page 111), Huevos Rancheros (page 97) to a Brunch-Worthy Vegetable Cheese Frittata (page 99). Our Portable Breakfast Sandwich (page 95) will get you out the door in record time.

Quinoa Oat Granola with Coconut

   E DF V VG   MAKES 8½ CUPS (1.5 KG) | SERVING SIZE ¼ CUP (31 G)

This granola has everything going for it: It is hardy, a little sweet, packed with nutrition, and equally great in a bowl with almond or lactose-free milk (do not use if following a dairy-free or vegan diet) or eaten out of hand as a snack. And prep time is 5 minutes! The recipe calls for oats as well as quinoa flakes, which are basically quinoa grains given the rolled-oat treatment. You can substitute the raw quinoa grain itself with no alteration in the preparation technique; the texture will just be much crunchier. Get ready to smell the most amazing aroma of the nuts, cinnamon, and coconut intermingling, which will also signal when the granola is done baking.

4 cups (396 g) old-fashioned rolled oats (use gluten-free if necessary)

1¼ cups (128 g) quinoa flakes (we love Ancient Harvest brand)

1 cup peeled, chopped hazelnuts (115 g) or natural sliced almonds (86 g)

⅔ cup (165 ml) coconut oil, in liquid form (warm gently if it is solid)

⅔ cup (165 ml) pure maple syrup

½ cup (57 g) unsweetened shredded coconut

1¾ teaspoons ground cinnamon

1 cup lightly packed raisins (166 g) or dried cranberries (160 g)

Position a rack in the middle of the oven. Preheat the oven to 300°F (150°C). Have a rimmed baking sheet handy.

Stir together the oats, quinoa flakes, nuts, coconut oil, maple syrup, coconut, and cinnamon in a mixing bowl until combined. Scrape out onto the rimmed baking sheet and spread into an even layer. Bake for 30 minutes, then toss the granola around with a large spatula to help all the surfaces bake and dry out. Bake for 20 to 30 minutes more, or until just beginning to take on some color. The granola will also begin to smell ridiculously toasty and enticing. Allow the pan to cool on a wire rack. Toss in the dried fruit. Store at room temperature in an airtight container for up to 3 weeks.

KATE'S NOTES

Portion size matters with granola, as many of the ingredients used to make it contain small amounts of FODMAPs that collectively can add up to be too much for your sensitive tummy. For instance, we find oats are best tolerated when limited to ¼ to ½ cup (25 to 50 g), measured dry, and some dried fruits, such as raisins and dried cranberries, have a 1-tablespoon FODMAP limit per serving. So, start incorporating some of our granola into your diet in ¼-cup (25 g) servings during the elimination phase. We love it as a great topping for lactose-free yogurt or as a crunchy layer in your fruit and lactose-free yogurt parfait (do not use dairy-based lactose-free yogurt if following a dairy-free or vegan diet; substitute coconut yogurt instead). During the challenge phase, you may learn your body can tolerate a larger serving; if so, in a serving larger than ¼ cup, this granola makes a hearty and nourishing breakfast.

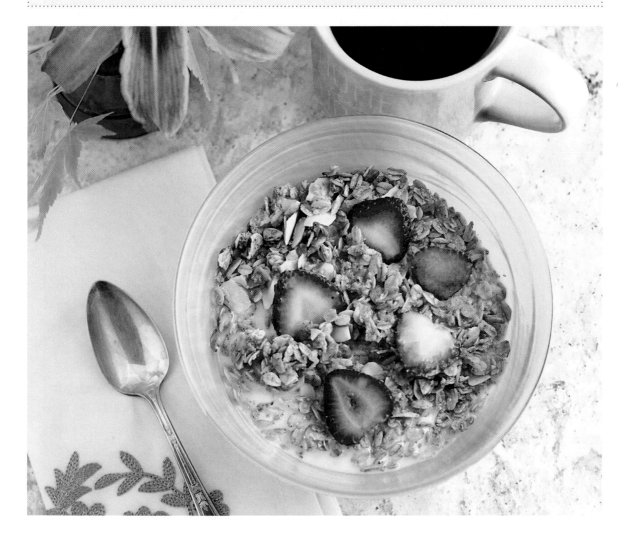

Overnight Oats with Fruit

  MAKES 1 SERVING

Cooked oatmeal and cold soaked muesli-type cereal recipes have been around for ages, but recently the concept of soaked raw oats, or "overnight oats," is a hot trend. The technique offers do-ahead convenience as well as a protein- and fiber-rich breakfast for busy mornings—and portability if made in an airtight container. Your choice of fruit can be varied among low FODMAP options. If you use any of the recommended milks, you have the option of heating the oats in a microwave for a hot breakfast. Get the hang of the technique and you will be able to customize this recipe to your heart's content. The recipe may be doubled, tripled, or quadrupled for multiple servings.

¼ cup (25 g) old-fashioned rolled oats (use gluten-free if necessary) (see Dédé's Tips)

Pinch of salt (optional)

⅓ to ½ cup (75 to 120 ml) lactose-free milk (whole, 2%, 1%, or fat-free); unsweetened almond, hemp, macadamia, quinoa, or rice milk (use if following a dairy-free diet); or ½ cup (114 g) plain lactose-free yogurt

¼ ripe medium-size banana

1 tablespoon blueberries, raspberries, or hulled, sliced strawberries

1½ teaspoons dried cranberries or raisins (optional)

½ to 2 teaspoons pure maple syrup, granulated sugar, or light brown sugar (optional)

1½ teaspoons to 1 tablespoon chia seeds

Pinch of ground cinnamon (optional)

A few drops of pure vanilla extract (optional)

1½ teaspoons toasted chopped walnuts or pecans (optional)

1½ teaspoons unsweetened shredded coconut or coconut flakes (optional)

Use a 6- to 8-ounce (180 to 240 ml) airtight container if you want to take this with you in the morning, or simply have a similarly sized nonreactive bowl ready to use. Place the oats in your container or bowl and add the salt. Add the milk (use the larger amount if you are planning to add the chia seeds) or yogurt, then slice the banana right into the container. Add the berries and dried fruit, if using. If you want to add a sweetener, try ½ teaspoon for your first attempt. If using the chia seeds, add at this time. If you would like a bit of cinnamon and/or vanilla, add them now. Stir very well to thoroughly saturate the oats and distribute the fruit and flavorings. Cover the jar with its lid or the bowl with plastic wrap and refrigerate for at least 4 hours, or preferably overnight. You can make this up to 2 days ahead.

Stir well before eating. Crunchy add-ins, such as nuts or coconut, may be added right before serving. You can eat this cold right out of the refrigerator, or if you have used a microwave-safe container, you can heat in the microwave until hot (try 30 seconds to 1 minute on high). Serve immediately.

DÉDÉ'S TIPS

Old-fashioned rolled oats are best in this recipe. Steel-cut remain too chewy and tough and quick oats become gluey. You can certainly use rolled oats as they come out of the box or bulk bin, but a tasty alternative is to toast them lightly. Preheat the oven to 350°F (180°C). Spread out the oats in a single layer on a rimmed baking sheet and toast until just beginning to color and you sense a whiff of toasted oat fragrance in the air, for 5 to 8 minutes, depending on the amount. You can toast a whole bunch of oats at once and then store them, once cooled, in an airtight container until you need them later that week.

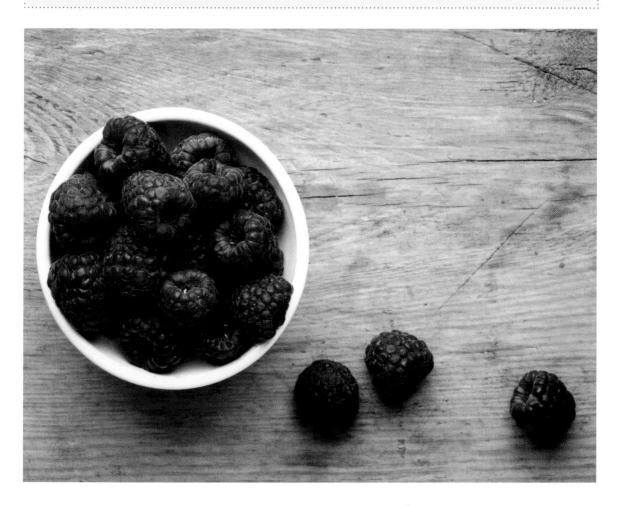

Hot & Creamy Buckwheat & Oats

    MAKES 4 SERVINGS

There is a world of whole grains out there that not only provides nutrition and flavor but is also approved for our low FODMAP diet. Buckwheat is actually a seed that is related to rhubarb (which is also low FODMAP). The form of buckwheat we are recommending here is a broken-down, cracked version of the whole grain. The whole-grain nutrition remains but the seed is smaller and therefore cooks much more quickly. The addition of fresh fruit, nuts, and/or dried fruit is up to you, but we suggest that you try some or all of them per our recommended limits instead of adding a sweetener, although a drizzle of maple syrup or brown sugar can be added.

4 cups (960 ml) water

1 cup (120 g) buckwheat cereal, such as Bob's Red Mill Organic Creamy Buckwheat Hot Cereal

½ cup (50 g) old-fashioned rolled oats (use gluten-free if necessary)

¼ teaspoon salt

Almond, hemp, macadamia, quinoa, or rice milk (use if following a dairy-free or vegan diet); or lactose-free milk (whole, 2%, 1%, or fat-free) (optional)

Ground cinnamon

Freshly grated nutmeg

Almonds, walnuts, or pecans, lightly toasted and chopped (optional) (limit up to 1 tablespoon almonds or 2 tablespoons walnuts or pecans)

Raspberries, blueberries, or sliced strawberries (about ½ cup [60 g] per serving), or raisins or dried cranberries (up to 1 tablespoon per serving) (optional)

Stir the water, buckwheat cereal, oats, and salt together in a medium-size saucepan. Bring to a boil over medium heat, lower the heat to low, cover, and simmer for about 10 minutes, or until the water is absorbed and the cereal is cooked. Divide among four bowls and allow everyone to customize their serving: A splash of milk will loosen up the mixture, if desired. A little bit of cinnamon and/or nutmeg can be stirred in at this point. Top with nuts and/or fresh or dried fruit, as preferred. Serve immediately.

POST-FODMAP FOOD CHALLENGE OPTIONS

Fructose: If you passed the excess fructose challenge, add ½ cup (83 g) of chopped fresh mango, or for a sweet infusion, drizzle with local honey (omit if following a vegan diet).

Portable Breakfast Sandwich

MAKES 6 SANDWICHES | SERVING SIZE 1 SANDWICH

This filling breakfast sandwich is packed with flavor and can be made the night before so that you can get out the door on time. This recipe makes a whole batch of sandwiches, which you can customize for each family member. Be creative: try orange marmalade, Gruyère, and bacon; a combo of Dijon mustard, ham, and Swiss cheese; or strawberry preserves and Cheddar (see ingredient notes concerning special diets). There is some assembly work required here, but you can make these when you have time and then be set up for the whole week because the finished breakfast sandwiches can be refrigerated overnight or even frozen and reheated when ready to eat.

Nonstick spray

10 large eggs, at room temperature

¼ cup (60 ml) lactose-free milk (whole, 2%, 1%, or fat-free)

¼ cup (60 ml) water

¾ teaspoon kosher salt

¼ teaspoon freshly ground black pepper

Herbs of choice: dried tarragon, herbes de Provence, or finely chopped fresh chives especially recommended (optional)

12 slices low FODMAP bread of choice (use gluten-free, vegan, or dairy-free if necessary)

OPTIONAL ADD-INS:

Condiments, such as mayonnaise, mustard (use gluten-free if necessary), orange marmalade, strawberry preserves, or other low FODMAP jam (optional)

Cooked, thick-cut bacon (1 slice per sandwich) or sliced ham (½ to ¾ ounce [15 to 20 g] per sandwich) (optional; use gluten-free if following a gluten-free diet; omit if following a vegetarian diet; check ham ingredients for FODMAP)

Cheese of choice (½ to ¾ ounce [15 to 20 g)] per sandwich; omit if following a dairy-free or vegan diet): Cheddar, Gruyère, Swiss, Muenster, and Monterey Jack are recommended. Thinly slice with a cheese plane or buy pre-sliced from the deli.

Position a rack in the center of the oven. Preheat the oven to 325°F (165°C). Coat a 13 x 9-inch (33 x 23 cm) ovenproof glass or ceramic dish with nonstick spray.

Whisk together the eggs, milk, and water in a mixing bowl until thoroughly combined. Season with salt and pepper and herbs, if using. Pour into the prepared pan and bake for 25 to 35 minutes, or just until the eggs are set: A toothpick inserted in the middle will come out clean and the edges will have begun to pull away from the sides of the pan. Remove from the oven and allow to cool in the pan on a wire rack.

Meanwhile, cook the bacon, if using, in a skillet on the stove top and drain on paper towels; set aside. Lightly toast the bread and set aside.

Once the eggs, bacon, and toast have cooled, cut the eggs into squares or rectangles to match the size of your bread. Any extras can be pieced together to make the last sandwich(es). Spread the toast slices with your choice of condiments. Place an egg portion on one piece of toast. Top with your choice of cheese, ham, or bacon, if using, trimmed to fit. Top with another piece of toast. Assemble the remaining sandwiches. Double wrap in plastic wrap and then place in a large, resealable plastic freezer bag and freeze for up to 1 month; or refrigerate one of them if you want a sandwich the following day.

To heat and eat, unwrap, place on a paper towel, and microwave on high for 1 to 2 minutes, depending on the power of your microwave. Eat immediately, or wrap in foil to get out the door and eat within 20 minutes or so.

POST-FODMAP CHALLENGE PHASE OPTION

Fructan: If you passed the fructan wheat challenge, sub in a wheat bagel, whole-grain wheat bread, or a traditional wheat English muffin (use gluten-free if necessary).

Huevos Rancheros

     MAKES 2 SERVINGS

Just because you are following a new diet doesn't mean that you should ignore basic nutritional guidelines—breakfast is important! Here we have eggs served with a roasted tomato salsa on top of corn tortillas and a sprinkling of feta. Take advantage of the fact that the salsa can be made a few days ahead, allowing this dish to come together quickly on a weekend morning. The salsa can also be doubled or even tripled to serve a larger crowd. None of these components is difficult, but you do need to multitask to get everything on the plates hot at the same time; read through the recipe so there are no surprises.

ROASTED TOMATO SALSA:

1 teaspoon Garlic-Infused Oil (page 68) made with vegetable oil, purchased garlic-infused vegetable oil, or plain vegetable oil

½ cup (32 g) chopped scallion, green part only

1 (14.5-ounce [411 g]) can diced fire-roasted tomatoes (without garlic or onion), such as Muir Glen brand

1 teaspoon ground cumin

1 teaspoon chopped Chipotle Chiles in Adobo Sauce (page 82), plus more to taste

Kosher salt

¼ cup (8 g) chopped fresh cilantro

2 tablespoons freshly squeezed lime juice

EGGS:

Vegetable oil

4 white or yellow corn tortillas

4 large eggs, at room temperature

¼ cup (29 g) crumbled feta cheese

2 tablespoons chopped fresh cilantro

¼ ripe Hass avocado, sliced (optional)

Prepare the salsa: Heat the oil in a medium-size saucepan over medium-low heat, add the scallion greens, and cook, stirring occasionally, for about 5 minutes, or until softened but not browned. Stir in the tomatoes, cumin, and chipotle chile in adobo. Increase the heat and simmer for 5 minutes, stirring often. Taste, add salt if needed, and add additional chipotle if more heat is desired. Remove from the heat. Stir in the cilantro and lime juice, taste again, and adjust the seasoning if needed. Use immediately, or allow to cool to room temperature and refrigerate in an airtight container for up to 4 days. Reheat before using.

Prepare the eggs: Very lightly brush a nonstick pan with vegetable oil and heat over medium heat. Lay one or two tortillas (depending on the size of the pan) completely flat in the pan and cook just until warmed but not browned, for maybe 30 seconds on each side. Remove from the pan and wrap in aluminum foil. Repeat with the remaining tortillas, and leave the pan on the stove top to use for cooking the eggs.

Have the salsa heating as you prepare the eggs. Brush the tortilla pan lightly with oil again and cook the eggs sunny-side up. Cover, if necessary, to help the whites set before the yolks cook through.

Place two tortillas on each plate and top each tortilla with an egg. Spoon the warm salsa around the eggs (you might have salsa left over), then sprinkle the cheese and cilantro on top. Add sliced avocado, if desired. Serve immediately.

POST-FODMAP CHALLENGE PHASE OPTIONS

Fructan: If you passed the fructan onion challenge, sub in ½ cup (71 g) of chopped white or yellow onion, or as tolerated, for the scallion greens.

GOS: If you passed the GOS challenge, consider adding a scoop of drained and rinsed canned black beans.

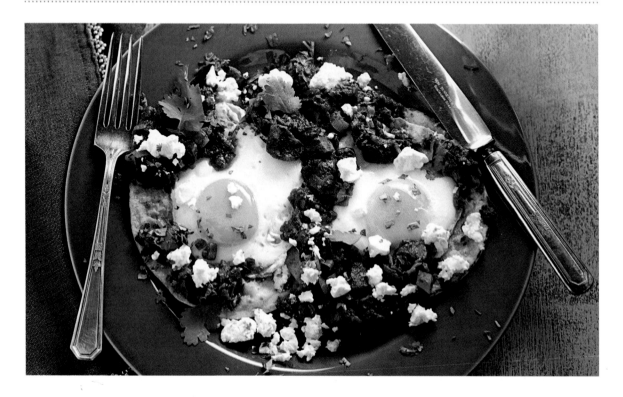

Brunch-Worthy Vegetable Cheese Frittata

  MAKES ONE 9-INCH (23 CM) FRITTATA | 10 TO 12 SERVINGS

Combining an assortment of colorful vegetables as well as two kinds of cheese and the heartiness of potatoes, you cannot beat this showstopper as a savory breakfast, brunch, or lunch option. We make it in a springform pan, as it stands tall. It also cuts beautifully and a wedge of leftover frittata makes a great room-temperature lunch box meal. The key to success with this frittata is to drain the sautéed vegetables very well, as they will throw off a lot of liquid, so take time with that step.

Nonstick spray

2 tablespoons Garlic-Infused Oil (page 68) made with olive oil, or purchased garlic-infused olive oil

¼ cup (16 g) chopped scallion, green part only

2 medium-size red bell peppers, cored, cut into ¼-inch (6 mm) strips

1 medium-size green bell pepper, cored, cut into ¼-inch (6 mm) strips

1 medium-size orange bell pepper, cored, cut into ¼-inch (6 mm) strips

1 medium-size yellow bell pepper, cored, cut into ¼-inch (6 mm) strips

2 medium-size yellow squash (summer squash), ends trimmed, cut into ¼-inch (6 mm) rounds

2 medium-size zucchini, ends trimmed, cut into ¼-inch (6 mm) rounds

1 pound (455 g) red, white, or Yukon gold potatoes, scrubbed and cut into 1-inch (2.5 cm) cubes

8 large eggs, at room temperature

2¼ cups (9 ounces; 255 g) finely grated Gruyère cheese

8 ounces (227 g) soft, mild goat cheese, such as Vermont Creamery brand

1 teaspoon dried thyme

Kosher salt

Freshly ground black pepper

Position a rack in the center of the oven. Preheat the oven to 325°F (165°C). Coat a 9-inch (23 cm) springform pan with nonstick spray. Line a baking sheet with parchment or aluminum foil and set aside.

Heat the oil in a 5-quart (4.7 L) Dutch oven or heavy-bottomed saucepan. Add the scallion greens and sauté over medium heat, stirring often, for about 5 minutes, or until softened. Add all the peppers, squash, and zucchini, stir to combine and coat with oil, cover, and cook over medium heat, stirring occasionally, until the vegetables soften but still retain a bit of texture, for 15 to 20 minutes. The vegetables will cook down in volume and begin to exude liquid. When done, scrape into a strainer set in the sink and use the back of a sturdy spoon or ladle to press as much liquid out of the vegetables as possible.

Meanwhile, cook the potatoes, covered with water, in a separate saucepan until just tender when pierced with a knife. Drain well.

Whisk the eggs in a large mixing bowl. Add the cooked vegetables, including the potatoes, and the cheese and thyme and toss to combine well and evenly distribute all the ingredients. Season liberally with salt and black pepper.

Scrape into the prepared pan and level the top. Place the pan on a baking sheet to catch any drips. Bake for about 1 hour, or until the filling is slightly puffed, set, and firm to the touch. It might take on some color around the edges. If at any point it is browning too quickly, simply cover with foil. Remove from the oven and let sit for 5 to 10 minutes before serving, to yield the cleanest slices. The frittata may be served warm or at room temperature. It may also be covered with plastic wrap and refrigerated overnight. Reheat, if desired, in a microwave (metal bottom of the springform pan removed) using the reheat function or at 50 percent power or a preheated 300°F (150°C) oven until heated through.

POST-FODMAP CHALLENGE PHASE OPTIONS

Polyols: If you passed the mannitol challenge, consider adding 1 cup (78 g) of chopped or sliced button mushrooms along with the other vegetables as they are being sautéed.

Fructan: If you passed the fructan onion challenge, consider adding ½ cup (71 g) of chopped white, yellow, or red onion, or as tolerated, along with the other vegetables as they are being sautéed.

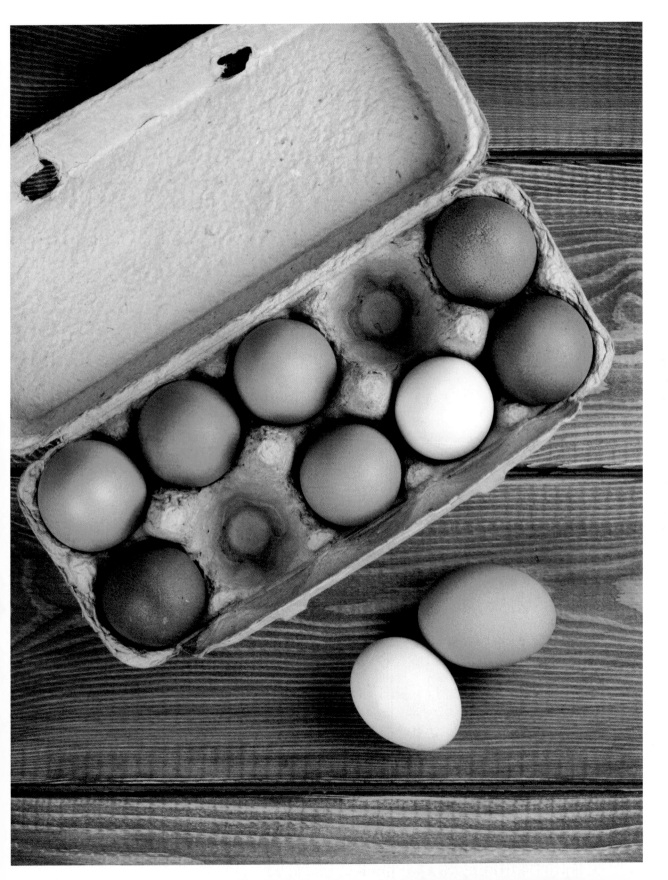

Buckwheat Pancakes

   MAKES TEN 4-INCH (10 CM) PANCAKES | SERVING SIZE 2 TO 3 PANCAKES

Pancakes make weekend appearances in our homes and a low FODMAP diet wasn't going to keep us from enjoying this beloved breakfast dish; these will keep you satisfied well into lunchtime. The addition of buckwheat adds nutrition and bold flavor (see Dédé's Tips); buckwheat, despite its name containing the word wheat, is wheat-free, gluten-free, and low FODMAP approved.

Pure maple syrup is a must alongside and we also like to add a handful of fresh blueberries or sliced bananas to our stack after cooking.

¾ cup (109 g) gluten-free all-purpose flour, such as Bob's Red Mill Gluten Free 1 to 1 Baking Flour

½ cup (60 g) buckwheat flour

1 tablespoon plus 1 teaspoon baking powder (use gluten-free if necessary)

1 tablespoon sugar

½ teaspoon salt

4 tablespoons (57 g) unsalted butter, cut into pieces

1 cup plus 2 tablespoons (270 ml) lactose-free milk (whole, 2%, 1%, or fat-free), plus more if needed

2 large eggs, at room temperature

Whisk together the flour, buckwheat flour, baking powder, sugar, and salt in a small bowl, to aerate and combine.

Melt the butter in a small saucepan over medium heat. Remove from the heat, add 1 cup plus 2 tablespoons (270 ml) of the milk, and whisk to combine. Check the temperature; it should be just warm. If not, let cool slightly. Whisk in the eggs.

Add the wet mixture to the dry and stir just until combined. If the mixture is too thick, add a bit more milk. It should be pourable but it will still have some heft.

Heat an electric griddle, or a heavy sauté pan, or nonstick pan over medium-low heat, brushing with a bit of melted butter and heating until a few drops of water flicked onto it dance. Dole out about ¼-cup (60 ml) amounts of batter at a time; we like to use an ice-cream scoop. You might need to help the batter spread out a bit with the back of the scoop. Cook until bubbles begin to appear here and there in the pancakes, for about 2 minutes. Check the bottoms, which should be golden brown. Flip over and cook for a minute or 2 more. Serve hot with real maple syrup and/or suitable portion sizes of low FODMAP fruit, if desired.

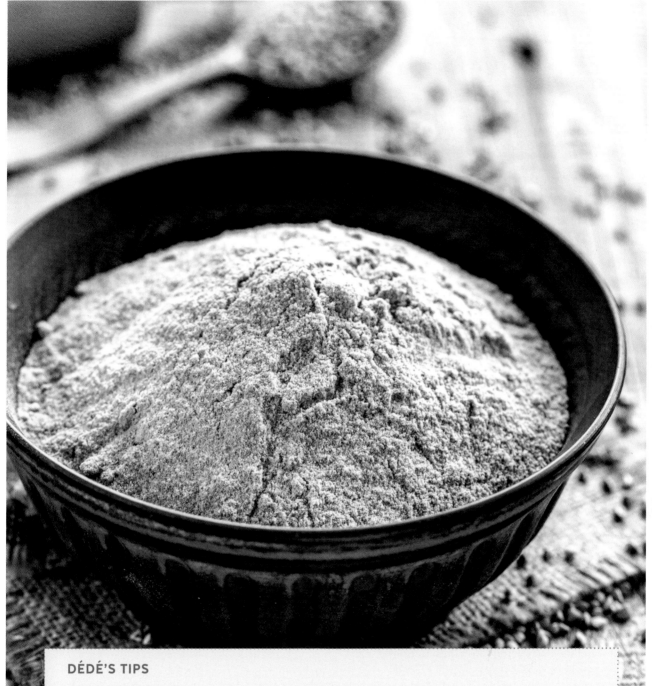

DÉDÉ'S TIPS

If the buckwheat flavor and texture is overwhelming for you, simply rework the ratios and try it with 1 cup (145 g) of suitable gluten-free all-purpose flour and ¼ cup (30 g) of buckwheat flour next time, for a lighter result.

Also, gluten-free flour mixes vary and you might need to add more milk if your pancake batter is too thick.

Crispy Outside, Tender Inside Waffles

  MAKES ABOUT THREE 8-INCH (20 CM) ROUND OR EIGHT 4-INCH (10 CM)
SQUARE WAFFLES | 4 TO 6 SERVINGS

Waffles depend on two things: the recipe itself and the waffle maker. Truth is that some waffle makers just make better waffles than others, so results will vary. Also, makers vary wildly in size and shape, so the yield is also hard to gauge. Deep wells in the waffle maker will help create the crispy outer texture that we love. This recipe makes a basic waffle: crispy on the outside, tender in the middle, and gluten-free. If you want to add fruit, we suggest serving it alongside. Cooking fruit into the waffle can create a soggy waffle and unmolding problems. The recipe may be doubled for guests—or frozen for later for quick weekday meals. Simply reheat in a toaster.

---

2 cups (290 g) gluten-free all-purpose flour, such as Bob's Red Mill Gluten Free 1 to 1 Baking Flour

2 tablespoons sugar

1 tablespoon plus 1 teaspoon baking powder (use gluten-free if necessary)

1 teaspoon salt

1½ cups (360 ml) lactose-free milk (whole, 2%, 1%, or fat-free), at room temperature

½ cup (1 stick, 113 g) unsalted butter, cut into pieces

2 large eggs, at room temperature

Nonstick spray

Preheat the waffle iron according to the manufacturer's instructions. Preheat the oven to 200°F (95°C) if you want to keep the waffles warm between batches.

Whisk together the flour, sugar, baking powder, and salt in a large mixing bowl, to aerate and combine. Make a well in the center, then set aside.

Heat the milk and butter together in a small saucepan over medium-low heat until the butter is melted. Whisk together, then pour into a small mixing bowl and allow to cool until just slightly warm. Alternatively, measure the milk in a 4-cup (960 ml) microwave-safe measuring cup, then add the butter and microwave on 50 percent power until the butter is melted and the milk is warmed. Allow the milk mixture to cool slightly. Whisk the eggs into the milk mixture until well combined, then pour into the well in the dry mixture and whisk gently until just combined.

Coat the waffle maker lightly with nonstick spray (you will probably only need to do this once). Scoop the waffle batter into the preheated waffle iron, making sure the batter covers the entire surface but does not overfill the waffle maker. Close the top and cook until the waffles are crispy on their top and bottom and are golden brown, probably for 4 minutes or so, depending on the waffle maker. Keep the cooked waffles warm by placing them directly on a rack in the preheated oven as you make the remaining waffles. Serve the waffles immediately with pure maple syrup and a pat of butter and suitable low FODMAP fruit alongside, if you like.

POST-FODMAP CHALLENGE PHASE OPTIONS

Lactose: If you passed the lactose challenge, use regular whole, 2%, 1%, or fat-free milk.

Fructan: If you passed the fructan wheat challenge, you can use regular unbleached all-purpose flour, or half all-purpose flour and half whole wheat pastry flour, which will make the waffles a bit heavier (do not substitute if following a gluten-free diet). Use weights of flour when making substitutions for best results.

(Recipe photo on page 88)

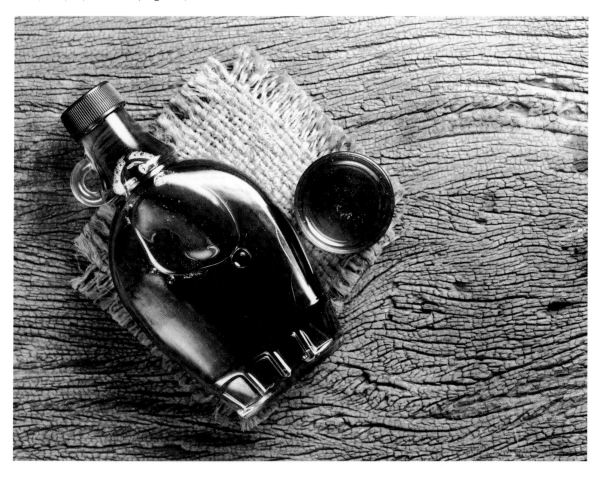

Buckwheat Oat Raisin Breakfast Cookies

    MAKES ABOUT 18 COOKIES | SERVING SIZE 1 TO 2 COOKIES

Warning: These are the ugly duckling of the book—with hidden attributes, so don't give up on them before you taste them. This cookie is portable, healthy, and just a tad sweet, making it a perfect breakfast for at home, on the run, or tucked into a lunch box for a midday snack. They have sustained us through many a morning and afternoon and we have found ourselves reaching for them in lieu of their sweeter brethren. Trust us; they become craveable in their own beguiling way. We used walnuts and raisins, but feel free to try pecans, almonds, or dried cranberries, keeping the amounts in check so as to keep the overall cookie low FODMAP. Don't leave out the carrot, as it contributes to a healthier and moister cookie.

---

2 cups (290 g) gluten-free all-purpose flour, such as Bob's Red Mill Gluten Free 1 to 1 Baking Flour

1 cup (99 g) old-fashioned rolled oats (not quick or instant; use gluten-free if necessary)

½ cup (60 g) buckwheat flour

½ cup (50 g) ground flaxseeds

2 teaspoons ground cinnamon

1 teaspoon baking soda

½ teaspoon salt

⅔ cup (165 ml) coconut oil, in liquid form (warm gently if it is solid)

⅔ cup (165 ml) pure maple syrup

4 large eggs, at room temperature

1 cup (99 g) packed finely grated carrot (from about 3 medium-size carrots)

⅔ cup (105 g) dark raisins

½ cup (64 g) walnut halves, lightly toasted and finely chopped

Position racks in the upper and lower thirds of the oven. Preheat the oven to 350°F (180°C). Line two baking sheets with parchment paper; set aside.

Whisk together the flour, oats, buckwheat flour, flaxseeds, cinnamon, baking soda, and salt in a large mixing bowl, to aerate and combine; set aside.

Whisk together the coconut oil and maple syrup in a medium-size mixing bowl. Whisk in the eggs, one at a time, allowing each to become incorporated before adding the next. Whisk in the carrot, raisins, and nuts.

Add the wet mixture to the dry and stir together just until combined. Drop by ¼-cup (60 ml) amounts, spaced about 2 inches (5 cm) apart, onto the prepared baking sheets. Press down gently to about ½-inch (12 mm) thickness or a little thicker. Bake for 13 to 17 minutes, rotating the pans front to back once during baking, until the cookies are dry to the touch and lightly colored on the bottom. They will have puffed slightly and give a bit when pressed, remaining soft in their center. Allow to cool on the pans set on wire racks. Store the cookies at room temperature in airtight containers for up to 4 days or freeze for up to a month.

POST-FODMAP CHALLENGE PHASE OPTIONS

Fructans and polyols: If you passed both the fructans and sorbitol challenges, sub in other dried fruit, such as dried blueberries or dried, chopped apricots, if they agree with you. Just stay with the recommended ⅔ cup (112 g) amount. Most dried fruit contains fructans and some contain sorbitol, too.

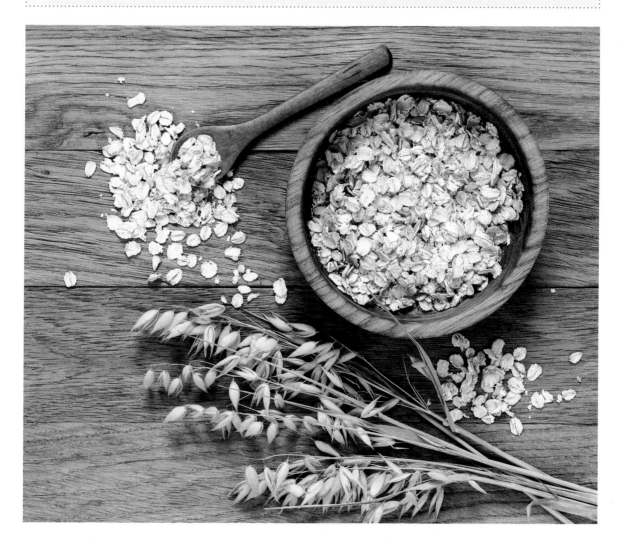

Green Extreme Smoothie

        MAKES ABOUT 2 CUPS (480 ML) | SERVING SIZE 1 CUP (240 ML)

In general, the order of ingredients makes a huge difference in how well your smoothies come out of your blender; put the liquid in first. Also, pulsing the ingredients initially will often give you better results; experiment. This green smoothie combines a variety of green veggies and fruit—green grapes, kale, spinach, cucumber, and lime—with fabulous results: a vivid, enticing green color and bright, fresh flavor. Drink right after blending, as it does separate upon sitting.

---

1 cup (170 g) seedless green grapes

1 (5-inch) piece unpeeled English cucumber, cut into chunks

1 cup (20 g) baby spinach

2 medium-size lacinato kale leaves, stemmed, washed, and dried

1 teaspoon freshly squeezed lime juice

1 cup ice cubes

Place the ingredients in a blender in the order listed. Pulse on and off to begin blending, then blend on high speed until pureed, blended, and smooth.

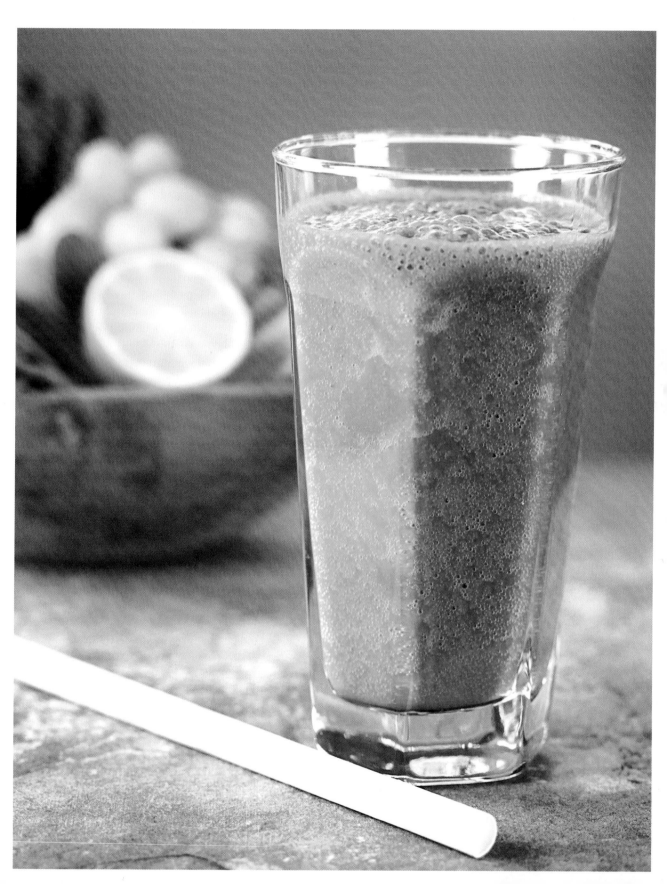

Almond Oat Berry Smoothie

    MAKES 1 SERVING

This is a perfect breakfast beverage, or follow Dédé's lead and have it for a midafternoon pick-me-up. It might seem odd to add raw oats to a drink, but they add healthy prebiotic fiber and thicken this pretty pink smoothie up quite nicely. The maple syrup is not necessary; taste the smoothie without before assuming you need it. If you use frozen berries, you won't need the ice cubes. If the smoothie is too thick, add some almond milk to thin out or next time use partially defrosted fruit. The recipe may be doubled.

½ cup (120 ml) unsweetened almond milk

2 tablespoons old-fashioned rolled oats (use gluten-free if necessary)

5 (23 g) raspberries

5 (70 g) medium-size strawberries, hulled

½ teaspoon to 2 teaspoons pure maple syrup (optional)

2 to 4 ice cubes

Place the almond milk and oats in a blender and let soak for 10 minutes. Add the berries and blend until smooth. Taste and add the maple syrup, if desired. Add as many ice cubes as you like and blend until frosty. Serve immediately.

KATE'S NOTES

Adding a bit of raw oats provides a nice dose of resistant starch, which is associated with feeding gut microbes that produce butyrate, a short-chain fatty acid associated with colon health.

Mix & Match Fruit Smoothies

 MAKES 1 SMOOTHIE

We love these for breakfast and as a midday pick-me-up snack. Smoothies begin with frozen ingredients pureed in a blender, then grains, greens, veggies, nut butters, sweeteners, and the like can be added. Note that you do have to have fruit already frozen before you begin, so plan accordingly. Also pay close attention to the serving size and recommended ingredient amounts: it is easy to overload with fruit (a common FODMAPer newbie mistake), and if you are sensitive to fructose and/or polyols, this can be an issue.

LIQUIDS:

Depending on the amount of body and thickness that you want, you might use up to 1 cup (240 ml), total, of liquid. Feel free to mix and match your liquids, such as part almond milk and part tea.

½ cup to 1 cup (120 to 240 ml) of one or two of the following (totaling no more than 1 cup): unsweetened almond milk, hemp milk, macadamia milk, quinoa milk, unsweetened rice milk, canned pure light coconut milk, cold, brewed tea (white, green, or black), cold, brewed coffee, pure cranberry juice (without high-fructose corn syrup or added other fruit juices), lactose-free plain yogurt (whole milk or low-fat; omit if following a dairy-free or vegan diet), plain lactose-free kefir (without chicory root or inulin; omit if following a dairy-free or vegan diet), and/or water

1 tablespoon freshly squeezed lemon or lime juice

FROZEN PORTION:

Add one of the following fruit additions, half of two choices or a third of three choices. Make sure you stick within the amounts and do the math carefully to stay within low FODMAP guidelines:

⅓ (33 g) ripe medium-size banana, peeled and frozen, then cut into chunks, 20 frozen blueberries, 10 frozen (unsweetened) raspberries or strawberries, 1 cup (150 g) frozen grapes, 1 cup (140 g) frozen papaya chunks, 1 cup (140 g) frozen pineapple chunks, ½ cup (90 g) frozen cantaloupe or honeydew melon chunks, 2 small (150 g) peeled kiwi (fresh or frozen)

GRAIN OPTION:

1 to 2 tablespoons old-fashioned rolled oats or oat bran (use gluten-free if desired or necessary), or quinoa flakes

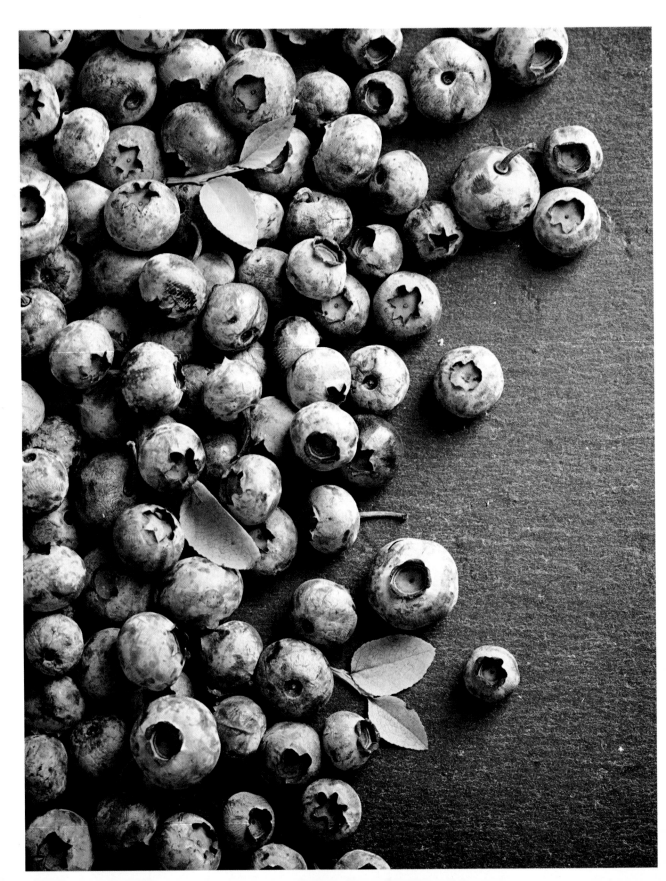

VEGETABLE OPTIONS:

¼ cup to ½ cup (55 to 110 g) baby spinach, baby kale, or chopped kale, ½ cup (50 g) shredded carrot

NUT, SEED, AND NUTRITION BOOSTERS OPTION:

1 to 2 tablespoons peanut butter, or 1½ teaspoons to 1 tablespoon almond butter

Up to 2 tablespoons chia seeds or raw, toasted or pumpkin seeds; up to 1 tablespoon pine nuts or raw or toasted sesame seeds; up to 2 teaspoons raw, toasted or sunflower seeds; or up to 2 teaspoons flaxseeds, whole or ground

SWEETENER OPTION:

1 to 2 teaspoons pure maple syrup

FLAVOR BOOSTERS:

1 to 2 teaspoons unsweetened natural or Dutch-processed cocoa powder

¼ to 1 teaspoon ground or grated fresh ginger, and/or ¼ to ½ teaspoon ground cinnamon or turmeric, and/or a pinch to ¼ teaspoon freshly grated nutmeg

Ice cubes (optional)

Most blenders work best if you add liquid first. Begin with ½ cup (120 ml) of your chosen liquid (the lemon and/or lime juice that are used for flavor would be added at this time in addition to your main liquid). Quickly add your frozen fruit(s) of choice. Blend until well combined and smooth, adding additional liquid as needed to create a thick but pourable mixture. Now add the grains, greens, vegetables, nut butter, and/or extra additions and blend until smooth. Add your desired sweetener and/or flavor and texture options, if using. Add ice at this time if you want it frostier. Serve immediately.

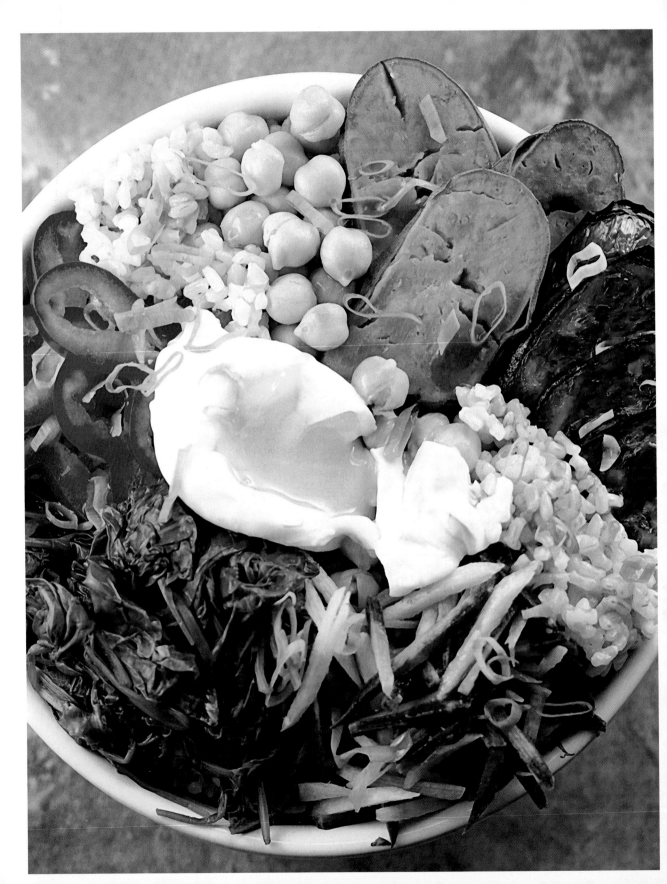

Chapter 7

WHAT'S FOR LUNCH?

EATING A WELL-BALANCED LUNCH will keep you feeling energized and nourished. Truth be told, when you are a FODMAPer, you do have to prepare ahead, so we made sure that most of the recipes in this chapter pack well. We know you want standbys such as tuna salad (page 116), egg salad (page 117), and chicken salad (page 118), but we want to expand your ideas of what lunch can be. How about a versatile Mason Jar Salad (page 124) or a deconstructed Maki Roll Bowl (page 127)? If you are at home during lunch, we highly recommend the super yummy Best Grilled Cheese with mix-and-match ingredient options to take it from basic to spectacular (page 121), or the simple yet elegant Spinach & Goat Cheese Lunch Frittata (page 120).

Best Ever Low FODMAP Tuna Salad

 MAKES ABOUT 2 CUPS (408 G) TUNA SALAD |
ENOUGH FOR 3 TO 4 SANDWICHES

There are many ways to make tuna salad. Most classic versions involve mayonnaise, but then folks go any manner of ways with such additions as celery, onion, and pickle relish. FODMAPers need to limit celery to about 2 inches (5 cm) of stalk per serving due to its moderate amounts of the FODMAP mannitol, but if you're thinking, "What else can I add to my tuna for crunch?" we have a delicious solution: add chopped bok choy stems for crisp texture and the fresh, green flavor (plus it's a great source of calcium). Note that tuna brands vary hugely in quality and will affect the final result; Dédé recommends Whole Foods 365 Everyday Value brand. This recipe may be doubled.

---

2 (5 ounce [142 g]) cans tuna, preferably 1 can chunk light and 1 can white albacore

¾ cup (107 g) diced bok choy stems (or up to 6 inches (15 cm) celery stalk, diced, with the remainder made up of diced bok choy)

⅔ cup (150 g) mayonnaise

1½ teaspoons freshly squeezed lemon juice

½ teaspoon dried dill, or to taste

Freshly ground black pepper

Place the tuna in a wire-mesh strainer set over a bowl and squeeze out as much liquid as possible, using the back of a wooden spoon. Discard the liquid. Place the tuna in a mixing bowl, stir in the chopped bok choy (and celery, if using), mayonnaise, lemon juice, and dill, and generously season to taste with pepper. The tuna is ready to use in sandwiches or as part of a salad plate. Refrigerate in an airtight container for up to 3 days for multiple lunches and high-protein snacks.

POST-FODMAP CHALLENGE PHASE OPTIONS

Fructan: If you passed the fructan onion challenge, consider adding ¼ cup (36 g) of finely chopped white, yellow, or Vidalia onion to the tuna salad. If you passed the fructan wheat challenge, you can use wheat bread to make a sandwich (use gluten-free and/or dairy-free bread if necessary).

Egg Salad

     MAKES ENOUGH FOR 2 SANDWICHES OR SERVINGS

Why include a recipe for egg salad? Well, first of all, we have the most perfect, foolproof method for making hard-boiled eggs and we want to share. Also, since we are limited to one quarter of a stalk of celery, we wanted to provide options. As in our tuna salad (page 116), we sometimes like to use chopped bok choy stems or chopped and seeded English cucumbers. Enjoy this egg salad as sandwich filling or scoop up with veggies, corn tortilla chips, or gluten-free pretzels.

---

2 large eggs, at room temperature

2 to 3 tablespoons mayonnaise

2 tablespoons finely chopped celery, bok choy stems, or peeled and seeded cucumber

½ teaspoon Dijon mustard (use gluten-free if following a gluten-free diet)

¼ teaspoon dried dill

Kosher salt

Freshly ground black pepper

Place the eggs in a saucepan and cover with cold water by 1 to 2 inches (2.5 to 5 cm). Cover the pot and bring to a full, rolling boil over high heat. Turn off the heat, cover the pan, and allow to sit for 12 minutes.

Drain, then plunge the eggs into a bowl of ice water and allow to sit for 1 to 2 minutes, or until cold to the touch. The hard-boiled eggs may be refrigerated for up to 1 week. Crack the eggs on a hard surface and peel. The shells should release easily.

Either chop the eggs on a cutting board or simply place in a mixing bowl and mash with a fork (this is what we do). Add the mayonnaise (the lesser amount yields a drier result), chopped celery, mustard, and dill. Season to taste with salt and pepper. Use the egg salad as a sandwich filling, serve with veggies or chips, or eat with a spoon! Refrigerate in an airtight container for up to 3 days for multiple lunches and high-protein snacks.

POST-FODMAP CHALLENGE PHASE OPTIONS

Fructans: If you passed the fructan onion challenge, consider adding ¼ cup (36 g) of finely chopped white, yellow, or Vidalia onion to the egg salad. If you passed the fructan wheat challenge, you can use wheat bread to make a sandwich (use gluten-free and/or dairy-free bread if necessary).

Tarragon Chicken Salad with Grapes & Pecans

    MAKES 3 TO 4 SANDWICHES OR SERVINGS

This is a perfect lunch dish for the whole family. If you can tolerate whole-grain bread, enjoy this as a sandwich filling. For those who are on the elimination phase, simply serve as a salad, with a side of corn tortilla chips or gluten-free pretzels, or use low FODMAP approved bread (use gluten-free if necessary). Versatile, easy, and delicious.

---

2 cups (250 g) diced or shredded, cooked chicken

¼ cup (57 g) mayonnaise

2 tablespoons minced fresh tarragon, or 1 tablespoon dried

1 tablespoon Dijon mustard (use gluten-free if necessary)

2 teaspoons freshly squeezed lemon juice

Salt

Freshly ground black pepper

½ cup (50 g) red seedless grapes, halved

2 tablespoons lightly toasted pecans, chopped

In a large bowl, combine the chicken, mayonnaise, tarragon, mustard, and lemon juice, folding the ingredients together until well mixed. Season with salt and pepper, then fold in the grapes and pecans. The salad is ready to serve, or refrigerate in an airtight container for up to 3 days.

DÉDÉ'S TIPS

Pre-FODMAP, I would often buy a rotisserie chicken to have around; now I have to be mindful of seasonings and additives, such as onion or garlic, which might trigger IBS symptoms, so I often make our Whole Roast Chicken with Lemon & Herbs (page 276) once a week so that I have leftovers for dishes such as this. Alternatively, you could poach skinless, boneless chicken breasts and use those.

POST-FODMAP CHALLENGE PHASE OPTIONS

Fructans: If you passed the fructan onion challenge, consider adding ¼ cup (36 g) of finely chopped white, yellow, or Vidalia onion to the chicken salad.

If you passed the fructan wheat challenge, you can use wheat bread to make a sandwich (use gluten-free and/or dairy-free bread if necessary).

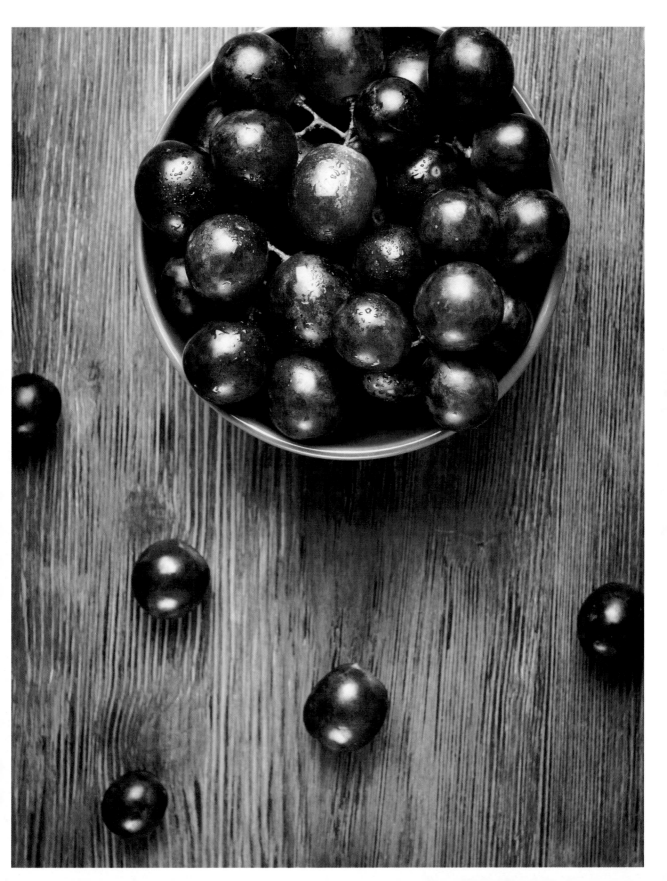

Spinach & Goat Cheese Lunch Frittata

  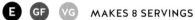 MAKES 8 SERVINGS

This simple, quick-to-prepare egg dish reheats well in the office microwave, so if you haven't already had eggs for breakfast, this makes a satisfying protein-filled lunch. It packs neatly, too. You could use 10 ounces (280 g) of fresh baby spinach (steam it and squeeze dry), but we like using frozen here for convenience. We want to make breakfasts and lunches as simple as possible for all of us following a low FODMAP lifestyle. If you pack low FODMAP-approved food, you will be less likely to slip up and pay for it with tummy troubles.

Nonstick spray

9 large eggs, at room temperature

Kosher salt

Freshly ground black pepper

½ teaspoon dried dill or tarragon (optional)

2 cups (450 g) lactose-free cottage cheese

5 ounces (140 g) medium or sharp Cheddar, finely shredded (about 1⅔ cups)

4 ounces (115 g) soft goat cheese, such as Montrachet, crumbled

1 (10-ounce [280 g]) package frozen chopped spinach, thawed

½ dry pint (142 g) cherry or grape tomatoes, quartered

Preheat the oven to 350°F (180°C). Coat a 13 x 9-inch (33 x 23 cm) ovenproof glass or ceramic baking dish with nonstick spray; set aside.

Whisk the eggs in a large bowl and season liberally with salt and pepper. Whisk in the dill or tarragon, if using. Whisk in the cottage cheese, Cheddar, and goat cheese.

Place the spinach in a colander and press out any excess water with the back of a large, sturdy spoon—or use your hands! Drain it as much as possible. Stir the spinach and tomatoes into the egg mixture and pour into the prepared pan.

Bake for 30 to 40 minutes, or until the eggs are set. The frittata will be puffed and golden around the edges. The frittata is ready to serve immediately, or let cool, cut into squares, and double wrap in plastic wrap and refrigerate for up to 2 days. The tomatoes get a bit watery upon longer storage. If you use just spinach, it can last an additional day in the fridge. The refrigerated frittata may be served at room temperature or reheated in a microwave.

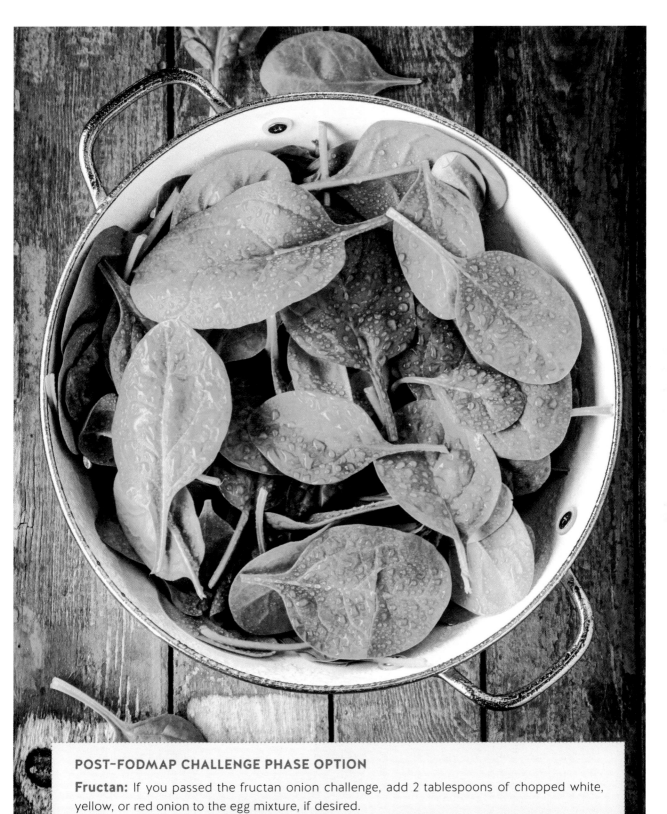

POST-FODMAP CHALLENGE PHASE OPTION

Fructan: If you passed the fructan onion challenge, add 2 tablespoons of chopped white, yellow, or red onion to the egg mixture, if desired.

The Best Grilled Cheese

  MAKES 1 SANDWICH | SERVING SIZE 1

Did you think a gooey grilled cheese sandwich was a thing of the past once you started eating a low FODMAP diet? You are about to learn how to make the best grilled cheese sandwich, period. See "Choosing Low FODMAP Bread" (page 45) for suitable breads. If you are slicing the bread yourself, keep the pieces to ½ inch (12 mm) thick. By choosing your bread and cheese appropriately—and then following our special technique using mayonnaise—you will be rewarded with the crispiest bread with the meltiest cheese in less than 10 minutes for the best comfort food lunch ever. Dig in.

---

2 slices of your choice of low FODMAP bread (use gluten-free bread if necessary), at room temperature

2 ounces (55 g) thinly sliced or grated cheese, such as Cheddar, Colby, Swiss, Gruyère, Monterey Jack, or Muenster, at room temperature (see Dédé's Tips)

2 tablespoons mayonnaise

1 tablespoon unsalted butter (optional; see Dédé's Tips)

OPTIONAL ADD-INS:

Freshly sliced tomato, drained on paper towels

Crisp cooked bacon (use gluten-free if necessary; omit if vegetarian)

Slices of ham or prosciutto (use gluten-free if necessary, and select option without other FODMAP additives); omit if vegetarian)

Schmear of orange marmalade (without high-fructose corn syrup)

Schmear of strawberry jam (without high-fructose corn syrup; we love it with Brie)

Dijon mustard (use gluten-free if necessary)

Soft, spreadable goat cheese

Brie cheese

Place the cheese and any optional add-ins on one slice of bread. Top with the second slice of bread and spread the top of that slice with half of the mayonnaise. Heat a small nonstick or cast-iron skillet over low-medium-low heat and melt half of the butter, if using. Place the sandwich, mayonnaise side down, in the pan, then coat the top of the sandwich with the remaining mayonnaise.

Increase the heat to medium—the bread should sizzle gently—and cook until the bottom is golden brown and crispy. Lift the sandwich with a spatula, slip the remaining butter, if using, into the pan, swirl the pan quickly to help it melt, then flip over and place back in the pan. Press the sandwich down gently with the spatula to compress it a bit and cook the second side until it is golden brown and crispy and the cheese is thoroughly melted. The sandwich is ready to eat and should be served hot. Whether you slice it in half crosswise or on the diagonal is up to you.

DÉDÉ'S TIPS

Breads vary in porosity and toast up differently. I opt for butter when I'm using very porous bread slices. You will learn through trial and error whether you need it or not.

The cheese should be brought to room temperature, and if you refrigerate your bread, take that out of the fridge, too. This approach will allow your cheese to melt and the bread to turn crispy golden brown at the same time, which is the whole point.

POST-FODMAP CHALLENGE OPTION

Fructan: If you passed the fructan wheat challenge, feel free to sub in wheat bread for the sandwich (use gluten-free and/or dairy-free bread if necessary).

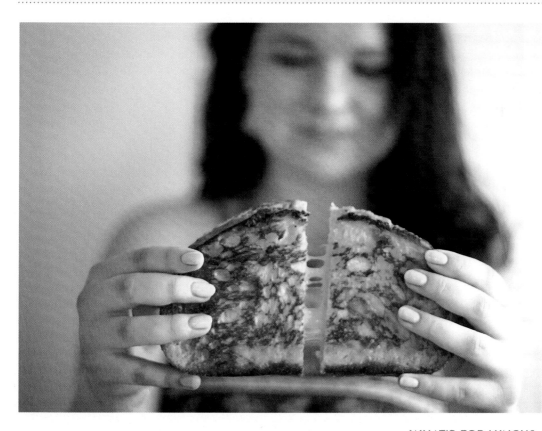

Mason Jar Salad

MAKES 1 SALAD | SERVES 1 TO 2

Type "mason jar salad" into your favorite search engine and just look at all of the gorgeous, inspiring images. Colorful, fresh, and healthy combos of protein, grains, veggies, and dressings abound. But how can you create a portable mason jar salad that is low FODMAP? Here we give you five of our favorite combinations, but feel free to refer to the charts on pages 12–14 to create your own versions, paying attention to the serving sizes of the ingredients and whether they are suitable for a special diet. In general choose, at least one protein, one green, one grain, at least two veggies, possibly a fruit, something crunchy such as nuts or seeds, and perhaps also a cheese. As you plan and shop, think about color, texture, and, of course, flavor. The dressing goes on the bottom, to keep the upper layers fresh and crisp. Simply empty into a bowl, toss, and dig in. If you have a large enough jar and leave headroom, it is possible to shake the covered jar and then eat right out of it.

TACO SALAD

corn (scant ¼ cup [31 g] per serving), bell peppers, cooked rice, and cumin in a simple red wine vinegar and vegetable oil salad dressing, plus avocado (max. ⅛ avocado [20 g] per serving), shredded Monterey Jack and Cheddar cheese, greens, crumbled corn chips, and a spoonful of lactose-free sour cream. A dollop of Salsa Fresca (page 80) would be perfect.

SALADE NIÇOISE

tuna, tomato, hard-boiled egg, green beans, salad greens, and sliced radishes with an olive oil and vinegar dressing (using low FODMAP vinegar).

BLT PASTA SALAD WITH CHICKEN

rice pasta, cooked chicken breast, tomatoes, crumbled bacon (use gluten-free if necessary), mozzarella balls, fresh baby spinach, and our Green Goddess Dressing (page 79).

EAT THE RAINBOW

canned chickpeas (max. ¼ cup [42 g] canned, drained and rinsed, per serving), red cabbage, red bell pepper, carrots, cooked quinoa, salad greens, and Carrot Ginger Dressing (page 78).

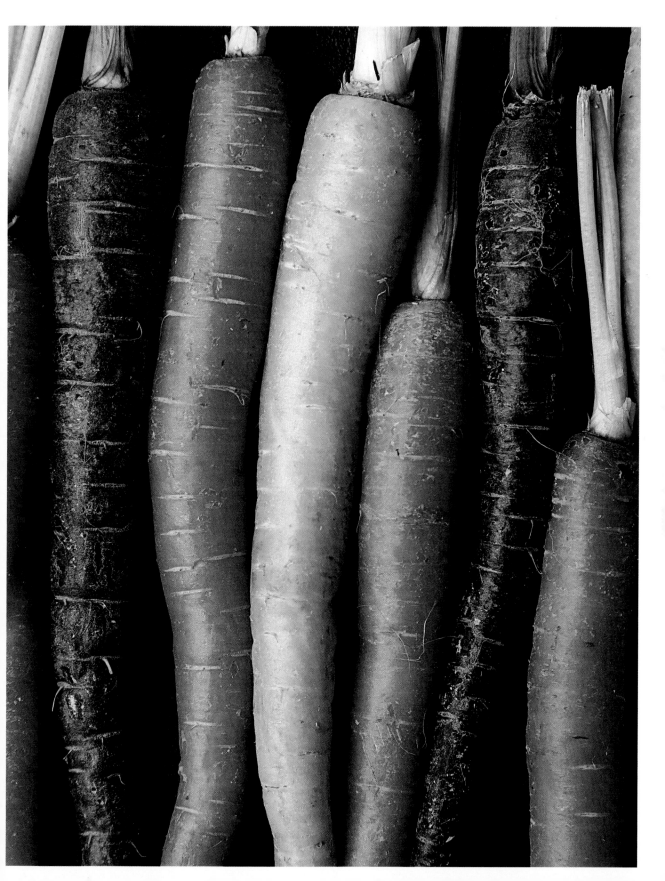

BUFFALO CHICKEN Ⓠ Ⓔ

shredded chicken from the Baked Buffalo Chicken Wings (page 149) plus tomatoes, blue cheese (not all blue cheese is gluten-free; omit if necessary), scallions (green parts only), and low FODMAP hot sauce (we like Texas Pete's).

Start with a wide-mouth mason jar; we like the 1-quart (960 ml) size.

Have all the ingredients ready to assemble.

There are certain rules for the order of layers that will help keep the ingredients as fresh tasting as possible. We always put the dressing first on the bottom (try 2 to 3 tablespoons). We recommend that sturdier items go in next, which could be chopped tomatoes or cucumbers, cooked diced potatoes, corn, or grains. Whatever you would like to marinate a little bit in the dressing is what you will add at this time; this can vary depending on your mood and ingredients.

The next layer can be grains, if not added already, and then softer, more tender or smaller vegetables or fruit, such as shredded carrot, raspberries, avocado, or sliced radishes.

Then come your proteins and cheeses, if using, in either order.

Leave a good amount of space for a generous portion of greens near the top and add them at this time.

Finish with any garnishes, such as a sprinkling of nuts or seeds, dried fruit, olives, or a shower of fresh herbs.

Seal with a lid and refrigerate until ready to serve, for up to 2 days. To eat, empty into a bowl and toss ingredients and dressing together, or mix and eat right from the jar.

Maki Roll Bowl

  MAKES 4 SMALLER LUNCHES OR 2 LARGER DINNER SERVINGS

This salad has all the components of your favorite maki roll arranged in a bowl, is easy to make, and is portable, to boot. The vegetables can be varied as long as you stay within low FODMAP choices; consider this version a blueprint. Want sushi-grade tuna or salmon instead of shrimp? Swap it in. The avocado is a must for us. We love the buttery, rich texture it brings, but remember to keep the serving size to one eighth of a Hass avocado. The dressing combines soy sauce, rice vinegar, and sugar to add that little bit of sweetness that you expect to find in traditional maki rolls.

DRESSING:

3 tablespoons rice vinegar

2 tablespoons low-sodium soy sauce or tamari (use gluten-free if necessary, such as San-J Organic)

1 teaspoon sugar

RICE AND SHRIMP:

2 cups water (480 ml)

1 cup (200 g) uncooked sushi rice

Salt

12 medium-size or large raw shrimp, shelled and deveined

VEGETABLES (CAN BE VARIED WITH OTHER LOW FODMAP CHOICES):

¼ Hass avocado, peeled and sliced

¼ pound (115 g) green beans or yellow wax beans, lightly steamed and drained

10 cucumber slices, partially peeled, or peeled if skin is thick and waxy

1 medium-size carrot, peeled, cut crosswise, then cut lengthwise into large julienne

Red cabbage

Pickled ginger

Wasabi, limited to 1 teaspoon per serving

1 sheet toasted nori seaweed

4 scallions, green parts only, sliced into ¼-inch (6 mm) pieces

Prepare the dressing: Simply whisk together all the dressing ingredients.

Prepare the rice: Combine the water and rice in a medium-size saucepan, season with salt, and bring to a boil, covered. Lower the heat and simmer until the liquid is absorbed, for 12 to 14 minutes. Turn off the heat. Leave, covered, to dry out for about 5 minutes. Fluff with a fork, transfer to a serving bowl, and drizzle with about half of the dressing, tossing gently to season.

Meanwhile, prepare the shrimp: Bring a medium-size saucepan of water to a boil. Add the shrimp, turn off the heat, and watch carefully. As soon as the shrimp turn pink, drain and pat dry with a paper towel; set aside.

Place the rice and shrimp in serving bowls and top attractively with vegetables in groupings or scattered randomly. Don't forget the pickled ginger and up to 1 teaspoon of wasabi per serving. Use scissors to cut the nori into small bits and sprinkle over all, then scatter the scallion greens on top. Serve with extra dressing, if desired.

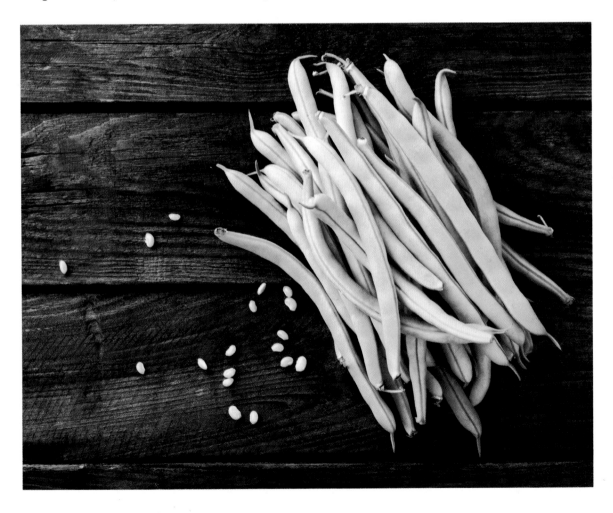

No-Recipe Grain & Veggie Bowls

 MAKES 1 BOWL

Whole grains, such as quinoa and rice, are a key part of the low FODMAP diet and provide well-tolerated and nutritious complex carbohydrates. They can also be the basis for a fabulous bowl with the addition of veggies, both raw and cooked, as well as other add-ins; feel free to make these vegan, vegetarian, or add a bit of animal protein, if you like. As you can see in the photo, our bowls are arranged with grain as the base and then the proteins, vegetables, and toppings are artfully arranged. Do not overlook leftover grains and veggies; they are perfect for repurposing! Hey, guys, feel free to get creative here: The five combinations we suggest contain some of our favorite grain and veggie bowl components, but any low FODMAP ingredients can be used. If your grains and proteins are cooked, then this dish fits within our Quick and Easy designations.

Note that certain ingredients have recommended amounts; we want to make sure that you don't go over recommended low FODMAP serving sizes.

BROWN RICE TOFU BOWL WITH POACHED EGG
Start with cooked brown rice; add cooked, cubed extra-firm tofu (sautéed in Garlic-Infused Oil (page 68) made with vegetable oil, plus soy sauce [use gluten-free if necessary] and ginger); then add a cooked green, such as broccoli (up to ½ cup [47 g] per serving), bok choy, or spinach over to the side. Add diced red bell pepper and a few slices of kabocha or cooked sweet potato (max. ½ cup [70 g] when diced raw). Top with a poached egg, crumbled nori, and a sprinkling of sesame seeds. Add a bit of suitable hot sauce on top, if you are so inclined and can tolerate.

GREEK RED QUINOA BOWL
Begin with cooked red quinoa, top with chickpeas (max. ¼ cup [42 g] drained and rinsed canned chickpeas per serving), sliced cucumber, halved cherry tomatoes, and kalamata olives. Dress with a lemony olive oil dressing, and top with chopped fresh mint and oregano and crumbled feta. You can also add some toasted walnuts or sunflower seeds (max. 2 teaspoons per serving) for crunch.

TURKEY DAY AFTERMATH BOWL
Place your choice of cooked rice in a bowl. Top with cooked turkey; cooked greens, such as kale or spinach; cooked green beans; a few slices of kabocha squash; and cranberry sauce (without high-fructose corn syrup; up to 1 tablespoon per serving).

SUPERFOOD BOWL (SHOWN ON PAGE 114)

cooked quinoa topped with chickpeas (max. ¼ cup [42 g] drained and rinsed canned chickpeas per serving), raw red bell pepper, and multi-colored carrots, cooked sweet potato (max. ½ cup [70 g] diced raw), roasted eggplant, and spinach, topped with a poached egg, sprinkled with scallion greens, and drizzled with low FODMAP hot sauce.

PIZZA MARGHERITA BOWL

Start with your grain of choice (use gluten-free if necessary). Top with halved cherry tomatoes, small fresh mozzarella balls, halved if necessary, and fresh basil leaves. Sprinkle with oregano, Parmigiano-Reggiano, and red pepper flakes.

Place the cooked grain, either hot or at room temperature, in your bowl of choice. Add the beans and/or protein, arranged in their own area. Now, add the cooked and raw vegetables in their own adjacent areas. Drizzle on the dressings or sauces, then sprinkle with the toppings, as desired. Serve immediately. If your ingredients will work well at room temperature or refrigerated, you may pack this in a portable airtight container for an easy-to-pack lunch.

KATE'S NOTES

When using the mix-and-match ingredients in mason jar salads and veggie grain bowls, this can lead to variable amounts of fat, fiber, and in some cases a slightly higher FODMAP amount in the final product. If you note one combo of ingredients doesn't settle as well, simply select another group of ingredients to try in your next creation.

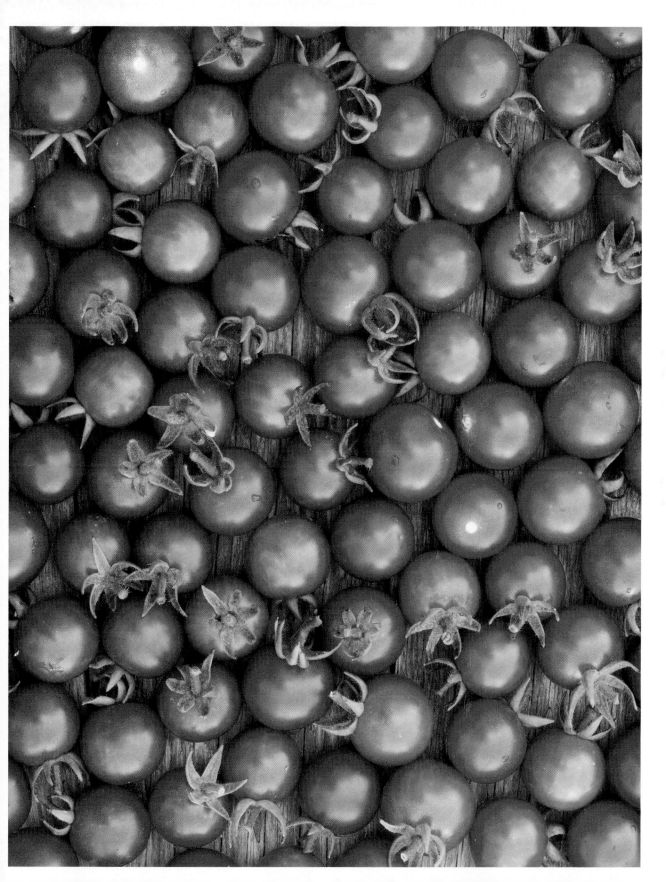

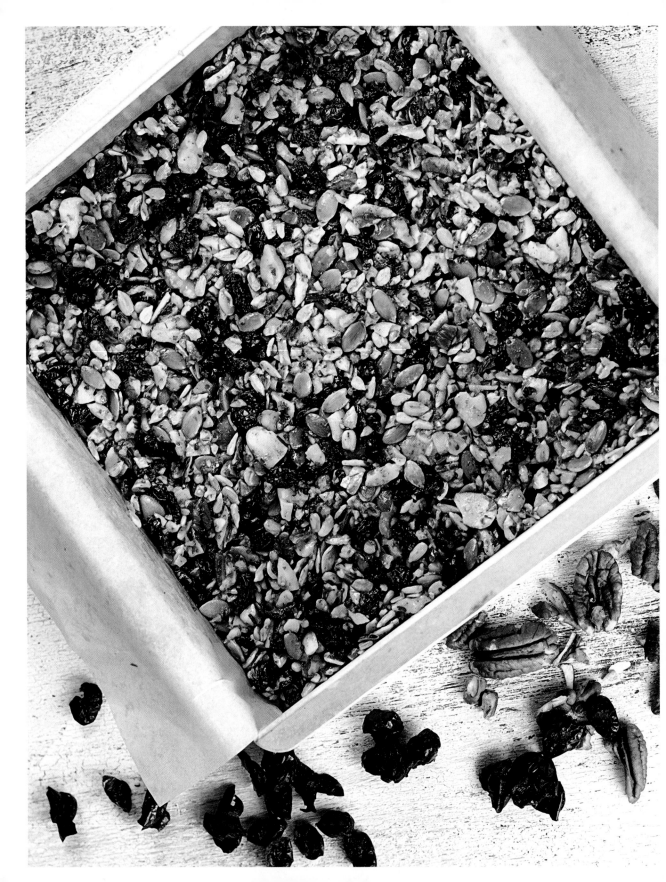

Chapter 8

LOW FODMAP SNACKS & TREATS FOR PARTIES & EVERY DAY

IF YOU'RE LIKE US, YOUR DAYS ARE BUSY. Sometimes we find ourselves running around for hours at a time, far from home, and all of a sudden hunger strikes. Finding low FODMAP food on the fly is not always easy, so we have learned to always pack a snack. Even if you have a 9-to-5 and are sitting in one place all day, that 3 p.m. slump can hit you hard. Here in this chapter you'll find our Fruit & Nut Protein Kinder Bars (our version of Kind brand bars) (page 134) that Dédé always keeps in her glove compartment, Kale Chips (page 140) and Seeded Whole-Grain Crackers (page 136). And we show you how to make the best low FODMAP Baked Buffalo Chicken Wings (page 149). Oh, yeah. Let the snacking begin.

Fruit & Nut Protein Kinder Bars

     MAKES 25 BARS | SERVING SIZE 1 BAR

When you start eating low FODMAP, it is not unusual to view an entire wall of snack bars and protein bars in the grocery store and find few to no options. This is our solution, packed with portion-controlled and low FODMAP-approved dried fruit, a variety of nuts and seeds, and just enough peanut butter to hold them together. They are a bit crispy, slightly chewy, and very gently sweetened with maple syrup.

Nonstick spray

½ cup (46 g) natural or blanched sliced almonds

½ cup (80 g) dried cranberries

½ cup (50 g) pecan halves, chopped

½ cup (83 g) raisins

½ cup (50 g) walnut halves, chopped (see Dédé's Tips)

⅓ cup (40 g) raw or toasted pumpkin seeds

2 tablespoons raw or toasted sunflower seeds

1 tablespoon flax- or chia seeds

¼ cup (60 ml) pure maple syrup

1 tablespoon natural peanut butter

Position a rack in the center of the oven. Preheat the oven to 325°F (165°C). Coat an 8-inch (20 cm) square pan with nonstick spray, then line with parchment paper cut to fit the width, but overhanging on two sides; the other two sides will be bare. Set aside.

Stir together the almonds, cranberries, pecans, raisins, walnuts, pumpkin seeds, sunflower seeds, and flaxseeds in a large, heatproof mixing bowl until evenly mixed.

Stir together the maple syrup and peanut butter in a small saucepan until combined. Bring to a boil over medium heat and boil for 1 to 2 minutes, or until visibly thickened, then immediately pour over the dry mixture and stir to combine thoroughly. (Using a silicone spatula coated with nonstick spray helps here.) The mixture will be thick; take your time and stir and fold until thoroughly mixed. Scrape into the prepared pan and press in evenly and very firmly (do not underpress—this step will determine whether your bars hold together once baked).

Bake for 15 to 17 minutes, or until dry and just beginning to take on some color. Allow to cool completely in the pan on a wire rack. Grasp the overhanging parchment with both hands and pull up to unmold. Peel away the parchment and place the solid square on a cutting board.

Use a long, sharp chef's knife to cut the square into a 5 x 5 grid, yielding twenty-five square bars. Store in an airtight container for up to 5 days. Refrigerate if your room temperature is very warm. You can also double wrap in plastic wrap, slip into a resealable plastic freezer bag, and freeze for up to a month.

DÉDÉ'S TIPS

You can double the recipe and divide it equally into two 8-inch (20 cm) pans to bake at the same time. The recipe does not work as well in a 13 x 9-inch (33 x 23 cm) pan because the center will not bake sufficiently and evenly.

KATE'S NOTES

These fruit-, seed-, and nut-rich bars are nutritious and yummy, but do limit them to one serving to stay within your meal and snack-time FODMAP limits.

(Recipe photo on page 132)

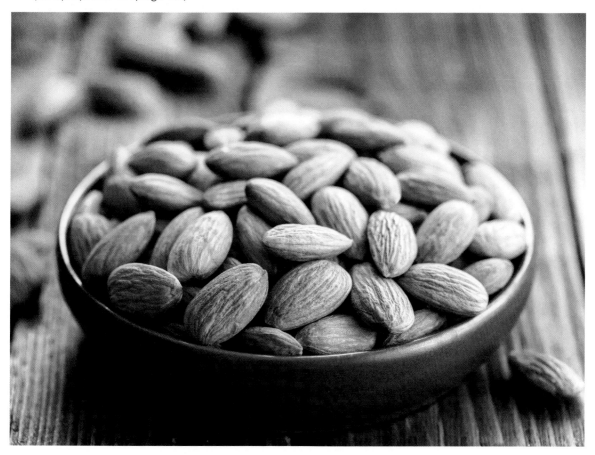

Seeded Whole-Grain Crackers

   MAKES 6 OUNCES (170 G) OF CRACKERS, ENOUGH FOR 8 GENEROUS SERVINGS

Who knew that low-fat, high-protein, delicious whole-grain crackers were so easy to make at home? You do need a food processor and parchment paper, but even the rolling pin is optional; we promise you will be amazed at the results—thin, crispy crackers that are wonderful alone or used with dips or served alongside a cheese platter. You will be combining a cooked grain, such as rice or quinoa, with soaked chia seeds and just a few other ingredients, to make a dough that comes together in less than 15 minutes (and 10 minutes of that is chia seed-soaking time!). These are also easy to customize; we like making a seeded version, but the choice is yours. Don't overlook a sweet version, such as sprinkling with cinnamon sugar.

¼ cup (60 ml) chia seeds

¼ cup (60 ml) water

2 cups (340 g) cooked short- or medium-grain brown rice or quinoa

1 tablespoon olive oil, Garlic-Infused Oil (page 68) or Onion-Infused Oil (see variation, page 68) made with olive oil, or purchased garlic-infused olive oil

½ teaspoon kosher salt

¼ teaspoon freshly ground black pepper

OPTIONAL SEASONINGS:

Cayenne pepper

Ground cinnamon

Ground cumin

Dried dill

Dried rosemary

Thyme

Additional freshly ground black pepper

Crumbled nori seaweed

Grated lemon zest

Parmigiano-Reggiano cheese (omit if following a dairy-free or vegan diet)

Low-sodium soy sauce or tamari (use gluten-free if necessary)

OPTIONAL TOPPINGS:

Pumpkin seeds

Sesame seeds

Sunflower seeds (up to 5 tablespoons
per entire recipe)

Fleur de sel, Maldon sea salt, or other
large-grain salt

Finely chopped almonds (up to 10 per
serving), hazelnuts (up to 10 per serving),
pecans, or walnuts

Granulated sugar or raw sugar

Position racks in the lower and upper thirds of the oven. Preheat the oven to 300°F (150°C). Have ready two large baking sheets and four pieces of parchment paper cut to fit pans.

Stir together the chia seeds and water in a small bowl or measuring cup and allow to sit for 10 minutes.

Place the rice (or quinoa, or a combination), soaked chia seeds (and any of their soaking water, not quite absorbed), olive oil, salt, and pepper in a food processor fitted with a metal blade, then pulse on and off to begin combining. Add your desired seasonings at this time, then process continuously until the mixture forms a very soft ball on top of the blades, 30 seconds to 1 minute.

Place one parchment paper sheet on a work surface and scoop half of the mixture onto it, using a silicone spatula. Place a second piece of parchment paper on top. Run your hands along the top parchment paper to smooth the dough out (you are aiming for it to eventually cover pretty much the entire bottom sheet of paper). Level out the dough as thinly as possible, to about ¹⁄₁₆ inch (2 mm) thick. If you have a rolling pin, it is helpful but not necessary. Don't worry if the dough is free-form around the edges. Peel back the top paper and scatter your desired toppings on top. If these include nuts and seeds. Place the loosened paper back on top of the dough and lightly press or roll again to compress the toppings into the dough. Peel off the top paper and slide the bottom paper and its dough onto one baking sheet. Repeat with the remaining dough, the clean pieces of parchment paper, and the second pan. Score both doughs with the tip of a sharp paring knife or a small pizza cutter in whatever shapes you would like the crackers to be; scoring is important, as it also helps the crackers bake evenly.

Bake for 12 minutes, then rotate the pans front to back and switch racks. Bake for 12 to 15 minutes more, or until the crackers feel dry but are still somewhat pliable. (Texture is much more important than time here; see Dédé's Tips). Hold the edge of each paper to slide the crackers off the pan and onto a work surface. Cut the crackers along the score lines, peel off the paper, and place the crackers back on the bare pans, spaced evenly apart; it's okay if they are touching here and there. Continue to bake for 5 minutes, rotate the pans front to back and switch racks again, then bake for 5 minutes more, or until the crackers are thoroughly dry and crisp and just beginning to take on some color. They will crisp up even more upon cooling. Allow the pans to cool on wire racks. Store the crackers at room temperature in an airtight container for up to 1 week.

DÉDÉ'S TIPS

If you use grain that has been cooked and refrigerated, the dough will be much drier than if you use just cooked. If the latter is the case, you might have to bake the crackers for up to twice as long, as the grain will still be very moist. Just bake the crackers until they are pliable but definitely dry and not rubbery in any way.

POST-FODMAP CHALLENGE PHASE OPTIONS

Fructans: If you passed the fructan garlic challenge add a sprinkle of garlic powder on the crackers as a seasoning option.

If you passed the fructan onion challenge, consider adding onion powder as a seasoning option.

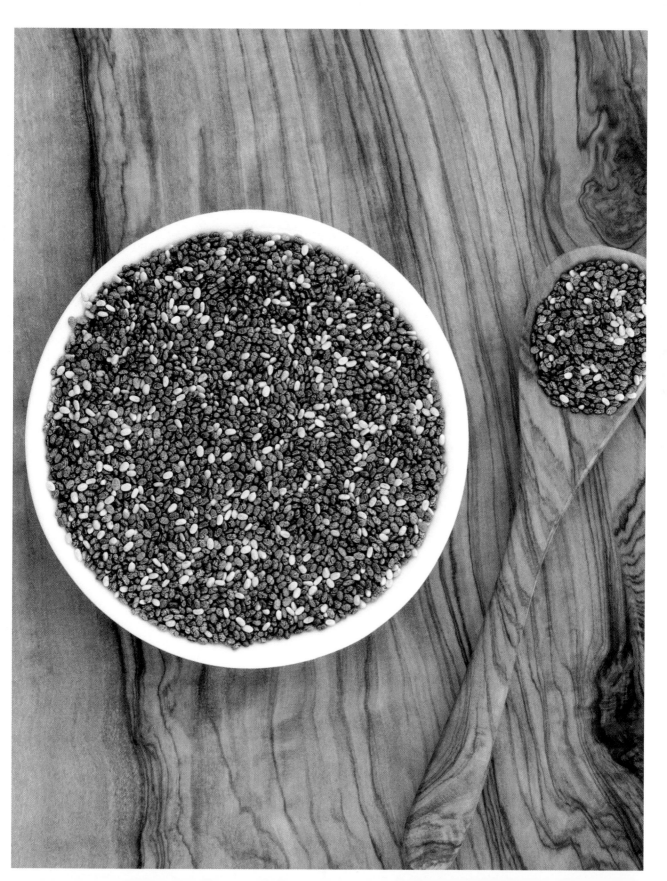

Kale Chips

      MAKES 2 TO 4 SERVINGS

Kale is a perfect green to add to your diet, as it provides a dose of well absorbed calcium, unlike the more popular leafy green, spinach, which contains calcium but it is not available to the body due to oxalic acid present in spinach, which interferes with its absorption. This recipe is simply seasoned kale baked at a low temperature until it is almost chiplike in its crunchiness. You can buy kale chips for crazy exorbitant prices, or take a bit of time to allow the oven to do the work and be rewarded with a healthy homemade snack. Note that bunches of kale vary widely in terms of size, so go by the weight when purchasing or harvesting the greens. See Dédé's Tips for flavor variations.

½ pound (225 g) curly fresh kale (about 1 small bunch or ½ large bunch)

1 tablespoon olive oil, Garlic-Infused Oil (page 68) made with olive oil, or purchased garlic-infused olive oil

⅛ teaspoon kosher salt, or more to taste

Position a rack in the center of the oven. Preheat the oven to 275°F (135°C). Line a rimmed baking sheet with parchment paper; set aside.

Wash and dry the kale thoroughly. Use a sharp paring knife to remove the larger parts of the kale stems and discard (or use for stock), then hand tear or cut the kale into pieces that are 2 to 3 inches (5 to 7.5 cm) across. Place the kale in a mixing bowl.

Drizzle the oil over the kale, using your other hand to toss the kale around as you drizzle. Sprinkle with the salt and use your hands to toss around until evenly coated. (Using your hands allows you to feel that the kale is uniformly coated with oil and salt.) Arrange the kale in an even, single layer on the prepared pan.

Bake for about 20 minutes, flipping the kale pieces over halfway through, or until crisp. Some of the edges might lightly brown, which is okay. Remove from the oven, allow to cool, and serve. These are best eaten the same day they are made; although you can store the chips in an airtight container at room temperature for up to 3 days, they will become a bit chewy.

DÉDÉ'S TIPS

Here are some flavor variations that you can try:

Use melted coconut oil instead of olive oil.

Sprinkle with 1 to 2 tablespoons of nutritional yeast while still in the bowl and mix well. We like the Bragg brand.

Try ⅛ to ¼ teaspoon of chipotle chile powder or cayenne pepper for a nice dose of heat, mixed in as above.

¼ to ½ teaspoon of paprika or smoked paprika adds color and flavor.

Add a sprinkling of Parmigiano-Reggiano and lots of freshly ground black pepper (do not use this variation if following a dairy-free or vegan diet).

Add 1 teaspoon of freshly squeezed lemon juice and ½ teaspoon of dill.

Add chipotle chile powder and freshly squeezed lime juice.

. . . you get the idea!

POST–FODMAP CHALLENGE PHASE OPTION

Fructan: If you passed the fructan garlic challenge, sprinkle with the kale with garlic powder as another creative flavor option.

Queso Dip

  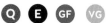   MAKES ABOUT 5 CUPS (1.2 L) | SERVES 10 TO 12 AS AN APPETIZER

If you grew up eating macaroni and cheese or cheese dips made with Velveeta, you probably thought all cheeses were that silky-smooth upon melting. They are not (at least, not without a little help). Velveeta and American cheese are manufactured cheese products that contain additives to make them more meltable. But they are not the sorts of cheeses we recommend eating on a healthy low FODMAP diet or otherwise. So, how do we get a smooth, creamy cheesy dip using real cheese, such as Cheddar and pepper Jack? It's all in the technique. Melt the cheeses slowly, follow our directions, and get ready to dig into this hot cheese dip with tortilla chips, gluten-free pretzels, or suitable low FODMAP bite-size raw vegetables.

---

10 ounces (280 g) extra-sharp Cheddar cheese, grated, at room temperature

4 ounces (115 g) pepper Jack cheese, grated, such as Cabot Creamery brand, at room temperature (see Dédé's Tips)

1 tablespoon cornstarch

¼ cup (60 ml) lactose-free milk (whole, 2%, 1%, or fat-free), at room temperature

2 plum tomatoes, cored, seeded, and diced

1 (4 ounce [115 g]) can diced mild green chiles

¼ teaspoon ground cumin

FOR SERVING:

Tortilla chips

Bite-size raw veggies, such as carrots, cucumber, and broccoli florets (limit broccoli to no more than 1 cup [90 g] per serving)

Gluten-free pretzels, such as Snyder's of Hanover

OPTIONAL GARNISH:

Chopped cilantro, Salsa Fresca (page 80), more chopped tomato, and/or pickled jalapeño peppers (see Dédé's Tips)

Toss the cheeses with the cornstarch in a medium-size, heavy-bottomed saucepan. Add the milk and heat over very low heat, stirring occasionally and very gently until the mixture is smooth. The mixture will not come together quickly and the whole melting period might take 10 minutes or more. At first the mixture will look separated; just keep cooking over low heat, stirring gently, until smooth. If you think the sauce is still too thick, add more milk, 1 tablespoon at a time.

Stir in the tomatoes, chiles with any juices, and cumin and transfer to a slow cooker set on low or a fondue pot, or place the cooking pot on a warming tray. Add some of the garnishes on top, if you like. Serve immediately with your choice of dippers.

DÉDÉ'S TIPS

Check labels, as some pepper Jack cheeses might have ingredients high in FODMAPs; check the labels on pickled jalapeños and look for those with no garlic, onion, high-fructose corn syrup, or other high-FODMAP ingredients.

Do not use preshredded cheeses. They have anticaking and antimolding additives that are not only unnecessary for our purposes but can also prevent the mixture from melting smoothly.

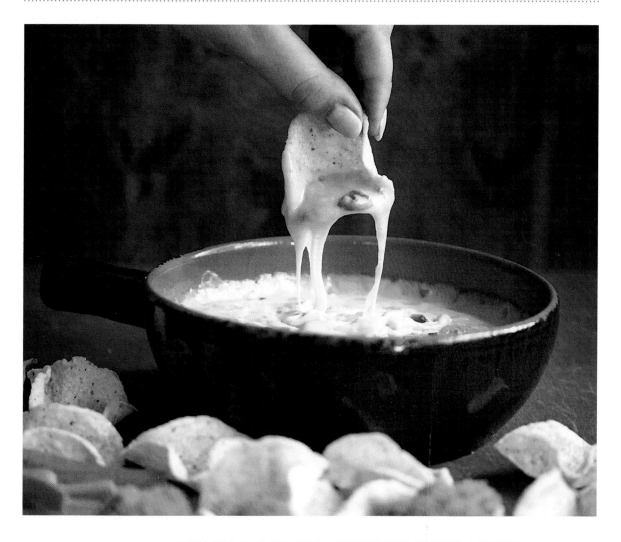

Protein-Packed Trail Mix

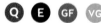 MAKES ABOUT 13 CUPS (ABOUT 52 SERVINGS) |
RECOMMENDED SERVING ¼ CUP (25 G)

Although you can buy trail mix from a variety of sources, they never seem to meet our low FODMAP needs: too many unapproved dried fruits or nuts, too much chocolate or candy, and they are always more expensive than making your own. And with homemade we can add protein-dense ingredients. Finding yourself with plummeting blood sugar while following a low FODMAP diet is something to avoid. This recipe makes a large amount: stash some at work, at home, in your gym bag—wherever it might be helpful to have on hand when hunger strikes, but remember to keep to our low FODMAP ¼-cup (38 g) serving size. You may use raw or toasted seeds in lieu of sprouted, but we love these for their extra digestibility. Toast the nuts separately for best results (see Dédé's Tips).

½ cup (80 g) dried cranberries

½ cup (83 g) dark or light raisins

2 cups (120 g) large flaked unsweetened coconut, toasted or untoasted

1 cup (86 g) toasted almonds, sliced or slivered or whole, natural or blanched

1 cup (225 g) finely chopped semisweet or bittersweet chocolate, preferably 70% to 80% cacao (use dairy-free if following a dairy-free or vegan diet)

1 cup (142 g) toasted peanuts

1 cup (99 g) toasted pecan halves

1 cup (118 g) raw or toasted pumpkin seeds

1 cup (140 g) raw or toasted sunflower seeds

1 cup (99 g) toasted walnut halves

4 cups (104 g) unsweetened puffed millet

Toss all the ingredients together in a bowl. Store in airtight container(s) at room temperature up to 2 weeks.

DÉDÉ'S TIPS

To toast nuts, preheat the oven to 350°F (180°F). Spread the nuts, one kind at a time, in a single layer on a rimmed baking sheet. Bake just until starting to color and you begin to smell their aroma, anywhere from 5 to 10 minutes, depending on the type and amount of nut and whether they were at room temperature. Allow to cool on the pan, and then they are ready to use.

Chicken Satay

  MAKES ABOUT 20 SKEWERS | SERVES 8 TO 10

This easy finger food features strips of boneless chicken marinated in a sauce packed with the Asian flavors of peanut, coconut, ginger, and coriander. You can use boneless, skinless chicken breasts, but we prefer the richness that chicken thighs provide. Make sure to use pure (canned) coconut milk, not sweetened cream of coconut or a coconut beverage. While these are often served as hors d'oeuvres, they also make a flavorful light dinner entrée or lunch.

½ cup (120 ml) canned pure full-fat or light unsweetened coconut milk, such as Thai Kitchen brand

½ cup (32 g) finely chopped scallion, green parts only, divided

¼ cup (68 g) smooth peanut butter (see Dédé's Tips)

¼ cup (60 ml) low-sodium soy sauce or tamari (use gluten-free if necessary)

2 tablespoons firmly packed light brown sugar

2 tablespoons freshly squeezed lemon juice

2 (1-inch [2.5 cm]) slices fresh ginger; no need to peel

¼ teaspoon ground coriander

¼ teaspoon ground cumin

⅛ teaspoon cayenne pepper

1½ pounds (680 g) boneless, skinless chicken thighs

¼ cup (8 g) finely chopped cilantro

Flavorless oil, such as canola or rice bran oil

EQUIPMENT:
20 (8-inch [20 cm]) bamboo skewers

Combine the coconut milk, ¼ cup (16 g) of the scallion greens, and the peanut butter, soy sauce, brown sugar, lemon juice, ginger, coriander, cumin, and cayenne in a blender and process until smooth. Set aside ½ cup (120 ml) of the sauce, then pour the remaining sauce into a mixing bowl.

Cut the chicken into strips about 1 inch (2.5 cm) across and 3 to 4 inches (7.5 to 10 cm) long. Add the chicken to the larger amount of sauce, toss to coat, cover, and refrigerate at least 4 hours or overnight. Cover and refrigerate the reserved ½ cup (120 ml) of sauce as well.

When ready to cook, either prepare a medium-hot charcoal or propane grill or have a grill pan ready for indoor cooking. If using a grill pan, heat over medium heat. Brush the grill or grill pan with oil.

Remove the marinated chicken from the refrigerator. Thread the chicken onto the skewers down the length of the chicken strip, weaving the skewer in and out of the chicken so it stays in place during cooking. The chicken should take up about half the length of each skewer. Discard any marinade left over from marinating the chicken and remove the reserved sauce from the refrigerator.

Place the chicken on the grill or grill pan, situating it so that only the chicken and not the bare skewers are in contact with the hot surface. Cook for 3 or 4 minutes, then flip over and cook for 3 or 4 minutes more, or until the chicken is just cooked through.

Remove from the grill or grill pan and immediately brush with the reserved sauce not previously used for marinating. Sprinkle with the chopped cilantro and reserved ¼ cup (16 g) of scallion greens and serve immediately.

DÉDÉ'S TIPS

You can use the newer styles of creamy peanut butter made with palm oil or a natural-style peanut butter; avoid those made with honey, high-fructose corn syrup, or other high-FODMAP ingredients. If you opt for the all-natural, use a commercially prepared version and not the type you grind to order in the store. Those are too dry for this sauce.

Double Coconut Shrimp with Sweet Chili Sauce

  MAKES 4 TO 6 APPETIZER SERVINGS

This fried shrimp appetizer is way better than any you can find in a restaurant—and it is low FODMAP approved! We like to use half unsweetened shredded coconut and half sweetened coconut shreds. The unsweetened coconut keeps the sweetness level in check, while the sweetened coconut adds a really nice chew. If you want to streamline the recipe, feel free to use just one or the other. Results will be different, but still quite tasty. The dipping sauce is a simple three-ingredient recipe that comes together in a flash. If you can tolerate small amounts of garlic, see the Post-FODMAP Challenge Options for a ready-made dipping sauce suggestion.

SWEET CHILI SAUCE:

½ cup (120 ml) orange marmalade (without high-fructose corn syrup)

¼ cup (60 ml) Dijon mustard (use gluten-free if necessary)

¼ teaspoon crushed red pepper flakes, or more to taste

SHRIMP:

¾ pound (340 g) large (26/30) shrimp, deveined and shelled

2 large egg whites, at room temperature

⅓ cup (38 g) gluten-free plain bread crumbs, such as Gillian's Foods Plain Bread Crumbs

⅓ cup (29 g) sweetened long shredded coconut (sometimes called "angel flake")

⅓ cup (38 g) unsweetened shredded coconut (sometimes called grated or dessicated; very fine in texture)

¼ teaspoon kosher salt

Pinch of cayenne pepper

Vegetable oil, such as canola or rice bran

Prepare the sweet chile sauce: Simply stir the marmalade and mustard together in a small bowl, then season to taste with red pepper flakes.

Prepare the shrimp: Pat the shrimp dry with a paper towel and set aside. Whisk the egg whites in a small bowl until frothy. Combine the bread crumbs, both coconuts, and the salt and cayenne in another bowl.

Heat 4 inches (10 cm) of oil in a large saucepan and bring to 365° to 375°F (185°C to 190°C) over medium-high heat. Line a tray with a double layer of paper towels and place nearby, but away from the flame. While the oil is heating, place the shrimp, a few at a time, in the egg whites and toss to coat, then coat completely in the bread crumb mixture. Have all the shrimp coated and ready to go.

Once the oil comes to temperature, fry a few shrimp at a time, allowing plenty of room for them to fry without touching. Maintain the oil temperature by adjusting the heat as necessary. Fry for about 3 minutes, tossing around with a spider or slotted spoon, or until golden brown. Remove from the pot, allowing any excess oil to drip back into the pot, and drain on the paper towels while you cook the rest. Serve immediately with the sweet chili sauce.

POST-FODMAP CHALLENGE PHASE OPTION

Fructan: If you passed the fructan garlic challenge, consider subbing in purchased sweet chili sauce, a sweet and slightly spicy option that you can use right out of the bottle. It does contain a small amount of garlic, so only use if you can tolerate it. And before you think this must be a specialty store item, know that you can even find it at Walmart!

Baked Buffalo Chicken Wings

 MAKES 24 PIECES | SERVES 10 TO 12

To make low FODMAP chicken wings, you must use a hot sauce without any added garlic or onion. This will take some label reading, but we have found it pretty easy to find versions, such as Texas Pete's, containing just hot peppers, vinegar, and salt. We bake and broil these, as opposed to deep-frying; the maple syrup in the sauce encourages such a wonderfully rich caramelization that you won't miss the texture created by frying. We bypassed the classic celery stick accompaniment because it would be too easy to overindulge, but carrot sticks make a great, fresh, crunchy addition. (If you can hold yourself to a 2-inch [5 cm] piece of celery, be our guest). By the way, chicken wings vary hugely in weight and some are sold with tip attached (3-part wings), whereas others are trimmed (2-piece "party wings").

WINGS:

12 medium-size chicken wings, without tips, a.k.a. party wings (about 3½ pounds [1.6 kg])

Salt

Freshly ground black pepper

¾ cup (180 ml) hot sauce, such as Texas Pete's (if using other brands, check labels for approved low FODMAP ingredients)

3 tablespoons pure maple syrup

3 tablespoons unsalted butter

FOR SERVING:

½ recipe Blue Cheese Dressing (page 75; do not use if following a gluten-free diet)

24 (3-inch [7.5 cm])-long carrot sticks or "baby" carrots

Prepare the wings: Position a rack in the center of the oven. Preheat the oven to 400°F (200°C). Line a rimmed baking sheet with foil and place a wire rack on top.

Halve the chicken wings at the joint. Season the wings well with salt and pepper.

Place the chicken wings on the rack and roast for 30 to 40 minutes, or until the skin is dry and crispy and the meat is just cooked through (the time may vary, depending on the size of the wings).

Meanwhile, combine the hot sauce, maple syrup, and butter in a small saucepan and heat over medium heat, stirring occasionally, until the butter melts. Pour off about ¼ cup (60 ml) to reserve for finishing.

When the wings are just cooked through, remove from the oven and place the pan on the stove top (with the heat turned off). Adjust an oven rack so that it is about 4 inches (10 cm) from the broiler. Preheat the broiler. Brush the wings with some of the sauce from the larger portion of sauce and broil for 2 to 3 minutes, or until the wings get a nice caramelized char. Flip, brush with more of the brushing sauce, and broil for 2 to 3 more minutes (discard any leftover brushing sauce). When completely cooked, brush the wings with the unused, reserved sauce and serve immediately with the blue cheese dressing and carrot sticks.

KATE'S NOTES

Some assume all spicy foods are a problem for those with a sensitive tummy, but that is simply not the case. If spicy foods consistently trouble your GI symptoms, then by all means stay clear of them, but many can tolerate foods with a bit of heat without an issue.

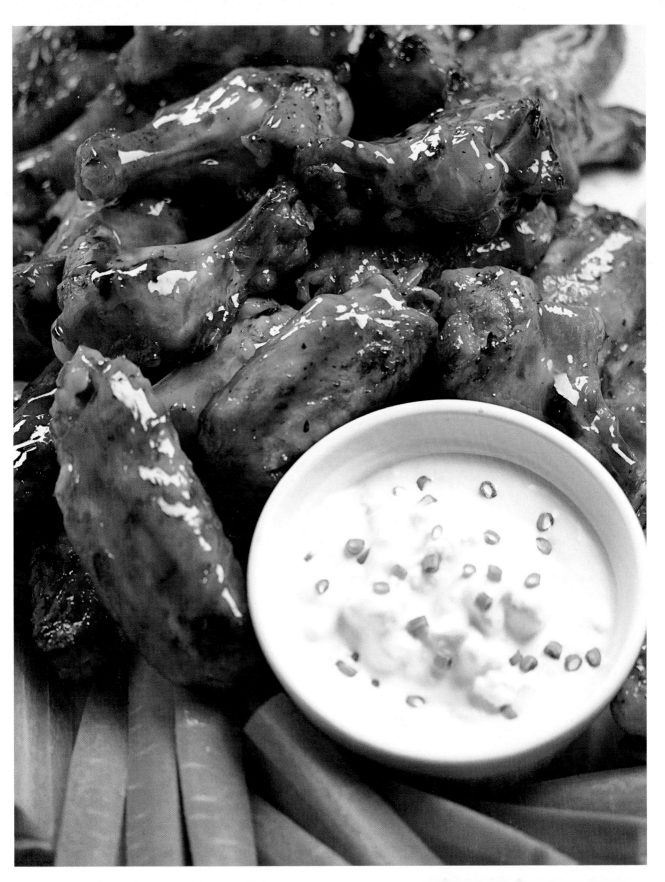

Teriyaki Meatballs

    MAKES 26 COCKTAIL-SIZE MEATBALLS | SERVING SIZE 3 OR 4 MEATBALLS

These are a great low FODMAP hot hors d'oeuvre, fancy enough for a swanky party. They are also great for everyday: Tuck a few in a Boston lettuce leaf for a light lunch or pack them in a thermos for a nice warm lunch. They are best served right after cooking, when their texture is lighter and the sauce is hot and silky. However, you can form the raw meatballs a day ahead of time, so take advantage of that helpful step. Use all beef or a blend of beef and pork; your choice. And don't skimp on the sesame seed and scallion garnishes; they truly add flavor and texture and finish off the dish in a more complete way.

---

1 pound (455 g) ground beef (80% lean), or ½ pound (225 g) ground beef and ½ pound (225 g) ground pork

1 tablespoon peeled and grated fresh ginger (grate with a coarse Microplane or rasp-style grater)

5 tablespoons (20 g) very finely chopped scallion, green parts only

½ teaspoon kosher salt

2 teaspoons Garlic-Infused Oil (page 68) made with vegetable oil, or purchased garlic-infused vegetable oil

2 teaspoons toasted sesame oil

2 tablespoons pure maple syrup

2 tablespoons low-sodium soy sauce or tamari (use gluten-free if necessary, such as San-J Organic)

1 tablespoon plus 1 teaspoon rice vinegar

½ teaspoon cornstarch

2 tablespoons cold water

1 tablespoon white hulled sesame seeds

Combine the meat(s), ginger, 3 tablespoons of scallion greens, and the salt in a mixing bowl and use your hands to mix together well. Form into twenty-six small meatballs, each about 1¼ inches (3.2 cm) across. Take your time making smooth, round balls. This step will affect the attractiveness of the finished dish, so don't rush. Place the balls on a plate (we use a pie plate), cover with plastic wrap, and refrigerate for at least 1 hour or overnight to firm up.

Heat a 12-inch (30.5 cm) nonstick pan over medium heat. Add the garlic-infused oil and sesame oil. Add all the meatballs, which should sizzle when they hit the pan. Adjust the heat as necessary. Cook through, tossing the pan frequently for even cooking and browning, for 6 to 8 minutes. Transfer the meatballs to a clean plate. Discard any excess fat in the pan but do not wipe out the pan.

With the pan still over medium heat, add the maple syrup, soy sauce, and vinegar and boil for about 15 seconds, stirring with a silicone spatula or wooden spoon. The mixture should look slightly thickened and bubbling all over. Quickly dissolve the cornstarch in the cold water and add to the hot sauce. Stir the mixture and continue to cook for about 30 seconds, or until the sauce is thick and glossy. Add the meatballs back to the pan and toss around to reheat and coat completely in the sauce. Place the meatballs on a serving platter and sprinkle with the sesame seeds and reserved scallion greens. Serve immediately with toothpicks for spearing.

POST-FODMAP CHALLENGE PHASE OPTION

Fructan: If you pass the fructan garlic challenge, add 1 to 2 garlic cloves, finely chopped, to the raw meatball mixture.

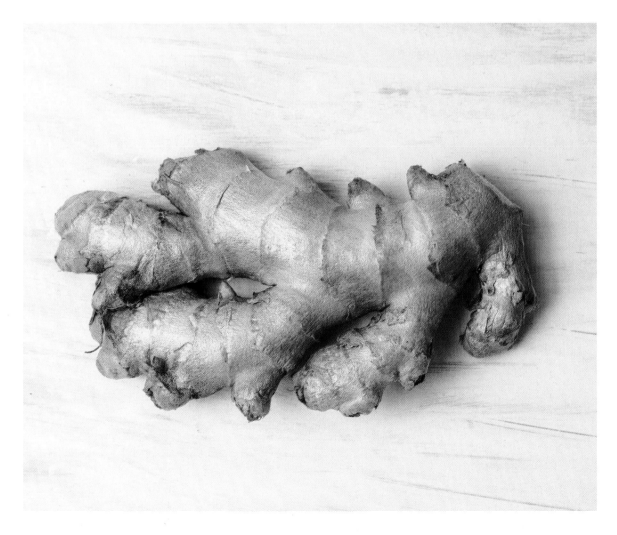

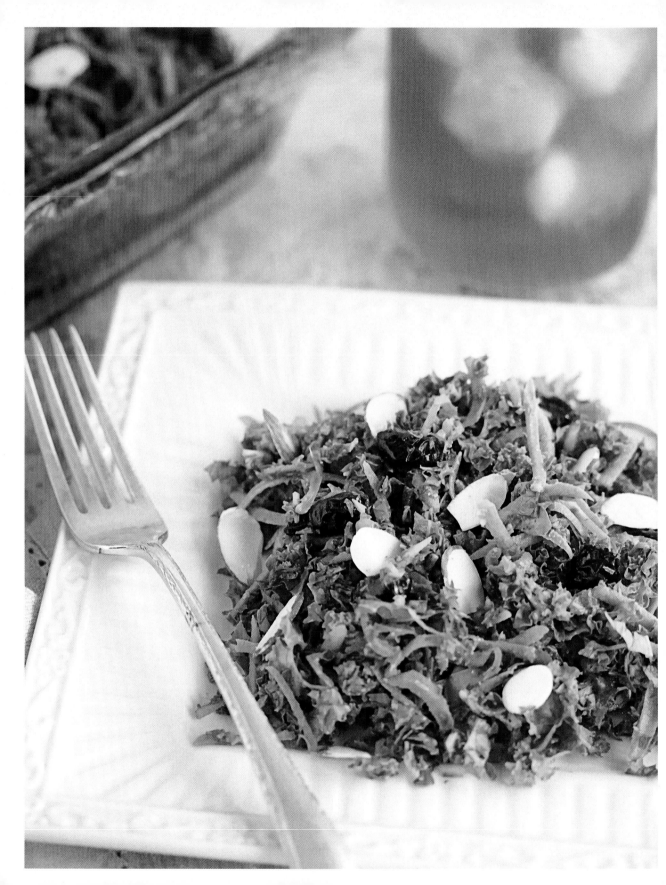

Chapter 9

SALADS & SIDES

WE DON'T GO A DAY WITHOUT SOME kind of salad, and thankfully our low FODMAP diet allows for a bevy of choices. From Kale Carrot Salad with Citrus Vinaigrette and Almonds (page 156), Rainbow Chopped Salad (page 163), and Quinoa Tabouli (page 184) to a substantial Oven-Roasted Chicken Caesar Salad (page 170), there are plenty to choose from. Side dishes round out our main meals and this chapter brings you everything from Garlic Mashed Potatoes (page 173) and Cheesy Grits (page 172) to fancier fare, such as Roasted Eggplant, Zucchini, Potato & Tomato Gratin (page 166), which looks beautiful enough to present table-side. Hankering for a Spinach Salad with Hot Bacon Dressing? It's here on page 159.

Kale Carrot Salad with Citrus Vinaigrette & Almonds

    MAKES 8 SERVINGS

The first few kale salad recipes Dédé ever encountered spoke of "massaging" the raw kale to soften its hardy texture, and frankly, the process sounded laborious. Turns out that a food processor breaks down the texture very well, and very quickly, and you may want one for this recipe (if you don't have one, we provide by-hand directions as well). Kate loves kale as it is one of the few leafy greens that contain well absorbable calcium—and calcium intake can take a hit while on the low FODMAP diet. This recipe will help you add kale to your menu more often. Not only is this a very nutritious salad but it also keeps for days in the refrigerator. Make a big batch over the weekend and have kale salad for several lunches throughout the week.

DRESSING:

3 tablespoons extra-virgin olive oil

1 tablespoon Dijon mustard (use gluten-free if necessary)

1 tablespoon freshly squeezed lemon juice

1 tablespoon sherry vinegar, rice vinegar, or red wine vinegar

Kosher salt

Freshly ground black pepper

SALAD:

1 navel orange

1 pound (455 g) bag washed curly kale, or enough leaves, stemmed and torn into pieces, to equal 1 pound

4 medium-size carrots, scrubbed or peeled if desired

⅓ cup (29 g) lightly toasted sliced almonds, natural or blanched

⅓ cup (70 g) dried cranberries

Prepare the dressing: Combine the olive oil, mustard, lemon juice, and vinegar in a jar and season with salt and pepper to taste. Cover the jar and shake vigorously. Set aside.

Prepare the salad: Cut the peel and white pith from the orange. Cut between the membranes to release the segments into a large mixing bowl, reserving all the juice in the bowl as well.

Remove any large pieces of kale stem, if present. Chop the kale in batches, in a food processor fitted with a metal blade, until finely chopped (use photo for guidance; see Dede's Tips for making by hand), adding as it is chopped to the orange. After all the kale is chopped, remove the metal blade and insert the shredding disk, shred the carrots, then add them to the kale mixture. Toss in the almonds and cranberries. Add the dressing, a little at a time, folding it in. Do not overdress the salad. The kale salad is ready to serve, or refrigerate in an airtight container for up to 4 days.

DEDE'S TIPS

If you prefer to chop by hand, there will be a little more prep work. Dump the torn pieces of kale into a roomy bowl and literally massage the leaves. Use a kneading action with your fingers, firmly manipulating each leaf, squeezing again and again. This will help break down the very fibrous texture (which the food processor does so beautifully). Once the kale pieces are softened, chop as finely as possible with a very sharp chef's knife and proceed with the recipe.

(Recipe photo on page 152)

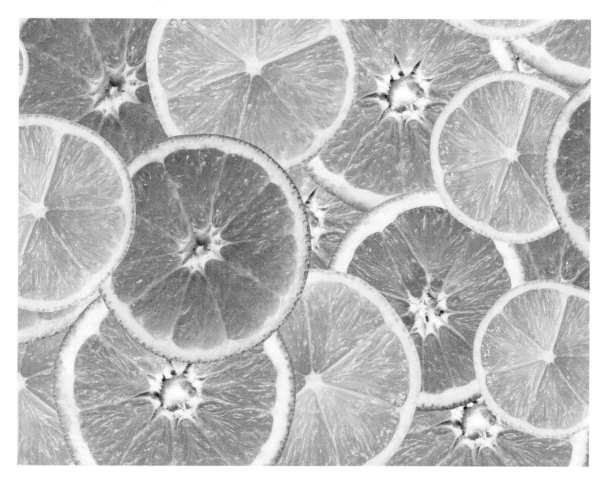

Cucumber, Tomato & Feta Salad

     MAKES 5 TO 7 SERVINGS

During her many years of catering, Dédé made this salad in huge batches almost year-round. The original had a hefty amount of red onion added, so it needed a low FODMAP facelift. Scallion greens make a fine substitute; feta cheese is low in lactose, so it is low FODMAP friendly as well. This salad pairs particularly well with grilled main dishes or anything vaguely Mediterranean in flavor. Although the salad can be made up to a day ahead, it begins to get watery and loses its freshness on day two, so plan accordingly.

---

2 medium-size beefsteak tomatoes, 3 plum tomatoes, or ¾ dry pint (213 g) cherry or grape tomatoes

1 medium-size cucumber or ½ English cucumber

1 green, yellow, orange, or red bell pepper, cored and cut into bite-size pieces

½ cup (32 g) chopped scallion, green parts only

1 tablespoon chopped fresh flat-leaf parsley

4 ounces (115 g) feta cheese, roughly crumbled or cubed

½ cup (120 ml) extra-virgin olive oil

¼ cup (60 ml) red wine vinegar

1 teaspoon chopped fresh oregano, or ½ teaspoon dried

Salt

Freshly ground black pepper

⅓ cup (48 g) pitted kalamata olives, drained and halved (optional)

If using beefsteak tomatoes, core, cut in half crosswise, squeeze, and discard some of the extra juice and seeds, then chop the flesh into bite-size pieces. Plum tomatoes can be cored and chopped; cherry or grape tomatoes should be halved. Place the tomatoes in a medium-size mixing bowl.

If using a standard cucumber, peel, cut off and discard the ends, quarter lengthwise, and then cut into ½-inch (12 mm) chunks; English cucumber can be cut up unpeeled. Add to the tomatoes.

Add the peppers, scallion greens, parsley, and feta and toss to combine. Whisk together the oil, vinegar, and oregano in a small bowl, pour over the salad, and stir to coat. Season with salt and black pepper to taste. Add the olives, if desired. The salad is ready to serve, or refrigerate in an airtight container for up to 1 day. Bring to a cool room temperature before serving.

Spinach Salad with Hot Bacon Dressing, Blue Cheese & Grapes

 MAKES 2 LARGE OR 4 SMALL SERVINGS

Classic spinach salads call for more mature spinach leaves, but we like the more tender baby spinach; it is your choice! As the contrast of cold veggies and hot dressing is one of the joys of this salad, timing is paramount. Read the recipe through so that you can proceed from beginning to end as swiftly as possible. The savoriness of the bacon; saltiness of the blue cheese; crisp cool texture of the spinach; and sweetness from the grapes come together in a marvel of textures and flavors.

SALAD:

4 ounces (115 g) baby spinach, or washed, dried, stemmed mature spinach leaves torn into bite-size pieces

½ cup (76 g) seedless red grapes, halved

2 ounces (55 g) blue cheese, crumbled (not all blue cheese is gluten-free; omit if following a gluten-free diet or substitute feta cheese)

2 tablespoons chopped scallion, green parts only

DRESSING:

2 slices thick-cut bacon

2 tablespoons red wine vinegar

1 teaspoon Dijon mustard (use gluten-free if necessary)

1 teaspoon sugar

Extra-virgin olive oil, if necessary

Kosher salt

Freshly ground black pepper

Prepare the salad: Toss together the spinach, grapes, cheese, and scallion greens in a mixing bowl; set aside.

Prepare the dressing: Cook the bacon in a skillet until crisp; leaving the fat in the pan, drain the bacon on paper towels and set aside. Whisk the vinegar, mustard, and sugar into the hot bacon fat. Taste and add olive oil, if desired. Season to taste with salt and pepper.

While the dressing is still warm, pour it over the salad, crumble the bacon over all, toss well, and serve immediately.

> **POST-FODMAP CHALLENGE PHASE OPTION**
> **Fructan:** If you have passed the fructan onion challenge, sub in sliced red onion for the scallion greens to taste and tolerance.

Kale Cabbage Coleslaw with Creamy Poppy Seed Dressing

   MAKES 12 TO 14 SERVINGS

We like a good coleslaw, especially in the summer to accompany grilled meats and burgers. Green cabbage is low FODMAP as it is, but we have added some finely shredded kale for extra nutrition, color, and flavor. Although you can refrigerate this dish overnight, the texture is best the day it is made. You can, however, make the salad and the slightly sweet, slightly tangy Sweet Poppy Seed Dressing (page 74) the day before and store them separately, then combine the day of serving. This recipe yields a good amount and is a great party dish.

DRESSING:

⅔ cup (165 ml) Sweet Poppy Seed Dressing (page 74)

⅔ cup (150 g) lactose-free plain yogurt

SALAD:

1 pound (455 g) green cabbage (do not use savoy; see Kate's Notes), cored, outer leaves removed, and finely shredded

½ pound (225 g) red cabbage, cored, outer leaves removed, and finely shredded

½ pound (225 g) lacinato kale, large ribs removed and finely shredded

2 medium-size carrots, scrubbed (peeled, if desired) and finely shredded

Prepare the dressing: Simply whisk together the Sweet Poppy Seed Dressing and the yogurt in a small bowl until well blended; set aside.

Prepare the salad: Toss together the cabbage, kale, and carrots in a large mixing bowl. Drizzle with the dressing, tossing as you go, only using enough to moisten and flavor the vegetables. You might not use all the dressing and you do not want to oversaturate the salad with it. The salad is ready to serve or may be refrigerated covered in an airtight container for up to 6 hours.

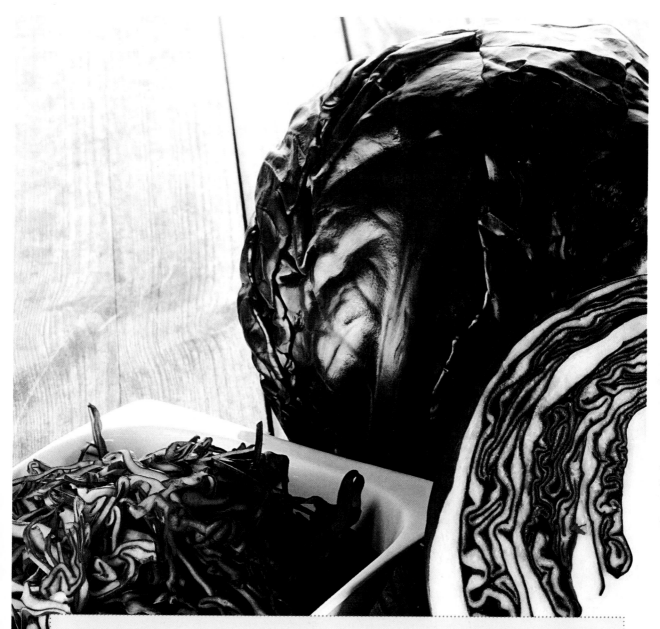

KATE'S NOTES

 When it comes to the low FODMAP diet, not all cabbage is alike! Common green cabbage, with the round and smooth head, is considered a low FODMAP option. Red cabbage is low FODMAP, too. Savoy cabbage, a round cabbage with a noticeably crinklier leaf, is a source of fructans, so try that during the challenge phase to test your tolerance.

POST-FODMAP CHALLENGE PHASE OPTION

Fructose: If you passed the excess fructose challenge, sub in honey for the maple syrup in the Sweet Poppy Seed Dressing.

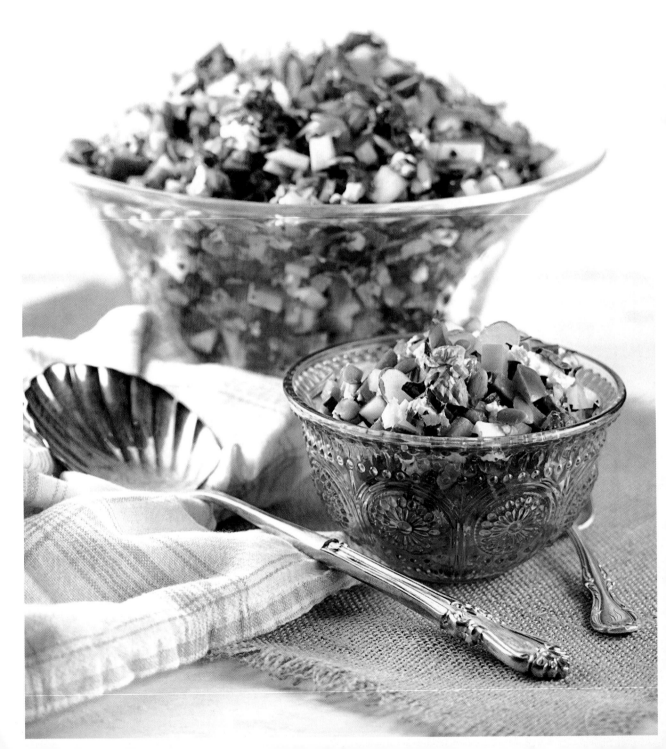

Rainbow Chopped Salad

    MAKES ABOUT 24 SERVINGS

This recipe embodies what *The Low FODMAP Diet Step by Step* is about: an accessible recipe, every bite filled with flavor and nutrition, a dish versatile enough to accompany some protein for lunch, serve a side salad at dinner, or bring to a large potluck party. Visually it is overflowing with a sense of colorful and textural abundance! Every bite is packed with flavor and crunch and will leave you feeling great. The success of this dish depends on the quality of the vegetables and the small, even sizes of all the veggies, so take your time while prepping; you want to able to eat this with a spoon. Ultimate veggie comfort food. This makes a large amount, as it actually keeps quite well, and we have provided do-ahead information for your convenience. You may halve the recipe, if you wish.

SALAD:

2 cups (134 g) very finely chopped lacinato kale

2 cups (134 g) very finely chopped romaine lettuce

1 cup (100 g) diced bok choy stems and leaves

1 cup (89 g) very finely chopped red cabbage

1 English cucumber, ends discarded, halved lengthwise, seeded, then diced

1 medium-size green bell pepper, cored and diced

1 medium-size red bell pepper, cored and diced

1 medium-size yellow or orange bell pepper, cored and diced

1 cup (180 g) plum tomatoes, cored and diced

1 (6- to 8-ounce [170 to 225 g]) celery root (a.k.a. celeriac), peeled, ends discarded, and diced (¾ to 1 cup [180 to 240 ml])

6 ounces (170 g) chopped slender, raw green beans

3 medium-size carrots, peeled, ends discarded, and finely julienned

½ cup (32 g) chopped scallion, green parts only

¼ cup (8 g) finely chopped fresh flat-leaf parsley

3 cups (450 g) crumbled feta cheese

¾ cup (89 g) raw or toasted pumpkin seeds

¾ cup (69 g) raw or toasted sliced natural almonds

DRESSING:

6 tablespoons to ½ cup (90 to 120 ml) Balsamic Dijon Dressing (page 73) or
Sweet Poppy Seed Dressing (page 74), or use the following mustard vinaigrette:

MUSTARD VINAIGRETTE:

3 tablespoons red wine vinegar

1 teaspoon Dijon mustard (use gluten-free if following a gluten-free diet)

6 tablespoons (90 ml) extra-virgin olive oil (see Dédé's Tips)

Kosher salt (optional)

Freshly ground black pepper (optional)

Prepare the salad: Simply toss the veggies together in a large mixing bowl. If not serving right away, at this time you may transfer to airtight containers and refrigerate for up to 3 days. Make your dressing of choice when you plan to serve the salad.

Prepare the dressing: If using the mustard vinaigrette, whisk the vinegar and mustard together in a small bowl. Slowly whisk in the oil until smooth and combined. You can also shake the ingredients together in a covered jar. Season to taste with salt and black pepper, if desired.

When ready to serve, toss the veggies, feta, pumpkin seeds, and almonds together and dress to taste (don't overdress; allow the veggies to shine). Serve immediately. See Dédé's Tips for variations and serving tips if not using all at once.

DÉDÉ'S TIPS

This makes a lot, but it keeps well; with this in the fridge, you will have an easy-to-grab low FODMAP snack, lunch, or salad at your fingertips.

You can vary the taste of this salad by using different dressings. In the mustard vinaigrette, try rice vinegar instead of red wine vinegar; or walnut oil, Garlic-Infused Oil (page 68), or purchased garlic-infused olive oil instead of plain olive oil.

Zucchini & Summer Squash Salad

        MAKES 10 SERVINGS

This salad is a low FODMAP beauty, even in its simplicity. It sports few ingredients, but the ribboned visual, the tender crunch of the raw veggies, and the simple dressing come together to be more than a sum of the parts. The ribbons are fun to make, look unexpected, and allow the dressing to permeate the squash perfectly, creating a raw salad that has both a crunchy and a velvety quality.

---

1 pound (455 g) small to medium-size zucchini (about 3)

1 pound (455 g) small to medium-size yellow summer squash (about 3)

3 tablespoons extra-virgin olive oil

1 tablespoon freshly squeezed lemon juice

Salt

Freshly ground black pepper

Dried oregano (optional)

Wash and dry the zucchini and summer squash. Cut off and discard both ends of each veggie. Use a sharp vegetable peeler to peel broad ribbons of the veggies right into a large mixing bowl. Once you get near the center of each squash, you will see seeds. At that point, flip the squash over and begin peeling from the opposite side. When you see seeds from this side, simply stop and discard the center portion, or save for another use (for example, chop, sauté, and put into an omelet). Whisk together the oil and lemon juice in a small bowl and drizzle over the ribbons. Season to taste with salt, pepper, and oregano, if using, and toss evenly to coat. Serve immediately. The salad may sit for up to 4 hours, covered with plastic wrap, at a cool room temperature. Best eaten within 4 hours.

DÉDÉ'S TIPS

If your squash are too large, they will make unwieldy ribbons and their texture could verge on being cottony; the center seedy parts of thinner squash can also be cottony, hence our directions above. Also, in addition to being more tender, with smaller squash you will be able to use more of each veggie for this salad. Your best bet is to make this when zucchini and summer squash are at their peak, when you can buy them as fresh as possible.

Roasted Eggplant, Zucchini, Potato & Tomato Gratin

    MAKES 6 TO 8 SERVINGS

With its array of thinly sliced veggies, this is a very pretty dish. The thin slices are more than pretty, though: thinly slicing the vegetables allows them to cook at the same time. If you have a mandoline, use it. Otherwise, using a very sharp knife will do the trick. We like this dish hot or even at room temperature alongside fish, chicken, and lamb in particular. It is also very forgiving; Dédé has even made this in a cast-iron skillet in her covered grill. The mélange of hearty potatoes and eggplant with the juicy tomato and garden-fresh zucchini works very well. No need for an additional starch or veggie—it's all here in one dish. Note that this recipe is somewhat elastic, with regard to the quantity of the ingredients: We use a 3-quart (2.8 L) shallow gratin dish. If you have a dish that's a little larger or smaller, simply adjust the amount of veggies and oil as need be.

---

1 (11- to 12-ounce [312 to 340 g)]) eggplant, stem end removed

3 medium-size firm, ripe beefsteak tomatoes (5 or 6 ounces [140 to 170 g] each), stems removed

2 medium-size Yukon gold potatoes (about 1 pound [455 g] total), scrubbed

2 small to medium-size zucchini, ends removed

About ¼ cup (60 ml) extra-virgin olive oil, Garlic-Infused Oil (page 68) made with olive oil, or purchased garlic-infused olive oil

Salt

Freshly ground black pepper

A few sprigs of herbs, such as thyme, oregano, or marjoram (optional)

Position a rack in the center of the oven. Preheat the oven to 400°F (300°C).

All the vegetables need to be sliced to about ⅛-inch (3 mm) thickness, using a mandoline or a sharp knife. The eggplant, tomatoes, and potatoes can be cut crosswise into rounds. Cut the zucchini on a slight angle to create ovals so that the slices are approaching the same size as the other vegetables.

Brush the bottom and sides of a 3-quart (2.8 L) shallow, ovenproof dish with oil. Lay alternating and overlapping slices of vegetables in the pan, either in rows or concentric circles; use your pan to guide the shape. Brush the top of the vegetables with more oil and season with salt and pepper. If using herbs, sprinkle here and there on top.

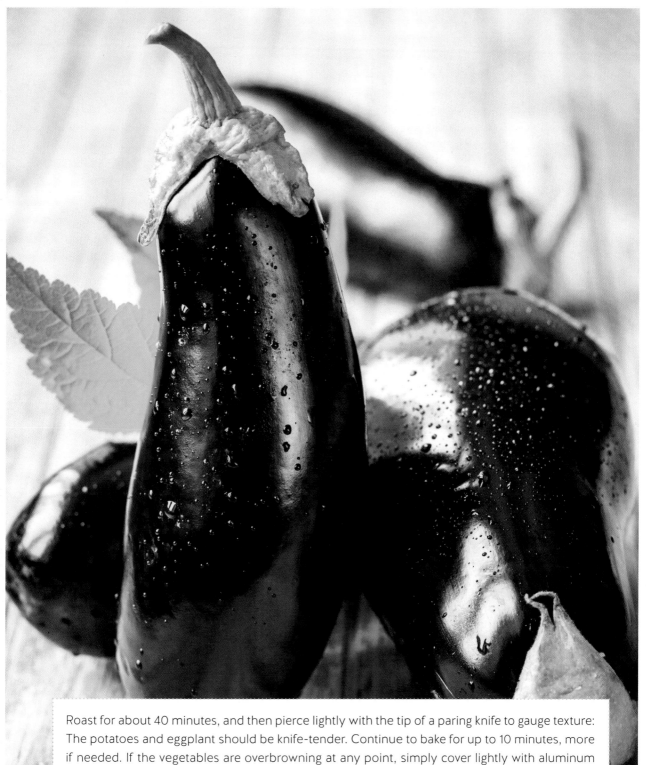

Roast for about 40 minutes, and then pierce lightly with the tip of a paring knife to gauge texture: The potatoes and eggplant should be knife-tender. Continue to bake for up to 10 minutes, more if needed. If the vegetables are overbrowning at any point, simply cover lightly with aluminum foil. Serve hot or at room temperature. Any leftovers can be covered in plastic wrap and refrigerated for up to 2 days.

Asian Chicken Salad

 MAKES 6 TO 8 SERVINGS

When fast-food restaurants offer a version of something, you know it has gone mainstream, which is the case with Asian Chicken Salad. Adaptations abound. Ours doesn't strictly adhere within any one Asian cuisine but instead plays with the "fusion" concept by combining peanut butter, fish sauce, soy sauce, and lime for a most flavorful dressing. Any cooked chicken breast (or for that matter, dark meat) will work. You can use some from our Whole Roast Chicken with Lemon & Herbs (page 276) or simply poach raw chicken breasts. Although we use this dressing over a combo of chicken, shredded cabbage, and fresh veggies and garnish with peanuts, feel free to use the sauce in whatever way you desire. Have some on hand and you will definitely think of uses.

SAUCE:

6 tablespoons (102 g) peanut butter, either natural or no-stir style (see Dédé's Tips, page 146)

3 tablespoons firmly packed light brown sugar

3 tablespoons rice vinegar

3 tablespoons low-sodium soy sauce or tamari (use gluten-free if necessary)

1½ tablespoons Asian fish sauce (use gluten-free if necessary)

1½ tablespoons freshly squeezed lime juice

1½ tablespoons Garlic-Infused Oil (page 68) made with vegetable oil, or purchased garlic-infused vegetable oil

⅛ to ¼ teaspoon hot sauce, such as Texas Pete's, or more to taste (use gluten-free if necessary)

CHICKEN SALAD:

1 pound (455 g) shredded cooked chicken breast, warm or at room temperature

4 cups (280 g) finely shredded green cabbage (do not use savoy)

1 cup (110 g) shredded carrot

1 red bell pepper, cored and finely sliced

¾ English cucumber, partially peeled vertically, cut vertically, seeded, and sliced into ½-inch (12 mm) half-moons

½ cup (32 g) chopped scallions, green parts only

½ cup (73 g) chopped roasted peanuts (without onion or garlic)

⅓ cup (11 g) chopped fresh cilantro

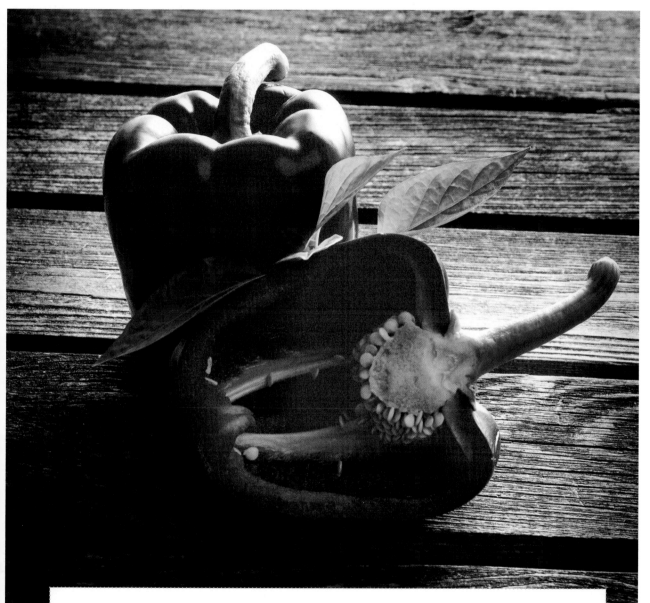

Prepare the sauce: Combine the peanut butter, brown sugar, vinegar, soy sauce, fish sauce, lime juice, oil, and hot sauce in a blender and blend until smooth and combined. Scrape down the blender as needed and add up to 2 tablespoons of water, if needed, to create a flowable sauce. Taste and add more hot sauce, if desired.

Make the chicken salad: Toss together the chicken, cabbage, carrot, bell pepper and cucumber in a large mixing bowl. Add some of the sauce and toss to coat; tongs make this easy. You might not use all the sauce; add more as needed. Serve garnished with the scallion greens, peanuts, and cilantro. The salad may be refrigerated in an airtight container for up to 3 days. Bring to room temperature before serving. (It is best if you can garnish with the scallion, peanuts, and cilantro right before serving).

Oven-Roasted Chicken Caesar Salad

 MAKES 4 SERVINGS

When was the last time you didn't see chicken Caesar salad on a menu? It has become a common offering, but this version, featuring Parmigiano-Reggiano–coated chicken breasts and roasted romaine, is a revelation. A bit smoky, crunchy, delicious, and easily modified to be totally gluten-free.

DRESSING:

2 tablespoons Garlic-Infused Oil (page 68) made with olive oil, or purchased garlic-infused olive oil

1 tablespoon freshly squeezed lemon juice or red wine vinegar

½ teaspoon Dijon mustard (use gluten-free if necessary)

¼ teaspoon Worcestershire sauce (use gluten-free if necessary)

4 oil-packed, canned flat anchovy fillets, chopped, 1 teaspoon oil reserved

1 tablespoon Parmigiano-Reggiano cheese

Kosher salt

Freshly ground black pepper

CHICKEN SALAD:

½ cup (25 g) gluten-free panko, such as Aleia's Gluten Free Original Real Panko

½ cup (50 g) grated Parmigiano-Reggiano cheese

2 tablespoons Garlic-Infused Oil (page 68) made with olive oil, or purchased garlic-infused olive oil

1 teaspoon oil from anchovy fillets

Kosher salt

Freshly ground black pepper

4 (7- to 8-ounce [200 to 225 g] boneless skinless chicken breasts, pounded to ½ inch (12 mm) thick

2 large heads romaine lettuce, quartered lengthwise through the core

2 tablespoons chopped, fresh flat-leaf parsley

Prepare the dressing: Whisk together the oil, lemon juice, mustard, and Worcestershire sauce. Whisk in the chopped anchovies and cheese, then season to taste with salt and pepper; set aside.

Prepare the chicken salad: Position a rack in the center of the oven. Preheat the oven to 450°F (230°C).

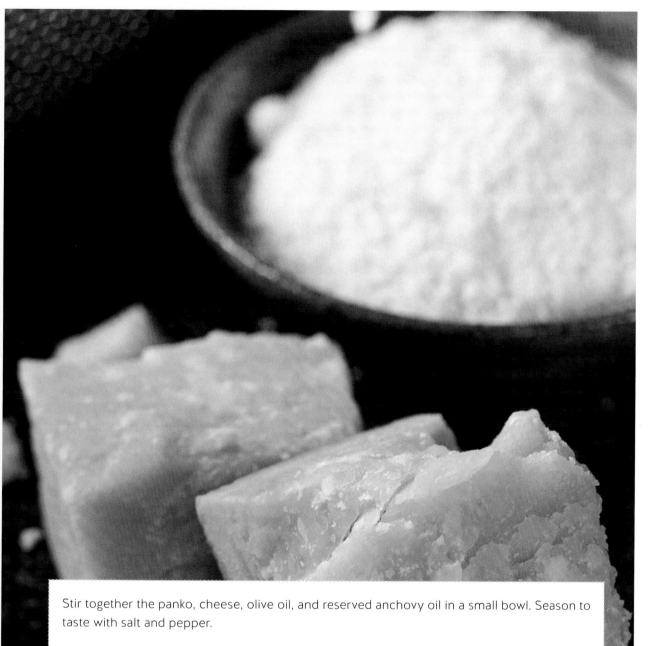

Stir together the panko, cheese, olive oil, and reserved anchovy oil in a small bowl. Season to taste with salt and pepper.

Place the chicken breasts on one half of a large, rimmed baking pan and pack the panko mixture on top of them, distributing evenly. Lay the lettuce quarters on the other half of the pan. Brush a generous amount of the dressing on the lettuce, saturating well, reserving some of the dressing.

Roast in the oven for 12 to 15 minutes, or until the chicken is cooked through; an instant-read thermometer inserted in the center of a breast should register 165°F (74°C). Remove from the oven and allow the chicken to rest for 5 minutes, then plate the chicken and lettuce, drizzle the reserved dressing over all, sprinkle with chopped parsley, and serve.

Cheesy Grits

   MAKES 4 TO 6 SERVINGS

Grits are simply cooked cornmeal and although they can be enjoyed plain, or perhaps with some butter, salt, and pepper, they become something very special with the addition of cheese. We like them as a side dish to Perfect Pot Roast (page 292) or as an integral part of our Shrimp & Grits (page 246). You can try different cheeses for varied results. We like sharp or extra-sharp Cheddar, but be sure to try smoked Gouda or aged Parmesan as well.

2 cups (480 ml) lactose-free milk (whole, 2%, 1%, or fat-free)

2 cups (480 ml) water

1 teaspoon kosher salt

2 cups (226 g) coarse ground yellow cornmeal (we prefer stone-ground)

¼ cup (½ stick; 57g) unsalted butter, cut into pieces

4 ounces (115 g) finely shredded extra-sharp Cheddar

Freshly ground black pepper

Place the milk, water, and salt in a large, heavy-bottomed saucepan over medium-high heat and bring to a boil. Very slowly sprinkle in the cornmeal, whisking all the while, until all is added and the cornmeal is combined with the liquid. Lower the heat to low until the mixture barely simmers; whisk frequently—almost constantly—until the mixture is thickened and smooth. The liquid will absorb and you will be able to see whisk marks in the grits, but the mixture should be fluid as well as thick. Grits firm up tremendously as they cool. The total cooking time will be 20 to 25 minutes.

Remove from the heat and whisk in the butter and cheese until incorporated. Taste and season generously with pepper. Place back over low heat for a few moments, whisking constantly, to heat through and make sure all the cheese is melted. Serve immediately.

> **DÉDÉ'S TIPS**
>
> Grits do have a tendency to stick to the pot. If you have a pot with rounded bottom corners, your whisk will be able to contact all of the grits, making your whisking easier and more efficient.
>
> Although freshly made grits are the best—they lose their flowy texture upon sitting—you can make them up to two hours ahead and reheat them if absolutely necessary. Add a bit of water to the grits and place over low heat. Stir to reloosen the grits and incorporate with the water and heat until hot all the way through. Serve immediately.

Garlic Mashed Potatoes

    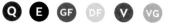   **SERVES 6 TO 8**

By now you know that Garlic-Infused Oil (page 68), either homemade or purchased, is one of our favorite ways to still enjoy garlic's pungent flavor, and it is used to great effect in these mashed potatoes. Freshly ground pepper is a must in this dish, but consider the optional whole peppercorns thrown into the cooking water. Just as when making a stock, they lend a perfume to the liquid that permeates the potatoes. Yukon gold potatoes impart a rich color and flavor; the extra-starchy russets, or baking potatoes, lend a more classic mashed potato texture. Feel free to use a total of 3 pounds (1.4 kg) of either, if you like. Potatoes are a great way to boost potassium and vitamins B6 and C. By the way, these are naturally dairy-free, as we use the cooking liquid instead of milk or cream, so do not drain all of it away! You need to reserve part of it.

1½ (680 g) pounds Yukon gold potatoes, peeled and cut into chunks

1½ (680 g) pounds russet potatoes, peeled and cut into chunks

6 whole peppercorns (optional)

Salt

¼ cup (60 ml) Garlic-Infused Oil (page 68) made with olive oil, or purchased garlic-infused olive oil

Freshly ground black pepper

Place the peeled potato chunks in a large pot and cover with water by at least 2 inches (5 cm). Throw the peppercorns into the pot, if using. Lightly salt the water as well. Cover and bring to a boil, then uncover, lower the heat to a simmer, and cook until tender when pierced with a knife, for 12 to 15 minutes (depending on the size of the potato chunks).

Drain well, reserving about 1 cup (240 ml) of cooking liquid. Place the potatoes back in the pot (no need to dirty another dish). Pick out the peppercorns and discard, if you want (Dédé usually leaves them in). Drizzle the garlic oil over the potatoes, season with salt and pepper, and begin to mash. Add enough cooking liquid as you mash to create the texture that you want. We go for not too thick, not too thin, and we even like a bit of chunky potato texture, but that is up to you.

> **POST-FODMAP CHALLENGE PHASE OPTION**
>
> **Fructan:** If you passed the fructan garlic challenge, add one to three garlic cloves to the cooking water and mash them right into the potatoes.

Rosemary Garlic Roasted Potatoes

      MAKES 4 SERVINGS

Roasted potatoes are so versatile and will be at home alongside grilled and roasted main dishes that range from roast chicken to a grilled steak. We couldn't imagine not having them in our repertoire, and thankfully, potatoes are low FODMAP approved. Rosemary, as with all herbs, is welcomed into our diet as well and our Garlic-Infused Oil (page 68) gets put to good use here for added flavor. The olive oil and the high oven heat are what make these roasted potatoes so luscious: crispy brown on the outside and tender and creamy on the inside. These are best when they are hot right out of the oven.

---

2 pounds (910 g) red, white, or Yukon gold potatoes, scrubbed and dried, unpeeled, cut into large bite-size chunks

2 tablespoons Garlic-Infused Oil (page 68) made with olive oil, or purchased garlic-infused oil

1 tablespoon crushed dried rosemary

Kosher salt

Freshly ground black pepper

Position a rack in the center of the oven. Preheat the oven to 400°F (200°C).

Toss the potatoes with the olive oil and rosemary and season very generously with salt and pepper. Spread out in a single layer on a rimmed roasting pan.

Roast for about 25 minutes, or until they begin to form a crust, at which point flip them over so that another side of the potato contacts the hot pan. Continue to roast for about 25 more minutes, or until well browned and crispy all over, flipping over one more time during this period. Taste, season additionally if necessary, and serve hot.

VARIATION:

Lemon Garlic Rosemary Potatoes: Add 1 tablespoon of freshly squeezed lemon juice and 1 tablespoon of finely grated lemon zest along with the olive oil and roast as directed.

> **POST-FODMAP CHALLENGE PHASE OPTION**
>
> **Fructan:** If you passed the fructan garlic challenge, add one to three garlic cloves, finely chopped, to the potatoes along with the olive oil before they go into the oven to roast.

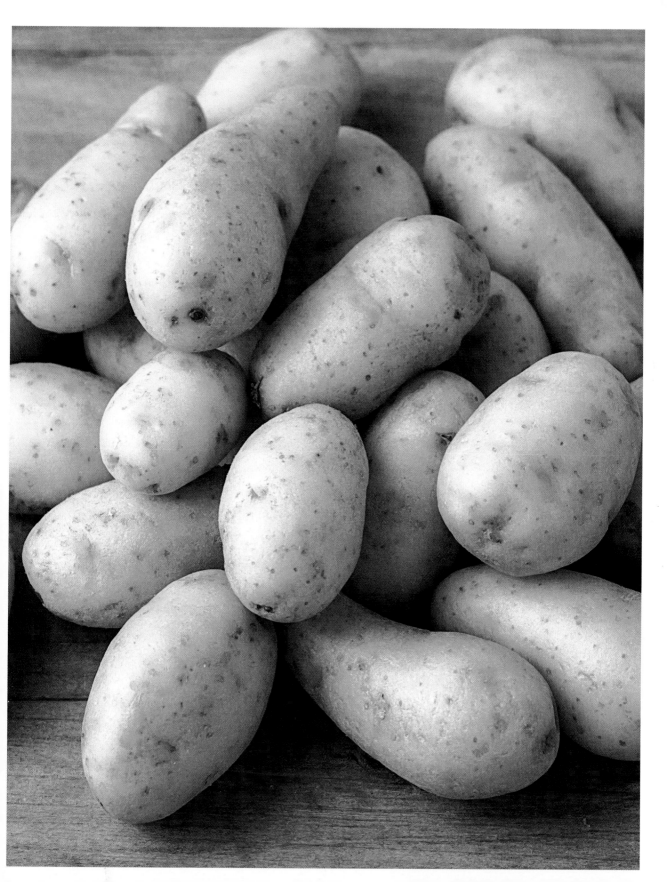

Potato Pancakes

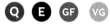 MAKES ABOUT TWELVE 3-INCH (7.5 CM) PANCAKES |
SERVING SIZE 2 TO 3 PANCAKES

Potato pancakes are one of the truly satisfying carb-filled recipes that we can still enjoy while eating low FODMAP. We enjoy these as a side dish or occasionally we make them a meal with a salad. These are one of those dishes that must be served as soon as they are made, so plan accordingly. **Note:** Although sour cream—a classic accompaniment—is available lactose-free, another, applesauce, is off-limits during the elimination phase.

---

2 cups (400 g) coarse-grated, peeled russet potatoes (about 2 medium-size potatoes)

2 large eggs, at room temperature

1¼ teaspoons kosher salt

1 tablespoon gluten-free all-purpose flour, such as Bob's Red Mill Gluten Free 1 to 1 Baking Flour

Heaping 1 tablespoon finely chopped scallion, green parts only, plus more for serving (optional)

Vegetable oil

Lactose-free sour cream (optional; omit if following a dairy-free or vegan diet)

Chives, finely chopped, for serving (optional)

Squeeze as much liquid as possible out of the potatoes. You can place them in a colander and press with the back of a large spoon or large silicone spatula, or Dédé likes to place the grated potatoes in a clean kitchen towel and squeeze as firmly as possible over the sink.

Whisk the eggs together in a large mixing bowl, then add the potatoes, salt, flour, and scallion greens, if using.

Preheat the oven to 300°F (150°C) and line a baking sheet with a wire rack if you want to keep the pancakes warm. Have several layers of paper towels nearby to receive the fried pancakes.

Heat about ¼ inch (6 mm) of vegetable oil in a heavy skillet, such as cast-iron, over medium-high heat (do not use nonstick). Create a mound of potatoes about 3 inches (7.5 cm) across and press down to about ¼ inch (6 mm) thick. Cook three or four potato pancakes at a time, depending on the size of the skillet, leaving room around each one. Fry until well browned and crisp on the bottom, about 3 minutes, lowering the heat to medium, if necessary. Flip the pancakes over and cook on the second side until well browned and crispy. Drain on paper towels. Place on the prepared rack and keep warm in the oven, if desired. Fry the remaining pancakes and serve as soon as possible. Serve with dollops of sour cream, if using, and/or a sprinkling of chives (and extra scallion), if desired.

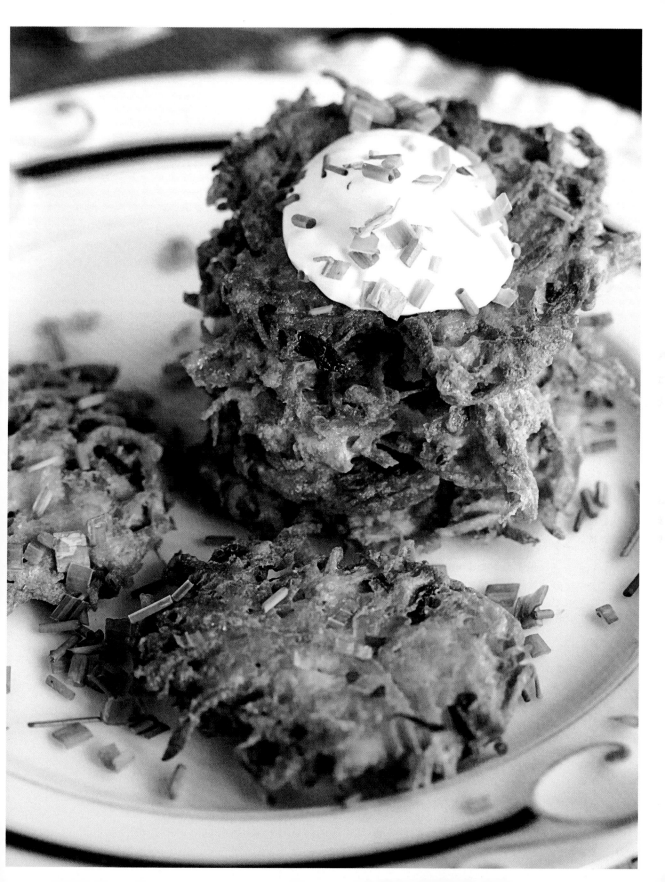

Peanut Noodles

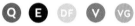 **MAKES 4 SERVINGS**

We love peanut noodles, but most classic recipes rely heavily on garlic. Our version adds garlic flavor with a small addition of our Garlic-Infused Oil (page 68). (Also see the Post-FODMAP Challenge Phase Option at the end of the recipe.) We have presented this recipe as a vegetable-based salad, but you can add shredded chicken or cubed raw or sautéed tofu to up the protein and hardiness. Pay attention to the timing of the preparation. The pasta begins cooking first so that you can use some of the cooking water to thin the peanut sauce. You will have to do a few things at once, but they are all easy steps.

PASTA:

12 ounces (340 g) gluten-free rice spaghetti or linguine pasta, such as Tinkyada brand

6 large boy choy stalks, sliced crosswise into ½-inch (12 mm) pieces (use both ribs and leaves)

4 medium-size carrots, peeled, top discarded, cut into 2-inch (5 cm) julienne

PEANUT SAUCE:

½ cup (135 g) peanut butter, either natural or no-stir style

¼ cup (60 ml) low-sodium soy sauce or tamari (use gluten-free if necessary)

4 (1-inch [24 mm]-diameter) slices peeled fresh ginger

2 tablespoons rice vinegar

2 tablespoons toasted sesame oil

1 tablespoon firmly packed light brown sugar

1 tablespoon Garlic-Infused Oil (page 68) made with vegetable oil, or purchased garlic-infused vegetable oil

½ teaspoon hot sauce, such as Texas Pete's, or more to taste (use gluten-free if following a gluten-free diet)

RAW VEGETABLES:

1 red bell pepper, cored, sliced into ¼-inch (6 mm) sticks

½ English cucumber, partially peeled vertically, cut vertically, seeded, and sliced into ½-inch (12 mm) half-moons

¼ cup (8 g) chopped fresh cilantro

¼ cup (16 g) chopped scallion, green parts only

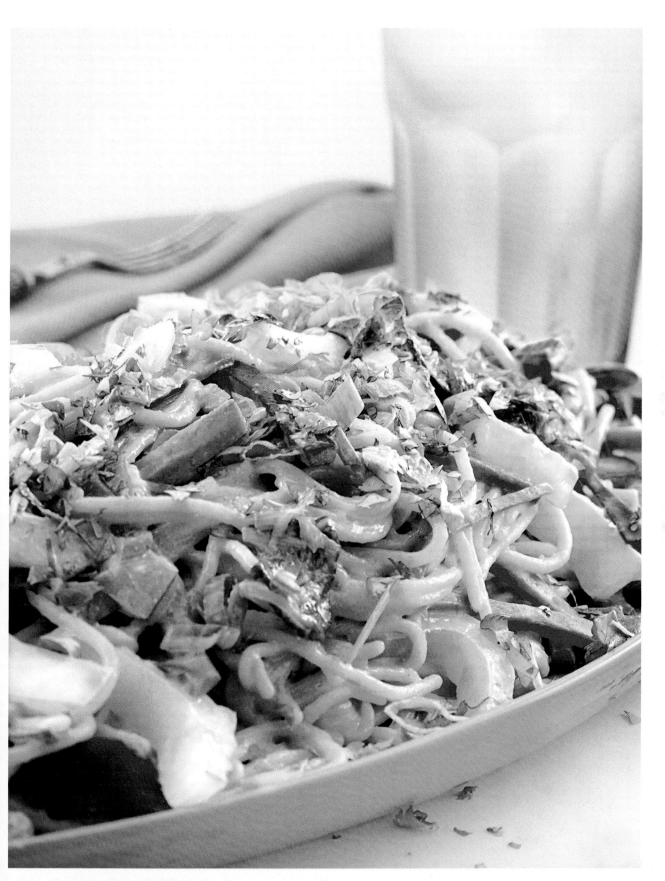

Bring 5 quarts (4.7 L) of salted water to a boil in a large pot and cook the pasta to a little softer than al dente (to more approximate the softer texture of Chinese noodles). While the water is boiling, remove about ½ cup (120 ml) of the pasta cooking water and reserve. During about the last minute of cooking, add the bok choy and carrots to the pot, to lightly cook. Drain the noodles and veggies well.

Meanwhile, prepare the sauce: Combine the peanut butter, soy sauce, ginger, vinegar, sesame oil, brown sugar, oil, and hot sauce in a blender and blend until smooth. Scrape down the blender as needed and add the reserved cooking water, if needed, to create a flowable sauce. Taste and add more hot sauce, if desired.

To assemble: Toss the warm noodles and cooked veggies with about three quarters of the sauce in a mixing bowl; we like to use tongs. Add the bell pepper and cucumber and continue to toss, adding more sauce, if needed. Serve warm or at room temperature sprinkled with cilantro and scallion greens as a garnish. The noodles may also be refrigerated in an airtight container for up to 3 days. Bring to room temperature before serving. (It is best if you can garnish with the scallion and cilantro right before serving.)

POST-FODMAP CHALLENGE PHASE OPTION

Fructan: If you passed the fructan garlic challenge, add two to four garlic cloves to the sauce ingredients before blending.

Tomato Basil Pasta Salad

  MAKES 6 TO 8 SERVINGS

A freshly made pasta salad is a great way to combine a FODMAP-approved starch (in this case rice pasta) with fresh veggies, herbs, and creamy, tangy goat cheese. Timing is important. How inconvenient is this? Not at all! Prep the veggies, herbs, and dressing while the water boils and the pasta cooks. Toss everything together while the pasta is still a bit warm (the dressing absorbs beautifully that way) and you will have a very easy and quick salad or light main meal. Make sure to read the directions all the way through before beginning so that you can take advantage of the time-saving order of preparation.

---

1 (12 ounce ([340 g]) package brown rice spiral pasta, such as Tinkyada brand

¼ cup (60 ml) extra-virgin olive oil, Garlic-Infused Oil (page 68) made with olive oil, or purchased garlic-infused olive oil

2 tablespoons red wine vinegar

2 teaspoons Dijon mustard (use gluten-free if following a gluten-free diet)

Salt

Freshly cracked black pepper

1 dry pint (284 g) cherry or grape tomatoes, halved if large

4 ounces (115 g) soft, crumbly fresh goat cheese, such as Montrachet (see Kate's Notes)

1 cup (20 g) baby arugula

½ cup (8 g) lightly packed fresh basil leaves, torn

Bring 5 quarts (4.7 L) of salted water to a boil in a large pot and cook the pasta just until it is al dente (see Dédé's Tips). While the pasta cooks, whisk together the olive oil, vinegar, and mustard in a small bowl. You can also prep the veggies and basil at this time.

Drain the pasta in a colander and rinse with cool water; drain again. Transfer the pasta to a large mixing bowl. Drizzle with about one quarter of the dressing, lightly season with salt and pepper, and gently toss with a large silicone spatula to coat. Add the tomatoes to the pasta, crumble the goat cheese evenly over all, then add the arugula and basil. Drizzle with more dressing, tossing lightly to coat, adding only as much as is needed, to taste. Season again with salt and pepper, if desired. Serve immediately or cover with plastic wrap. The pasta salad will keep for about 3 hours. We do not recommend refrigerating.

DÉDÉ'S TIPS

Rice pasta can certainly be cooked al dente, which "means to the tooth," but it will overcook pretty quickly. Thirty seconds too long in the boiling water can make the difference between al dente and mush. It's also important to note that brands vary in the way that they cook, so there might be a slight learning curve. Do not go by the timing on the label; we find that often overcooks the pasta. Give the recipe a go and write down how long it took to cook so you know for future batches.

KATE'S NOTES

Avoid overly wet cheeses, such as ricotta and cottage cheese, which are higher in lactose, while on the elimination phase. If you are following a vegan, vegetarian, or dairy-free diet, you can omit the cheese and add 1 to 1½ cups (168 to 210 g) of drained and rinsed canned chickpeas for protein. Just remember to keep your portion size in check, using no more than the ¼-cup (42 g) canned chickpea limit per serving.

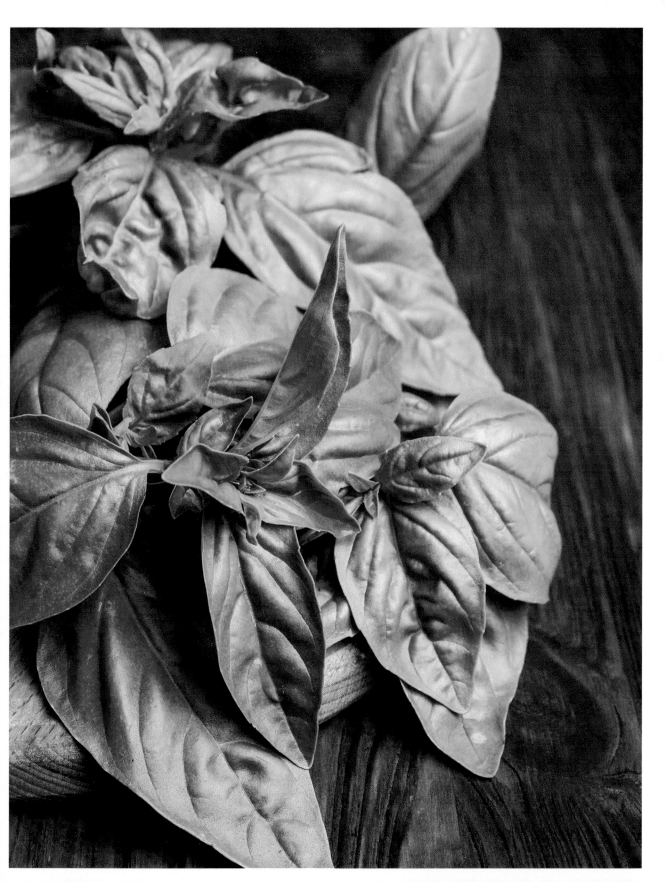

Quinoa Tabouli

   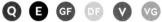   **MAKES 6 SERVINGS**

Authentic Lebanese tabouli has a very high proportion of parsley, giving it a refreshing flavor. In lieu of the traditional bulgur cracked wheat, we have subbed in a generous amount of red quinoa to up the protein factor. Quinoa can have a coating of saponin, a naturally occurring chemical that repels insects and can impart a bitter taste. Some quinoa comes "prewashed" and will say so right on the label. For best flavor, rinse your quinoa in water and drain before combining with fresh water to cook. This is a very simple salad and its bright, fresh quality depends on the freshness of the tomatoes, scallions, parsley, and mint, so buy as fresh as possible.

---

1 cup (170 g) red quinoa (see headnote)

1½ cups (360 ml) water

Kosher salt

3 tablespoons Garlic-Infused Oil (page 68) made with olive oil, or purchased garlic-infused olive oil

3 tablespoons freshly squeezed lemon juice

Freshly ground black pepper

2 beefsteak tomatoes, cored and diced

1 cup (32 g) chopped, fresh flat-leaf parsley

½ cup (32 g) finely chopped scallion, green parts only

¼ cup (10 g) finely chopped fresh mint

Stir together the quinoa, water, and ½ teaspoon of the salt in a medium-size saucepan. Bring to a boil over high heat. Lower the heat to low, cover, and simmer until the water is absorbed, for 10 to 15 minutes. Keep covered, remove from the heat, and allow to sit and steam for 5 minutes more. Fluff with a fork and allow to cool until it is barely warm.

Scrape the quinoa into a mixing bowl. Whisk together the oil and lemon juice in a small bowl, pour over the slightly warm quinoa, and toss to coat. Season to taste with salt and pepper and allow to cool completely. Stir in the tomatoes, parsley, scallion greens, and mint. Adjust the seasoning and serve. The tabouli may be refrigerated in an airtight container for up to 2 days, but it will begin to lose its very fresh flavor the longer it sits.

POST-FODMAP CHALLENGE PHASE OPTIONS

Fructans: If you passed the fructan onion challenge, sub in ½ cup (71 g) finely chopped red onion for the scallion. If you passed the fructan wheat challenge, use cracked wheat (bulgur) in place of the quinoa (do not substitute if following a gluten-free diet).

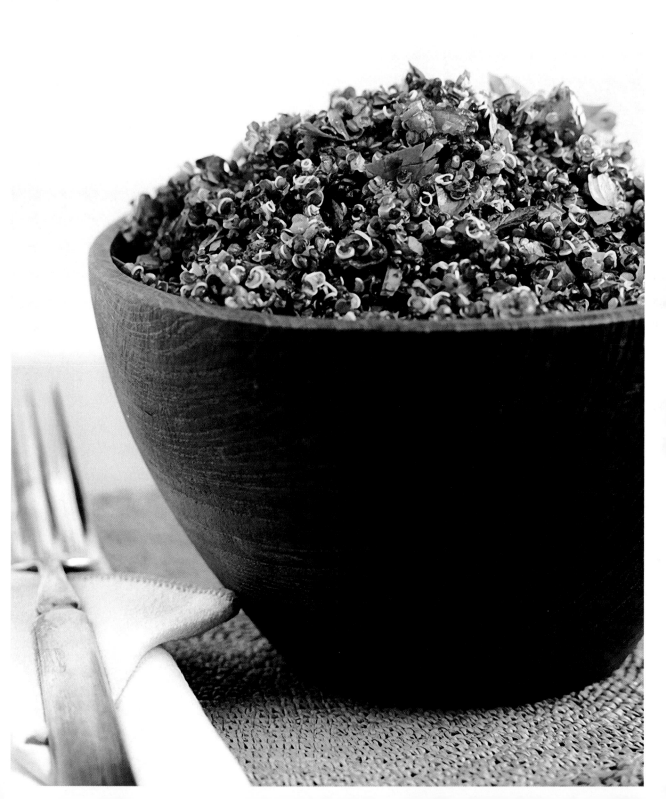

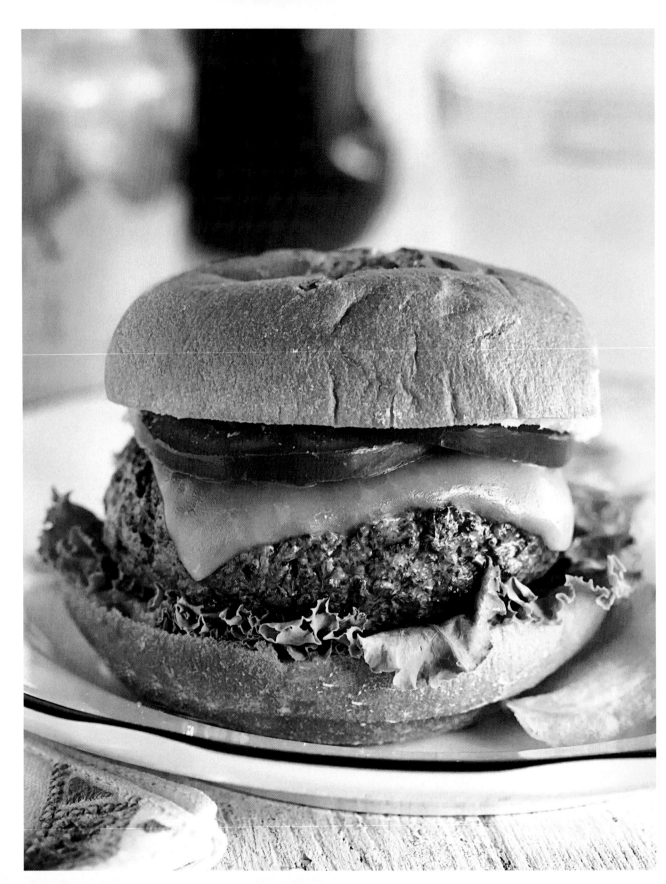

Chapter 10

MAIN DISHES FOR THE WHOLE FAMILY

KATE AND DÉDÉ BOTH FOLLOW a low-to-moderate FODMAP diet, yet not everyone in their household does. We are both very sensitive to the fact that we all have to get dinner on the table, often on a busy weeknight, and that most likely there is a blend of FODMAPers and non-FODMAPers alike waiting for a meal. These recipes, as with all the recipes in the book, were tested on a variety of diners, including non-FODMAPers. We know you and your friends or family will be thrilled with our delectable recipe offerings, from Weekday Meat Loaf (page 247), and Chicken Tostadas (page 226) to dishes elegant enough for company, such as Beef Tenderloin Stuffed with Goat Cheese, Spinach & Tomatoes (page 202) and Asian Chicken Lettuce Wraps (page 208).

Easy Oven "BBQ" Ribs

    MAKES 2 TO 4 SERVINGS

Before anyone gets in an uproar, yes, we know this is not true barbecue. We wanted to figure out a way to have ribs, made in the oven, with a relatively simple technique and to be able to enjoy some classic barbecue flavors, all while staying within the low FODMAP diet. You do need time as the oven temperature is low and the oven time long, which will yield tender, succulent, fall-off-the-bone ribs. Don't worry about the oven time, as it is largely unattended, freeing you up to make your side dishes, such as Corn Bread (page 337) and Kale Cabbage Coleslaw (page 160). Our approach combines a dry rub and a wet sauce, giving your diners options. Smoked salt is a specialty product and you might have to order it online, but also check specialty food and natural food stores.

---

2 (3-pound [1.4 kg]) racks (about 6 pounds [2.7 kg] total, give or take) St. Louis–style ribs

BBQ Sauce (page 84)

DRY RUB:

2 tablespoons firmly packed light brown sugar

2 tablespoons sweet paprika

1 tablespoon ground cumin

1 tablespoon freshly ground black pepper

1 tablespoon natural smoked salt, such as hickory or mesquite

1 teaspoon chipotle chile powder

Position racks in the upper third and lower thirds of the oven. Preheat the oven to 300°F (150°C). Have ready two heavy-duty rimmed half sheet pans and lots of aluminum foil.

Prepare the dry rub: Combine all the dry rub ingredients in a mixing bowl, use your fingers to break up any lumps of brown sugar, and mix everything together.

Use your hands to work the dry rub into both rib racks on both sides. Wrap each rib rack completely in aluminum foil and place each rack on a half sheet pan.

Bake for about 2½ hours. Unwrap and check for doneness. The meat should be fall-off-the-bone tender. You can check by wiggling a bone; it should slide away from the meat easily. Continue to bake for 10 to 15 minutes more if not yet tender enough.

Once the ribs are tender, unwrap and drain any moisture that might have accumulated within the foil packet. Spread out the foil on each pan with the ribs in the center. Now you have a choice: you can slather both racks with the BBQ sauce or leave one dry for those that prefer their ribs without. (If you are leaving one rack dry, remove from the oven now, cover lightly with foil, and allow to rest.) Increase the oven temperature to 450°F (230°C).

Coat the rib rack(s) with sauce on one side. Bake for about 10 minutes, or until the sauce darkens and becomes a bit sticky. Flip the rack(s) over, slather the other side with the sauce, and cook for an additional 10 minutes, or until that side is nice and sticky.

Remove from the oven, cover loosely with foil, and allow to rest for about 10 minutes. Use a sharp knife to cut the rack into individual ribs and serve immediately.

DÉDÉ'S TIPS

To make the dry rub even smokier in flavor, use smoked paprika instead of the sweet paprika (or half and half). Play with different smoked salts for a kaleidoscope of different flavors.

Shrimp Jambalaya

  MAKES 4 SERVINGS

This jambalaya highlights shrimp, and it also contains some ham (in lieu of sausage, which can be problematic for us FODMAPers due to many hidden fructan ingredients, such as onion and garlic). While the debates about Creole versions versus Cajun abound, we are not here to establish the most classic approach. We've modified the recipe by using Garlic-Infused Oil, scallion, and bell pepper, and minimized the amount of celery to make this suitable as a low FODMAP dish. The onion is sautéed in the oil to lend flavor and removed before proceeding with the recipe. If you are a classicist you might be cringing at our use of "jambalaya" in the title, but we think these flavors will satisfy your craving. This easy meal can be made in about forty-five minutes.

1 pound (455 g) large (26/30) shrimp, deveined, shells on

1 teaspoon paprika

1 teaspoon kosher salt

½ teaspoon freshly ground black pepper

½ teaspoon dried oregano

½ teaspoon dried thyme

¼ to ½ teaspoon cayenne pepper, depending on how hot you like it

2 tablespoons Garlic-Infused Oil (page 68) made with vegetable oil, or purchased garlic-infused vegetable oil

1 medium-size white or yellow onion, peeled and cut in half (make sure to follow the directions)

1 green bell pepper, cored, seeded, and diced

1 celery stalk, ends trimmed, diced

5 ounces (140 g) ham, sliced ¼ inch (6 mm) thick and diced (use gluten-free if necessary; without added FODMAP ingredients)

½ cup (32 g) chopped scallion, green parts only, divided

1 cup (200 g) long-grain white rice

1 (14.5-ounce [415 g]) can diced tomatoes, preferably fire-roasted (without garlic or onion), such as Muir Glen brand

1 bay leaf

Peel the shrimp, place in a mixing bowl, and set aside. Place the shells in a medium-size saucepan along with 3 cups (720 ml) of water. Bring to a boil, lower the heat, and simmer for 5 minutes.

While the shrimp shells are simmering, toss together the paprika, salt, black pepper, oregano, thyme, and cayenne in a small bowl. Sprinkle half of this spice mixture over the shrimp (do this by eye) and toss to coat. Reserve the remaining spice mixture.

After the shrimp shells have simmered, drain out 2 cups (480 ml) of stock for use in the recipe. Discard the shells and any excess stock, or save the stock for another use.

Heat the oil in a large skillet over medium heat. Place the onion halves, cut side down, in the skillet and sauté for a few minutes to infuse the oil with onion flavor; do not let the onion brown. *Remove and discard the onion.* This is very important to stay within low FODMAP guidelines. Add the bell pepper and celery and sauté for a few minutes, until beginning to soften. Add the ham and half of the scallion greens and sauté for a minute more. Add the rice and reserved spice mixture, toss to coat, and cook for 30 seconds, stirring frequently. Stir in the tomatoes, bay leaf, and the 2 cups (480 ml) of shrimp stock. Cover and bring to a simmer over medium-high heat. Lower the heat and simmer for 25 minutes, or until the liquid is absorbed and the rice is cooked through. Stir in the shrimp, cover, and cook for about 5 more minutes, or just until the shrimp are cooked through. Serve immediately, sprinkling with the reserved scallion greens.

POST-FODMAP CHALLENGE PHASE OPTIONS

Fructans: If you passed the fructan onion challenge, consider using ¼ cup (36 g) of finely chopped white or yellow onion for sautéing in the oil (and remaining in the oil, prior to adding the green pepper) and sprinkling another ¼ cup (36 g) on top of the dish, depending on your tolerance.

If you passed the fructan garlic challenge, consider adding one or two garlic cloves, finely chopped, to the oil (also remaining in the oil vs. removing) prior to adding the bell pepper.

Bouillabaisse

MAKES 4 SERVINGS

Bouillabaisse is a mixed fish stew. While it looks opulent—and it is—it is also very easy to make. You just have to have everything prepped and ready to go and the dish will come together in less than forty-five minutes. This stew does depend on the quality of your fish and shellfish. All the fish must be fresh, the one exception being the frozen shrimp. You can choose whichever white-fleshed fish you like. Just steer clear of oily or strong-flavored fish, such as salmon, tuna, bluefish, or mackerel. The toasted bread and garlicky roasted red pepper mayonnaise are optional but add hardiness to the dish that, along with a green salad, completes the meal. You can make the aioli a couple of days ahead, so take advantage of that convenience. See Dédé's Tips for a shortcut using prepared mayonnaise.

ROASTED RED PEPPER AIOLI:

1 large pasteurized egg yolk, at room temperature (see Dédé's Tips)

2 teaspoons freshly squeezed lemon juice

1 teaspoon cold water

¼ teaspoon Dijon mustard (use gluten-free if necessary)

½ teaspoon kosher salt, plus more as needed

1 cup (240 ml) Garlic-Infused Oil (page 68) prepared with olive oil, or purchased garlic-infused olive oil

½ cup (85 g) very finely chopped, jarred roasted red peppers

⅛ to ¼ teaspoon cayenne pepper

Freshly ground black pepper

TOAST:

1 low FODMAP French baguette, such as Udi's Gluten Free French Baguette or Against the Grain Original Baguettes (use gluten-free and/or dairy-free if necessary)

2 tablespoons Garlic-Infused Oil (page 68) prepared with olive oil, or purchased garlic-infused olive oil

FISH STEW:

¾ pound (340 g) large (26/30) shrimp, deveined, shells on

¼ cup (60 ml) Garlic-Infused Oil (page 68) prepared with olive oil, or purchased garlic-infused olive oil

1 cup (140 g) finely chopped leek, green parts only

1 cup (98 g) thinly sliced fresh fennel (bulb ends trimmed, bulb cut in half vertically, then cut into ½-inch (12 mm)

slices crosswise; reserve separately some fennel fronds–the delicate, feathery tops)

3 canned plum tomatoes (use brand without onion or garlic), drained of juice, chopped

2 tablespoons chopped fresh flat-leaf parsley

2 teaspoons finely grated orange zest (use a Microplane or rasp-style zester)

1 teaspoon chopped fresh thyme

½ teaspoon fennel seeds, crushed

24 small or medium-size clams or mussels or preferably a combination of both, scrubbed free of sand and grit; debeard the mussels if necessary

1½ pounds (680 g) white flesh fish, preferably more than one kind, such as cod fillets, cod loins, red snapper, halibut, haddock, monkfish, or striped bass, cut into chunks

¾ pound (340 g) scallops, preferably sea scallops (if very large, cut in half)

1 tablespoon chopped fresh basil

Kosher salt

Freshly ground black pepper

Prepare the aioli: Place the pasteurized egg yolk, lemon juice, cold water, mustard, and ½ teaspoon of salt in a medium-size nonreactive bowl. Whisk vigorously until blended. Very slowly, drop by drop, whisk in about a quarter of the olive oil, whisking all the while. This will take several minutes; go slowly, allowing the mayonnaise to thicken. Gradually add the remaining olive oil until the desired thickness is reached; you might not use all the oil, but you will need at least ¾ cup (180 ml). Gently stir in the chopped peppers and cayenne to taste. Season to taste with more salt and with black pepper, if desired. The aioli is ready to use, or refrigerate in an airtight container for up to 2 days.

Prepare the toast: Right before preparing the stew, slice the baguette into 1-inch (2.5 cm) slices, toast in a toaster or on a baking sheet in a 400°F (200°C) oven, then brush with the olive oil; set aside.

Prepare the stew: Peel the shrimp and set the shrimp aside. Place the shells in a medium-size saucepan with 4½ cups (1 L) of water. Bring to a boil, lower the heat, and simmer for 5 minutes.

While the shrimp shells are simmering, heat the oil in a deep 5-quart (4.7 L) pot, such as a Dutch oven, over medium heat. Add the leek greens and sliced fennel and sauté for 3 to 5 minutes, or until softened but not browned.

Strain and measure out 4 cups (960 ml) of the stock for the bouillabaisse. Discard the shells. Add the shrimp stock, tomatoes, parsley, orange zest, thyme, and fennel seeds to the leek mixture. Cover, increase the heat, and simmer for 10 minutes.

Add the clams and/or mussels, cover, and cook for about 5 minutes, or until the shells open, discarding any that do not open. Add the fish and large scallops (wait to add if using small scallops), cover, and cook for about 5 minutes, or until the fish is almost opaque. If using small scallops, add them next along with the shrimp and cook, covered, for about 5 minutes more, or just until the shrimp turn pink. Gently stir in the basil and taste the broth. Season with salt and pepper. Place a slice or two of garlic toast in each bowl and top with a generous dollop of aioli. Ladle the stew on top and garnish with fennel fronds, if you like. Serve immediately.

DÉDÉ'S TIPS

If making the mayonnaise at home, know that raw egg is considered a salmonella risk and not recommended for infants, elderly, pregnant women, and people with a weakened immune system. Please make sure to use a pasteurized egg yolk to eliminate this issue (pasteurized eggs can be found in many well-stocked supermarkets). Alternatively, combine ½ cup (113 g) of prepared mayonnaise, ¼ cup (85 g) of chopped jarred roasted red peppers, 2 teaspoons of freshly squeezed lemon juice, and ⅛ teaspoon cayenne pepper in a food processor and pulse until combined. Season to taste with salt and black pepper.

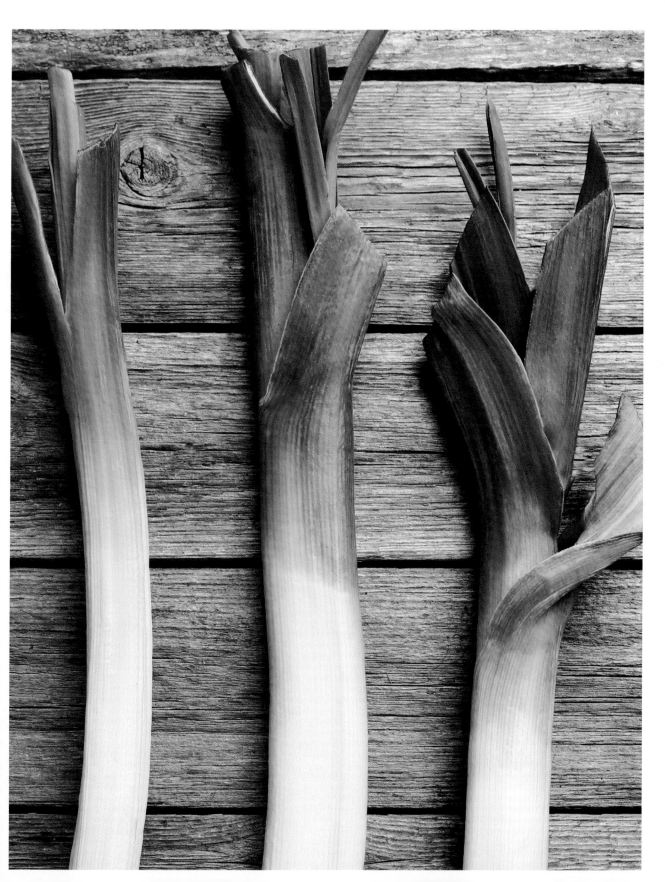

Lasagne the Low FODMAP Way

 MAKES 8 TO 10 SERVINGS

We really wanted to make sure to have a classic meat-based lasagne in this book because there are few dishes as comforting, satisfying, or fun to make. And versatile! (See Dédé's Tips.) Make the lasagne the day of, the day before, or even freeze and bake it up to a month later. It's portable enough to take to a party, reheats well in the oven or microwave, and feeds a crowd. We build our own layers of flavor from scratch: commercially prepared ricotta is not low FODMAP and so we use lactose-free cottage cheese instead (we like the flavor even better!). Pancetta, a salt-cured, unsmoked pork product, adds a savoriness to this dish that we love. If you can't find pancetta, you may substitute bacon (use gluten-free if necessary), but blanch it in boiling water first to reduce its smoky flavor. The ground pork, fennel seeds, and red pepper flakes bring the flavor that Italian sausage would.

---

1 (10-ounce [280 g]) box gluten-free lasagna noodles, such as Tinkyada
1 pound (455 g) mozzarella cheese (full-fat or low-fat), shredded

MEAT FILLING:

4 ounces (115 g) pancetta, minced

¾ pound (340 g) 80% or 85% lean ground beef

¼ pound (115 g) ground pork

2 teaspoons Garlic-Infused Oil (page 68) made with olive oil, or purchased garlic-infused olive oil

2 medium-size garlic cloves, smashed (make sure to follow the directions)

4 cups (960 ml) Quick Tomato Sauce (page 72)

½ teaspoon fennel seeds

½ teaspoon dried oregano

¼ teaspoon red pepper flakes

Kosher salt

Freshly ground black pepper

CHEESE FILLING:

1 pound (455 g) lactose-free cottage cheese, such as Lactaid brand

½ cup (50 g) grated Parmigiano-Reggiano cheese, divided

2 tablespoons chopped fresh flat-leaf parsley

1 large egg

Kosher salt

Freshly ground black pepper

Prepare the meat filling: Heat a large, non-reactive heavy saucepan, add the pancetta, and cook over medium heat, stirring frequently, until the fat renders and the pancetta begins to brown, about 3 minutes. Add the ground beef and pork and cook, stirring frequently, until the meats are cooked through, about 5 minutes. Drain away and discard any liquid and transfer the meat to a plate. Wipe the pan clean. In same pan, heat the oil and garlic cloves over medium-low heat, stirring frequently, for a minute or two, or until the garlic has softened. Remove all the garlic and discard. This is very important to stay within low FODMAP guidelines. Add the tomato sauce to the pan along with cooked meat, fennel seeds, oregano, and red pepper flakes and season with salt and black pepper to taste. Stir well to combine, then cook over medium-low heat at a simmer, covered, for about 15 minutes to blend the flavors. This filling may be made up to 2 days ahead and refrigerated in an airtight container.

Position a rack in the center of the oven. Preheat the oven to 350°F (180°C).

Meanwhile, bring a 5-quart (4.7 L) pot of well-salted water to a boil and cook the pasta, stirring frequently, until it is a bit firmer than al dente (do not overcook; it will cook more in the oven). Drain the pasta, rinse under cold water, and set aside.

While the pasta is cooking, prepare the cheese filling: Stir together the cottage cheese, ¼ cup (25 g) of the Parmigiano-Reggiano, and the parsley and egg in a mixing bowl. Season with salt and black pepper.

To assemble: Spoon a little bit of the tomato sauce into the bottom of a 13 x 9-inch (33 x 23 cm) ceramic or ovenproof glass baking dish or casserole and spread it around to cover the dish, to help release the pasta when serving. Lay three noodles lengthwise, touching but not overlapping, to cover the bottom of the dish. Cover the noodles with half of the cottage cheese filling, then one third of the sauce, then one third of the mozzarella. Repeat. Last, layer will be noodles, sauce, mozzarella, and then the reserved ¼ cup (25 g) of Parmigiano-Reggiano.

Bake for 55 minutes to 1 hour 5 minutes, or until the filling is bubbling and the mozzarella cheese is melted. Remove from the oven and allow to sit for 5 minutes before serving. The lasagne is ready to serve.

KATE'S NOTES

Although fennel tea was tested for FODMAP content and shown to be high in FODMAPs (an abundance of fructans), fennel seeds and whole fennel bulb are low FODMAP. Go figure! The FODMAP food analysis science is confusing at times. We have done the heavy lifting to ensure these recipes are low FODMAP, so you don't have to worry.

Yogurt-Marinated Grilled Lamb Kebabs

    MAKES 6 SERVINGS

This recipe offers huge flavor with very little effort: The yogurt in this marinade tenderizes and the cumin and coriander create spiciness without heat. Make sure your spices are fresh and fragrant to infuse maximum impact. By alternating the lamb and veggies on each kebab, you will have your vegetable side dish built in; we like to serve these with rice as well. Although you could make these inside on a grill pan, or on a propane-fueled grill, hardwood charcoal adds a smoky flavor that we highly recommend. By the way, after years of using soaked and unsoaked bamboo skewers, we haven't found much of a difference. So, save time and don't bother. Better yet, metal skewers are quite inexpensive and reusable; problem solved!

½ cup (114 g) plain lactose-free yogurt (whole-milk or low-fat), such as Green Valley Organics

½ cup (120 ml) Garlic-Infused Oil (page 68) or Onion-Infused Oil (see variation, page 68) made with olive oil, or purchased garlic-infused olive oil

2 tablespoons freshly squeezed lemon juice

1½ teaspoons ground cumin

1 teaspoon kosher salt

½ teaspoon ground coriander

Freshly ground black pepper

2 pounds (910 kg) boneless leg of lamb, cut into 1½-inch (4 cm) cubes

2 slender zucchini, cut crosswise into 1-inch (2.5 cm)-thick rounds

1 red bell pepper, cored, cut into 1½-inch (4 cm) pieces

1 green bell pepper, cored, cut into 1½-inch (4 cm) pieces

Olive oil

EQUIPMENT:
12-inch (30.5 cm) bamboo or metal skewers

Combine the yogurt, garlic-infused oil, lemon juice, cumin, salt, coriander, and a generous sprinkling of black pepper in a heavy resealable plastic bag or a nonreactive bowl. Add the lamb and toss to coat; if you are using the plastic bag, just add the meat and squish it around, using your hands on the outside of the bag. Seal the bag or cover the bowl with plastic wrap and refrigerate for at least 6 hours or overnight.

Preheat a grill or grill pan to medium-high.

You want all your meat and vegetables to be approximately the same diameter so that the entire kebab comes in contact evenly with the grill. Loosely thread the lamb and vegetables alternately on the skewers. Do not crowd the items on the skewer; they should barely touch one another, for the most even cooking. How many items you put on each skewer depends on the length of the skewer; just leave about 4 inches (10 cm) of one end of each skewer bare so that it can hang off the grill and allow you to flip the skewers easily. Discard any leftover marinade.

Brush the grill or grill pan with olive oil and cook the kebabs, spaced evenly apart on the grill, for 3 or 4 minutes on one side, then flip over and cook until medium rare or to your desired level of doneness. The kebabs are ready to serve.

POST-FODMAP CHALLENGE PHASE OPTIONS

Polyol: If you passed the polyol mannitol challenge, consider adding button or cremini mushrooms. Wipe the mushrooms clean, trim the stems flush with the caps, and thread the mushrooms onto the skewers.

Fructans: If you passed the fructan onion challenge, consider adding white or yellow onion to the skewer. Peel, halve crosswise, then cut each half into four to six chunks; these chunks can be further separated into thinner pieces, which can then be threaded onto the skewers.

If you passed the fructan garlic challenge, add one garlic clove, finely chopped, to the olive oil vs. using garlic-infused oil.

Lactose: If you passed the lactose challenge, consider using traditional yogurt versus lactose-free.

The 15-Minute FODMAP Dinner, a.k.a. Farfalle with Garlic Olive Oil, Parsley & Roasted Red Peppers

     MAKES 4 SERVINGS

You know by now that we are out to simplify your FODMAP journey. One way of doing that is by bringing you simple and quick dinners that will tantalize your taste buds as well as your eyes—this is, indeed, the recipe from the cover. Other than the fresh parsley, you might even have all of these ingredients in your pantry, making this a fabulous choice for those nights when you just don't know what to make, whether you are vegan, vegetarian, or simply following the low FODMAP diet. The timing is not a stretch; you can prep the ingredients while the water is coming to a boil and the pasta is cooking. Be sure to season well with salt and pepper, for balanced results. Fresh chopped tomatoes and fresh basil are perfect to add if making at the end of summer when these are at their peak.

---

12 ounces (340 g) gluten-free farfalle pasta, such as Jovial brand

8 ounces (225 g) jarred roasted red peppers, preferably fire-roasted (without garlic)

1 large bunch flat-leaf parsley

¼ cup (60 ml) Garlic-Infused Oil (page 68) made with olive oil, or purchased garlic-infused olive oil

Kosher salt

Coarsely ground black pepper

Bring 5 quarts (4.7 L) of well-salted water to a boil in a large pot. Add the pasta and cook, stirring frequently. While the pasta is cooking, drain the roasted peppers and cut into strips about ½ inch (12 mm) wide by 3 to 4 inches (7.5 to 10 cm) long and discard any seeds; set aside. Chop the parsley leaves and measure out ¾ cup (9 g); set aside.

Cook the pasta until it is al dente and still has a slight firmness. Drain well.

Place the pasta back in the pot. Add the oil, parsley, and roasted peppers and toss gently but thoroughly. Season liberally with salt and black pepper to taste as you toss; serve immediately.

Beef Tenderloin Stuffed with Goat Cheese, Spinach & Tomatoes

 MAKES 8 TO 10 SERVINGS

Beef tenderloin is very easy to prepare and the results are always party worthy. The final result looks fancy and complicated, but this recipe actually comes together in just a few minutes. The colorful slices are delicious hot or room temperature, making this a perfect buffet dish. Ask your butcher for an evenly sized piece of meat. However, if one end is smaller, that part will cook much faster, a way to end up with some meat more well done and some more rare, providing choices for everyone

---

2 plum tomatoes, cored, seeded, and finely chopped

1 tablespoon plus 1 teaspoon extra-virgin olive oil or Garlic-Infused Oil (page 68) made with olive oil, or purchased garlic-infused olive oil

1 teaspoon tomato paste

Kosher salt

Freshly ground black pepper

10 ounce (280 g) package frozen chopped spinach, defrosted, drained, and squeezed dry

8 ounces (225 g) mild, soft goat cheese, such as Montrachet

1 (4- to 5-pound [1.8 to 2.3 kg]) beef tenderloin, trimmed of fat

2 teaspoons herbes de Provence (see Dédé's Tips), or 1 teaspoon each dried rosemary and thyme

EQUIPMENT:
Kitchen twine

If planning to roast on the same day as assembling, position a rack in the center of the oven. Preheat the oven to 450°F/230°C.

Meanwhile, place the tomatoes in a saucepan, add 1 teaspoon of the olive oil, the tomato paste, and ⅛ teaspoon of salt. Bring to a simmer over medium heat, stirring and mashing occasionally, and cook until the liquid evaporates and the tomatoes are a thick paste, for 10 to 15 minutes. Season to taste with salt and pepper. Remove from the heat and allow to cool.

Stir together the spinach, goat cheese, and tomatoes in a medium-size mixing bowl until thoroughly combined.

Slice the tenderloin lengthwise down the center and about three quarters of the way through; do not cut all the way through. Open the beef as flat as possible. Season the interior well with salt and pepper and most of the dried herbs.

Spread the spinach mixture down the center of beef. Press the sides of the tenderloin back together, making sure no filling is protruding. Wrap with kitchen twine at 2-inch (5 cm) intervals. Rub the tenderloin all over with the remaining tablespoon of olive oil, then season with salt and pepper and the remaining herbs. Place the tenderloin on a rack in a roasting pan. (The meat may be prepared to this point up to 1 day ahead. Simply refrigerate until needed, then allow to come to room temperature and preheating your oven before proceeding.)

Roast the beef for 20 to 25 minutes, then check the temperature with an instant-read thermometer inserted into the meat (not the filling) in several places. You want a reading of 125°F (52°C) for medium rare. Remove from the oven, tent with foil, and allow to sit for at least 5 minutes.

Slice the tenderloin into ½- to ¾-inch (12 mm to 2 cm) slices and serve immediately, or allow to cool and serve at room temperature. If any pan juices remain in the pan, they may be drizzled over the slices.

DÉDÉ'S TIPS

Herbes de Provence is an herb blend combining a variety of herbs that can vary, but lavender is always included. A typical blend combines rosemary, fennel, thyme, savory, basil, French tarragon, dill, Turkish oregano, lavender, chervil, and marjoram. It is incredibly aromatic and can add sophisticated nuances to our low FODMAP dishes. Try it with roast chicken or even simple roast potatoes.

Baked Mac 'n' Cheese

 MAKES 10 TO 12 SERVINGS

We are determined to bring comfort foods to low FODMAP eating and good old homemade macaroni and cheese might be the #1 main dish in that category. It can be made ahead and it is endlessly customizable—do not miss our favorite variations, including a stove-top version. No need to even tell anyone that this is gluten-free and low FODMAP, including the crunchy bread crumb topping. No one will know—it is just ridiculously creamy, rich, and delicious. Don't leave out the mustard; it adds a welcomed tang. Many recipes call for dry mustard, but most of us have prepared Dijon on hand and it works perfectly.

TOPPING:

1 teaspoon unsalted butter

2¼ teaspoons Garlic-Infused Oil (page 68) made with olive oil or vegetable oil, or purchased garlic-infused olive oil or vegetable oil

¾ cup (84 g) gluten-free panko, such as Ian's Original brand

3 tablespoons finely grated Parmigiano-Reggiano cheese

⅛ teaspoon kosher salt

PASTA AND SAUCE:

1 pound (455 g) gluten-free elbow macaroni pasta, such as Tinkyada brand

½ cup (1 stick; 113 g) plus 1½ teaspoons unsalted butter, cut into pieces, divided

6 tablespoons (1.6 g) gluten-free all-purpose flour, such as Bob's Red Mill Gluten Free 1 to 1 Baking Flour

4½ cups (1 L) lactose-free milk (whole, 2%, 1%, or fat-free), such as Organic Valley, at room temperature

1 scant tablespoon Dijon mustard (use gluten-free if necessary)

2 teaspoons kosher salt

Freshly ground black pepper

16 ounces (455 g) finely grated extra-sharp orange Cheddar cheese

½ cup (50 g) finely grated Parmigiano-Reggiano cheese

If you are going to prepare and bake the mac 'n' cheese right away, preheat the oven now to 400°F (200°C) with a rack in the center of the oven. If you want to prepare the dish for baking later in the day or even the next day, do not preheat the oven and read through the recipe to understand do-ahead steps.

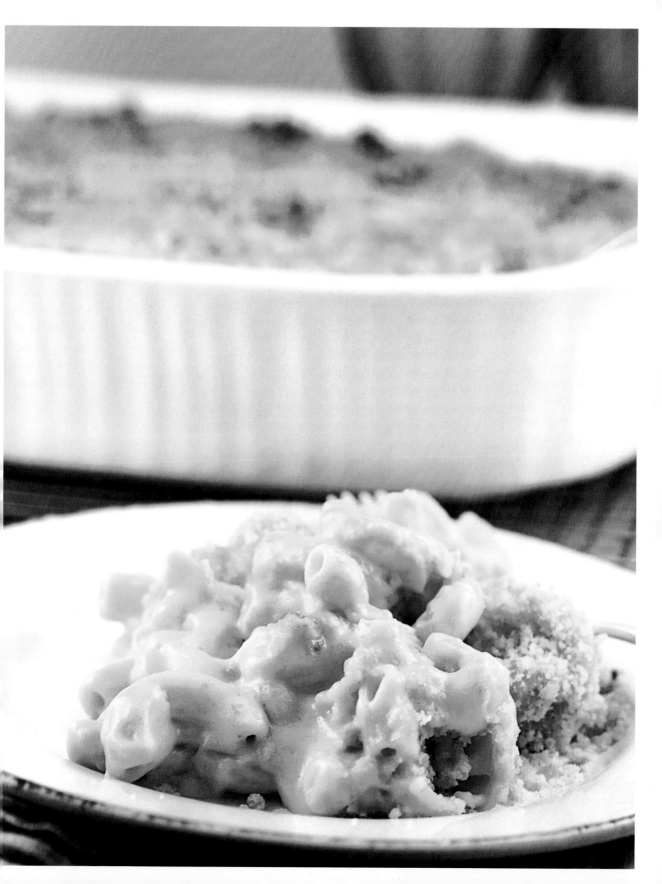

Prepare the topping: Melt the butter along with the oil over medium heat in a large sauté pan, preferably nonstick. Add the panko, toss to coat, and cook for a minute or two, just until the panko begins to take on color and smell fragrant (like garlic toast). Remove from the heat and stir in the Parmigiano-Reggiano and salt; set aside.

Prepare the pasta and sauce: Bring a 5-quart (4.7 L) pot of well-salted water to a boil and cook the pasta until it is al dente and still has a slight firmness (do not overcook; it will cook still more in the oven). Drain, rinse under cold water, and set aside. Wipe out the pot with a paper towel and use the same pot to make sauce.

Melt ½ cup (115 g) of the butter in the pot over medium heat, then whisk in the flour until combined to make a roux. Bring the roux to a boil over medium heat, whisking almost constantly, and cook for about 3 minutes, or just until the roux is very light brown. Slowly add the milk, whisking all the while. Continue to cook over medium heat, bringing back to a low boil, whisking all the while, for about 3 minutes, or until the sauce is thick and creamy. You should be able to see whisk marks for a moment before they dissolve back into the sauce. Remove from the heat, whisk in the mustard and salt, and season generously with pepper, then slowly add the grated Cheddar and Parmigiano-Reggiano, whisking them in as you go. The residual heat should melt the cheeses. Whisk gently until the cheeses are melted and incorporated and the sauce is thick and smooth. Only place back over low heat if needed to help melt the cheese and do not overcook at this point; if you do, the sauce will reduce and you will lose the satiny, creamy sauciness that you want in your finished dish.

To assemble: Use the remaining 1½ teaspoons of butter to coat the bottom and sides of a 13 x 9-inch (33 x 23 cm) baking dish.

Add the pasta to the cheese sauce and fold to coat, then scrape into the prepared baking dish. Sprinkle topping evenly over the pasta. The baking dish may be covered with aluminum foil at this point and held at room temperature for 2 hours before baking or being refrigerated overnight. Bring to room temperature before baking. When ready to cook, bake for 18 to 20 minutes, or until the edges are bubbling and the topping is light golden brown. The mac 'n' cheese is ready to eat. Leftovers may be covered with plastic wrap or placed in airtight containers and refrigerated for up to 3 days. Reheat in a microwave or in a 300°F (150°C) oven, covered with foil to prevent drying out.

VARIATIONS:

Bacon Jalapeño Mac 'n' Cheese: Cook ten slices of bacon until crisp (use gluten-free bacon if necessary) and drain on paper towels, reserving 1 tablespoon of the bacon fat in the pan. Seed and finely chop one jalapeño pepper and sauté in the reserved bacon fat just until it is soft. Crumble the bacon, then fold it and the sautéed jalapeño into the sauced pasta before you scrape it into the baking dish. Bake as directed.

Four-Cheese Mac 'n' Cheese: Use half romano cheese where the recipe calls for Parmigiano-Reggiano. Replace 8 ounces (225 g) of the extra-sharp Cheddar with 8 ounces (225 g) of grated Monterey Jack. Bake as directed.

Lobster Mac 'n' Cheese: Replace the 16 ounces (455 g) of the extra-sharp Cheddar with 10 ounces (280 g) of grated Gruyère cheese and 6 ounces (170 g) of grated medium or sharp Cheddar (Dédé likes to use white Cheddar for this one). Fold 1½ pounds (680 g) of cooked lobster meat and ½ cup (32 g) of finely chopped scallion greens into the sauced pasta before you scrape it into the baking dish. Bake as directed.

Stovetop Broccoli and Carrots Mac 'n' Cheese: When Dédé's kids were little, this was the superquick way to get dinner on the table. Don't make the crumb topping. Instead, have handy 1 cup (128 g) of chopped "baby" carrot and 2 cups (244 g) of tiny broccoli florets. About 2 minutes before the pasta is done cooking, throw the carrots into the pot. Make sure the water comes back to a boil quickly. About 1 minute before the pasta is done, add the broccoli. Drain the pasta and veggies, toss with the cheese sauce, and serve immediately.

POST-FODMAP CHALLENGE PHASE OPTION

Fructan: If you passed the fructan wheat challenge, you can sub in traditional wheat-based pasta for the gluten-free pasta in the recipe (do not use this substitution if following a gluten-free diet).

Asian Chicken Lettuce Wraps

 MAKES 4 SERVINGS | SERVING SIZE 2 WRAPS

These might sound exotic but they are quick to make and are a great low FODMAP week-day dinner. The original recipe used hoisin sauce but as of now, no low FODMAP version is approved, so we turned to another Chinese condiment that is approved—oyster sauce. It has a depth of flavor that adds dimension to this dish, as do the toasted sesame oil and soy sauce. You can also turn these into a turkey version by using ground turkey. The optional peanuts add a crunchy texture, which is most welcomed. Kids love assembling these and are encouraged to eat with their hands. Offer forks, but they probably won't be used! Lots of napkins will come in handy. The recipe may be doubled.

---

2 teaspoons Garlic-Infused Oil (page 68) made with vegetable oil, or purchased garlic-infused vegetable oil

2 teaspoons finely grated fresh ginger

1 pound (455 g) ground chicken or turkey

1 medium-size carrot, peeled and shredded

½ medium-size red bell pepper, cored and finely chopped

½ cup (115 g) canned water chestnuts, drained and finely chopped

¼ cup (16 g) chopped scallion, green parts only

2 tablespoons oyster sauce (we like gluten-free Kikkoman brand)

1 tablespoon low-sodium soy sauce or tamari (use gluten-free if necessary, such as San-J Organic)

1 teaspoon toasted sesame oil

2 heads butter or Boston lettuce, washed, dried, cored, the 8 largest leaves removed

⅓ cup (48 g) chopped roasted peanuts (optional) (without added high-FODMAP ingredients)

2 tablespoons chopped fresh cilantro

Heat the oil in a large skillet or wok over medium heat. Add the ginger and stir-fry, stirring constantly, for about 1 minute, or until fragrant. Crumble in the chicken and stir-fry until just beginning to lose its pink color, for about 2 minutes. Add the carrot, bell pepper, water chestnuts, and half of the scallion greens, and stir-fry for 1 minute to combine, then add the oyster sauce, soy sauce, and sesame oil and continue to stir-fry for several more minutes, until the chicken is cooked through.

Meanwhile, place the lettuce on plates, ready to be used as "bowls" for the cooked chicken. Once the chicken is cooked, divide among the lettuce leaves, sprinkle with the peanuts, if using, and garnish with the remaining 2 tablespoons of scallion greens and the cilantro. Serve immediately. Wrap up the chicken in the lettuce leaves and eat with your fingers.

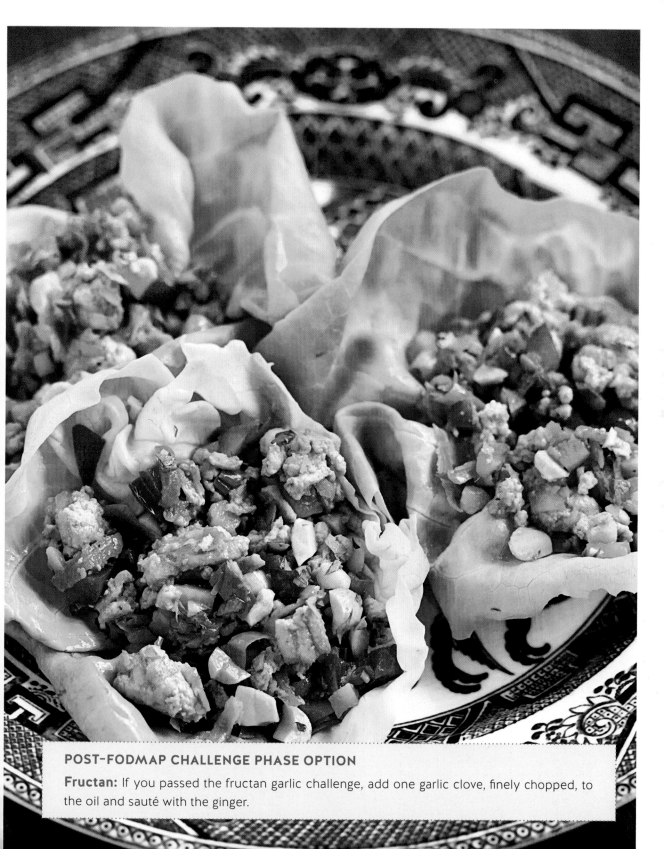

POST-FODMAP CHALLENGE PHASE OPTION

Fructan: If you passed the fructan garlic challenge, add one garlic clove, finely chopped, to the oil and sauté with the ginger.

Crab Cakes

MAKES ABOUT TEN 4-INCH (7 CM) CRAB CAKES | SERVING SIZE 2 TO 3 CRAB CAKES

The key to making great crab cakes is to start with large lump crabmeat and then to not do too much to it. You want to let the crab flavor and texture shine. Some binder—in this case, soft, white, gluten-free bread crumbs—provide some structure, but use just enough. Old Bay Seasoning is a classic flavor blend made in Maryland that accents the crab perfectly. You will see that there is a frying option and a broiling option, which uses about half the fat. Crab cakes make a great lunch or plated appetizer for a party. If you make them smaller, they can even be used as an hors d'oeuvres.

---

1 pound (455 g) lump crabmeat, fresh or refrigerated (not canned)

1 large egg, at room temperature

¼ cup (57 g) mayonnaise

1 tablespoon plus 1 teaspoon finely chopped fresh flat-leaf parsley

2 teaspoons freshly squeezed lemon juice

1 teaspoon Old Bay Seasoning

Dash of Worcestershire sauce (use gluten-free if necessary)

1 cup (42 g) finely ground, fresh low FODMAP white bread crumbs, such as from Udi's Gluten Free White Sandwich Bread (or other gluten-free if necessary)

2 tablespoons unsalted butter

1 tablespoon olive or vegetable oil

Lemon wedges

Drain the crab and pick over it for any shell or cartilage; set aside.

Whisk together the egg, mayonnaise, parsley, lemon juice, Old Bay Seasoning, and Worcestershire sauce in a mixing bowl. Gently fold in the crab and then fold in just enough of the bread crumbs to absorb some of the juiciness of the mixture (you will most likely need all of the bread crumbs or close to it). Cover the bowl with plastic wrap and refrigerate for at least 1 hour or up to 3 hours.

Line a baking sheet with aluminum foil. Use a ¼-cup (60 ml) measuring cup or scoop to create ten crab cakes, depositing the mounds, evenly spaced apart, on the prepared pan. Use your fingers and palms to gently press down to about ¾-inch (2 cm) thickness and use your fingers to press any loose pieces of crab into each cake.

If panfrying, melt the butter and oil in a large skillet over medium heat. Add a few crab cakes at a time, using a broad, sturdy spatula to transfer them to the pan. Cook the first side for 3 to

4 minutes over medium heat, allowing the bottom to lightly brown. Flip carefully and cook the second side for 3 or 4 minutes more, or until heated through.

If broiling, preheat the broiler to high and place a rack about 4 inches (10 cm) below. Melt half of the butter and the oil and brush over the crab cakes. Broil for about 5 minutes, or until lightly browned. Carefully flip over and broil the second side until browned. The timing will depend on the strength of the broiler. If browning too quickly, transfer to a lower rack.

Serve the crab cakes immediately with lemon wedges alongside.

KATE'S NOTES

The Old Bay Seasoning, a blend of celery seeds, red pepper, black pepper, and paprika, is a popular seafood seasoning in the United States. We find it is a perfect accent in this crab cake recipe and is well tolerated by FODMAPers.

Maple Dijon Pork Chops with Root Vegetable Mash

MAKES 4 SERVINGS

Pork chops are a quick and easy weeknight option. Here we have paired them with the slightly sweet mash-up of potatoes, sweet potatoes, and parsnips and a quick glaze of white wine, maple syrup, Dijon mustard, and thyme. The only thing to watch out for is to not over-cook the pork. Literally a minute or two too long can change a pork chop from supermoist to dry and tough, so follow our directions for juicy success. The first step toward this fabulous result is to buy chops that are bone-in and no thinner than ¾ inch (2 cm); a full inch (2.5 cm) thick is even better.

ROOT VEGETABLE MASH:

1 large russet potato, peeled and diced

1 small to medium-size sweet potato, peeled and diced

3 medium-size parsnips, peeled and diced

Kosher salt

¼ cup (60 ml) lactose-free milk (whole, 2%, 1%, or fat-free)

Freshly ground black pepper

PORK CHOPS:

¼ cup (60 ml) olive oil

½ cup (45 g) finely chopped leek, green parts only

4 center-cut bone-in pork chops, about ½ pound (225 g) each and at least ¾ inch (2 cm) thick (no thinner), at room temperature

Kosher salt

Freshly ground black pepper

½ teaspoon dried thyme

⅓ cup (75 ml) dry white wine or Chicken Stock (page 70)

2 teaspoons Dijon mustard (use gluten-free if necessary)

2 teaspoons pure maple syrup

Prepare the root vegetables: Combine all the diced vegetables in a medium-size saucepan and cover with water by 2 inches (5 cm). Salt the water lightly. Cover and bring to a boil over high heat, then lower the heat and simmer until the veggies are tender when pierced with a knife, for 15 to 20 minutes. Reserve ½ cup (120 ml) of the cooking water (you won't need all of it), then drain the vegetables and return them to the pot. Add the milk, season liberally with salt and pepper, and mash well with a potato masher. Add the reserved cooking water as needed to create a light, fluffy texture. Cover and keep warm while you make the chops.

Prepare the pork: Heat the oil in a large skillet over medium-low heat and add the leek. Sauté until very soft, but do not brown. Season the chops on both sides with salt, pepper, and the thyme. Increase the heat to medium and add the chops; they should sizzle. Cook for about 1½ minutes on each side. Meanwhile, whisk together the wine with the mustard and maple syrup. After the second side of the chops has cooked, add the wine mixture to the skillet; it should boil immediately when it hits the pan. Shake the pan a couple of times, cover, and cook for another 2 to 3 minutes, or just until the chops are cooked through. An instant-read thermometer should register between 140° and 145°F (60° and 63°C). Remove from the heat and allow to sit for a few minutes (the temperature will rise to 145°F [63°C]). Meanwhile, reheat the mash, if necessary.

Serve a mound of root vegetable mash and a chop on each plate with the pan juices poured over the top.

POST-FODMAP CHALLENGE PHASE OPTION

Fructan: If you passed the fructan onion challenge, sauté ¼ cup (36 g) of chopped white or yellow onion instead of the leek greens.

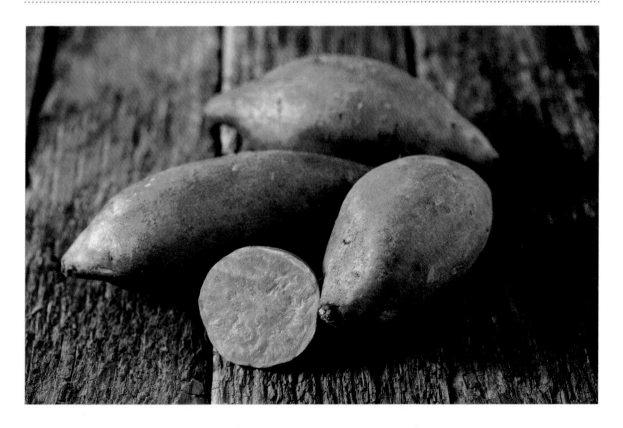

Main Dish Steak Salad

  MAKES 2 TO 4 SERVINGS

We love a good steak salad for lunch or dinner because it combines several elements to tantalize our senses: crisp cool lettuce, juicy tomatoes, salty cheese, hearty warm potatoes, rich and tender steak, and a sharp dressing. The colors and textures beckon even before the first bite. The dish is made of several components, but the whole dish can come together in less than half an hour. If you can grill outdoors, by all means do so, but we make this all the time using a grill pan or cast-iron pan indoors. Just turn on the hood fan.

Balsamic Dijon Vinaigrette (page 73)

¾ pound (340 g) small red or white potatoes, halved or quartered

1 pound (455 g) steak, such as rib eye, flank, or skirt steak

Kosher salt

Freshly ground black pepper

1 medium-size head romaine lettuce, cored, leaves washed and dried well

2 cups (40 g) baby arugula

⅓ dry pint (95 g) cherry or grape tomatoes

3 medium-size red radishes, stems removed, sliced into thin rounds

4 ounces (115 g) Gorgonzola cheese, crumbled (may contain gluten; omit if necessary)

Place the potatoes in a medium-large pot and cover with water by an inch (2.5 cm). Salt the water and bring to a boil over high heat. Lower the heat and simmer vigorously until just tender when pierced with a knife, 12 to 15 minutes. Drain well and set aside, keeping warm.

Meanwhile, season the steak with salt and pepper on both sides and cook to your desired doneness either on an outdoor grill (gas or propane) or indoors in a grill pan or cast-iron pan, 3 to 5 minutes per side, depending in thickness, for medium rare. Allow to rest for at least 5 minutes while you assemble the rest of the salad.

Tear the lettuce leaves into large bite-size pieces and place in a mixing bowl along with the baby arugula. Toss in the tomatoes, radishes, and Gorgonzola. Add the warm potatoes, cut into bite-size pieces if they aren't already. Drizzle with some of the dressing and toss gently to coat and flavor, but do not overdress. Divide the salad among individual plates, making sure each serving receives a bit of each ingredient. Slice the steak across the grain and place on top of the salads. Drizzle a little more dressing on top of the steak. Serve immediately.

Salade Niçoise

 MAKES 4 TO 6 SERVINGS

This classic French salad, which is hearty enough for a summer dinner, fits perfectly within our low FODMAP protocol. As a dietitian, Kate approves the balance to this recipe with protein (tuna, hard-boiled egg), starch (potatoes) veggies (green beans, tomatoes, lettuce), and flavorful healthy fats (olives, anchovies).

This is what is called a salade composée (composed salad), meaning that the ingredients are placed in groupings, to be combined upon serving. It makes a gorgeous buffet presentation. Tuna is the star in this dish, so make sure to use high-quality oil-packed tuna; it really makes a difference in this dish. Look for glass jars of high-quality imported tuna, or high-quality canned tuna such as Wild Planet brand.

VINAIGRETTE:

¾ cup (180 ml) Garlic-Infused Oil (page 68) made with extra-virgin olive oil, or purchased garlic-infused olive oil

¼ cup (60 ml) white wine vinegar

2 tablespoons minced fresh herbs; we used a combo of tarragon, chives, and parsley (dill and marjoram can work, too)

2 teaspoons Dijon mustard (use gluten-free if necessary)

¼ teaspoon kosher salt

SALAD:

1¼ pounds (680 g) small yellow waxy potatoes, scrubbed, left whole or halved depending on size

Kosher salt

3 tablespoons white wine

Freshly ground black pepper

12 ounces (340 g) slender green beans, stem ends trimmed

1 large head Boston or butter lettuce, cored, leaves separated, washed, and dried

½ dry pint (142 g) cherry or grape tomatoes or 2 medium-size beefsteak tomatoes, cored and quartered

10 to 12 ounces (280 to 340 g) oil-packed tuna; we used a combo of white albacore and light-fleshed chunk tuna

4 hard-boiled eggs, halved lengthwise

½ cup (121 g) olives, such as kalamata or niçoise, drained

1 (2-ounce [55 g]) tin oil-packed flat anchovy fillets, drained

Prepare the vinaigrette: Place all the vinaigrette ingredients together in a jar with an airtight lid and shake vigorously until combined; set aside. Reshake right before using if it separates.

Prepare the salad: Place the potatoes in a medium-large pot and cover with water by an inch (2.5 cm). Salt the water and bring to a boil over high heat. Lower the heat and simmer vigorously until just tender when pierced with a knife, for 12 to 15 minutes. Drain; place in a mixing bowl, drizzle with the white wine, season with salt and pepper, and toss to coat; set aside. This may be done early on the day of serving.

Use the same pot to bring 5 cups (1.2 L) of salted water to a boil. Add the beans and cook for a minute or two, until just crisp tender. Drain and rinse under cold water to halt the cooking. Pat dry with a paper towel; set aside. This may be done early in the day of serving.

Right before serving, arrange the components on a large platter as follows: Place a tablespoon or two of the vinaigrette in a large mixing bowl. Gently toss the lettuce leaves in the dressing and arrange on a large platter. Toss the cooked potatoes in the same bowl with a few additional tablespoons of dressing and arrange in a cluster or clusters on the lettuce leaves. Repeat the same process with the green beans, tomatoes, tuna, and hard-boiled eggs; scatter the olives over all; and arrange the anchovies as well. We like to put the anchovies to the side as not everyone likes them. Drizzle with extra vinaigrette right before serving, if desired, or pass alongside so that everyone can dress the salad to their taste. Serve family style.

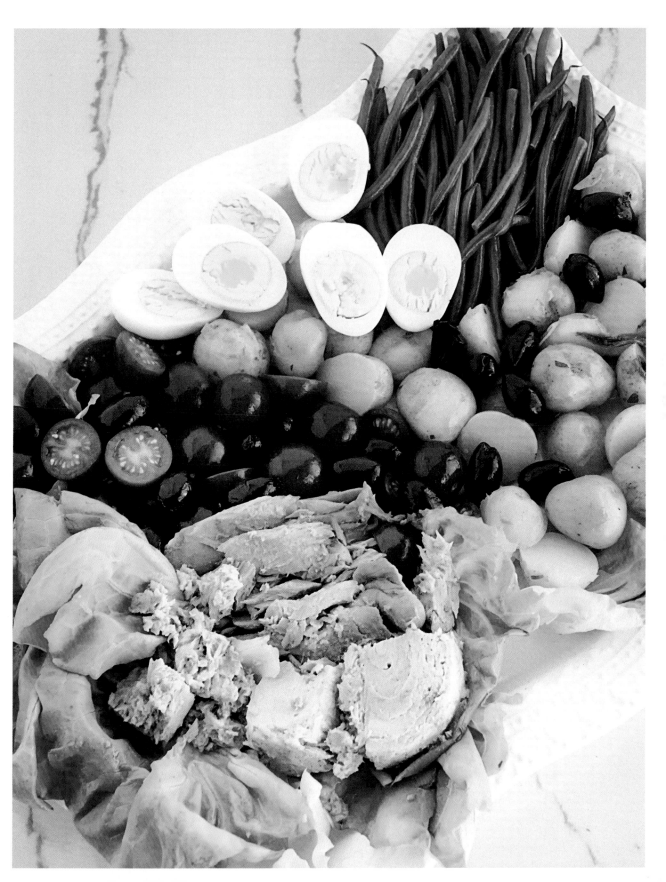

Turkey Skillet Dinner with Corn Bread Biscuits

MAKES 6 SERVINGS

If you don't have a cast-iron pan, we strongly urge you to get one now. Not only are they inexpensive (even the preseasoned ones we love from Lodge), but they will last your lifetime and beyond if cared for well. Here we use our versatile 10-inch (25 cm) cast-iron pan to make a one-pot meal that begins on top of the stove, goes into the oven, and then arrives at the table piping hot and ready to eat.

TURKEY:

1 tablespoon Garlic-Infused Oil (page 68) made with vegetable oil, or purchased garlic-infused vegetable oil

½ medium-size green bell pepper, cored and diced

¼ cup (23 g) finely chopped leek, green parts only

1½ pounds (680 g) ground turkey or chicken

½ teaspoon ground cumin

½ teaspoon dried oregano

Kosher salt

Freshly ground black pepper

1 (14.5-ounce [415 g]) can fire-roasted diced tomatoes (without garlic or onion), such as Muir Glen brand

1 tablespoon tomato paste

CORN BREAD BISCUITS:

½ cup (120 ml) lactose-free milk (whole, 2%, 1%, or fat-free)

1 teaspoon freshly squeezed lemon juice

3 tablespoons melted unsalted butter

1 large egg, at room temperature

⅔ cup (75 g) finely ground stone-ground yellow cornmeal

⅓ cup (1.7 g) gluten-free all-purpose flour, such as Bob's Red Mill Gluten Free 1 to 1 Baking Flour

1 teaspoon baking powder (use gluten-free if necessary)

¼ teaspoon baking soda

Pinch of kosher salt

2.5 ounces (70 g) sharp or extra-sharp Cheddar cheese, shredded

¼ cup (16 g) finely chopped scallion, green parts only (optional)

Prepare the turkey: Position a rack in the center of the oven. Preheat the oven to 400°F (200°C).

Heat the olive oil in a cast-iron pan and sauté the pepper and leek over medium heat until soft, for about 5 minutes. Crumble the turkey into the pan and cook, stirring often, until no longer pink, for about 5 minutes more. Add the cumin and oregano and season to taste with salt and black pepper. Stir in the tomatoes and tomato paste until the mixture is well combined and simmer for 5 minutes to blend the flavors. Taste and adjust the seasoning.

Prepare the corn bread: While the turkey is cooking, make the corn bread biscuits. Whisk the milk and lemon juice together in a 2-cup (480 ml) measuring cup or small bowl and allow to sit for 5 minutes. Then, whisk the melted butter and egg into the thickened milk mixture, set aside.

Whisk together the cornmeal, flour, baking powder, baking soda, and salt in a large mixing bowl, to aerate and combine. Make a well in the center and pour in the milk mixture. Fold together with a large rubber spatula until almost blended, add the cheese and the scallion greens, if using, and fold together until just combined.

The turkey mixture should be simmering and juicy. Dollop the biscuit batter on top—one scoop in the center and five around the edges. Place the pan in the preheated oven.

Bake until the biscuits are dry to the touch and lightly colored, for 15 to 20 minutes. The skillet dish is ready to serve and is best served immediately.

POST-FODMAP CHALLENGE PHASE OPTIONS

Fructans: If you passed the fructan garlic challenge, add one garlic clove, finely chopped, to the oil rather than use garlic-infused oil.

If you passed the fructan onion challenge, sub in ¼ cup (36 g) of finely chopped white or yellow onion for the leek greens.

Build-a-Better-Burger

   MAKES 4 BURGERS | SERVING SIZE 1 BURGER

Eating a burger out on the town might not be easy during the elimination phase, as many restaurants will flavor the meat with onion, garlic, or other ingredients that we need to steer clear of. Fear not, as you can make an even better burger at home and customize it to each diner's liking. Just follow our recommendations for selecting the meat, seasoning, handling, and cooking it, and you will be on your way to the best burger ever. For the juiciest burger, use the 80% lean. It you want to trim some calories and fat, use the 85%. Any leaner and you do risk ending up with a dry burger.

---

1 pound (455 g) 80% or 85% lean ground beef, well chilled

4 low FODMAP-approved gluten-free buns or English muffins, such as Against the Grain Original Rolls or Food for Life or Foods by George Plain Gluten Free English Muffins

Kosher salt

Freshly ground black pepper

YOUR CHOICE OF TOPPINGS:

Cheddar, Monterey Jack, mozzarella, Gruyère, or blue cheese (blue cheese may contain gluten; omit if necessary)

Lettuce (green or red leaf, Boston, or butter lettuce)

Tomato slices

Ranch Dressing (page 77, prepared gluten-free if necessary)

Cooked bacon (use gluten-free if necessary)

Mustard (we like Dijon; use gluten-free, if necessary)

Ketchup, in moderation (see Kate's Notes)

Buy freshly ground beef and use the day of purchase for best results. Only take out of the refrigerator right before you are ready to prep the meat and cook. Divide the beef into four equal portions, creating 4 x ½-inch (10 x 13 mm) patties on your work surface. Take care not to compress the meat. Some raggedy edges are okay; make a slight dimple in the center of each patty with your thumb (this will prevent the burgers from bulging vertically). Set aside.

Have your buns toasted, if desired, and any toppings ready to go. If you want cheeseburgers, have the cheese very thinly sliced with a cheese plane and ready to use.

Heat a large, cast-iron skillet over medium-high heat until it smokes slightly, for about 2 minutes. While the pan heats, season the meat by sprinkling liberally with salt and pepper on both sides of the patties. Once the pan is hot, add the patties and cook for about 3 minutes; do not press down with a spatula, which will squeeze out the delicious juices! Flip over and cook for about 3 minutes more for medium-rare, or cook to your liking.

If you are making cheeseburgers, add the cheese slices about 1 minute before the burgers are done. You can cover the skillet to help the cheese melt. Remove the burgers from the pan when done and place on a plate or platter to rest for about 1 minute to rest and redistribute the juices. Now, load up your buns any way you like and serve immediately.

KATE'S NOTES

US-made ketchup has been analyzed by the Monash University researchers and found to be suitable for low FODMAP diets in small quantity, about 1 tablespoon or less per meal. Note: New food companies are catering to the low FODMAP crowd and creating low FODMAP condiments and more. Check out FODY Foods for a tasty low FODMAP ketchup option. Most mustards are low FODMAP but be careful not to select one with added FODMAPs, such as honey mustard. Mayonnaise is usually low FODMAP but be on the lookout for varieties that sneak in added onion or garlic, as they would be off the table during the low FODMAP elimination diet.

(Recipe photo on page 186)

Fully Loaded Stuffed Potato Skins

 MAKES 6 TO 12 SERVINGS | SERVING SIZE 1 TO 2 POTATO HALVES

Did the recipe title get you? Sound decadent? These are, and while we do not suggest you eat these every day, they will definitely satisfy your desire for carbs. The combination of baking the potatoes and then broiling the halves provides the perfect texture for these enticing, flavor-packed spuds. You can serve these as they come out of the oven, but offering one of the dipping sauces—Ranch Dressing (page 77), Blue Cheese Dressing (page 75) (note that the these first two dressings may not be gluten-free), or Salsa Fresca (page 80)—makes these over-the-top fantastic.

6 small (about 3½ inches [9 cm] long) starchy baking potatoes, about 2 pounds (910 kg)

6 slices thick-cut bacon (use gluten-free if necessary)

1 tablespoon unsalted butter, melted

Kosher salt

Freshly ground black pepper

5 ounces (140 g) extra-sharp Cheddar cheese, shredded

¾ cup (171 g) lactose-free sour cream (optional; see directions)

⅓ cup (16 g) chopped fresh chives

⅓ cup (24 g) chopped scallion, green parts only

Blue Cheese Dressing (page 75), Ranch Dressing (page 77), or Salsa Fresca (page 80) (optional; see headnote)

Position a rack in the center of the oven. Preheat the oven to 400°F/200°C.

Scrub the potatoes well and dry them. Pierce with a knife in a few places. Place the potatoes directly on the oven rack and bake until tender, for about 45 minutes. Remove from the oven and allow to cool briefly.

While the potatoes are baking, cook the bacon until crisp, drain on paper towels, and reserve 1 tablespoon of the fat. Stir this bacon fat together with the melted butter. Chop or crumble the drained and cooled bacon into small bits; set aside.

Preheat the broiler to high and place a rack 3 to 4 inches (7.5 to 10 cm) below the broiler. Halve the potatoes lengthwise. Use a teaspoon or a small scoop to remove most of the potato flesh from each potato, leaving about a ¼-inch (6 mm) wall of flesh still attached to the skin (we like to collect the potato innards in a bowl, mash them with a bit of lactose-free milk, add salt and

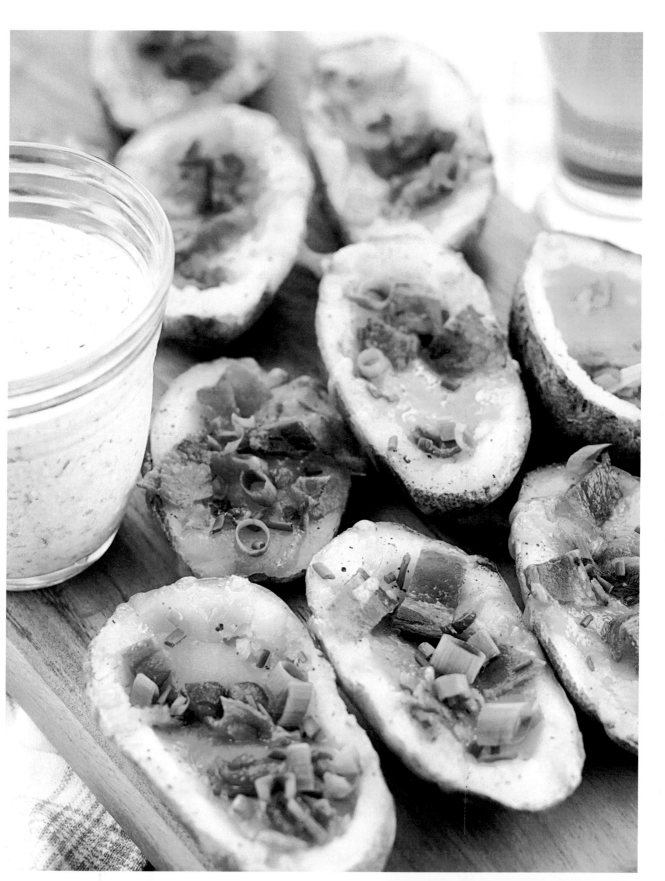

pepper, and have it as a snack or alongside dinner). Place the potato skins on a rimmed baking sheet and brush both sides, inside and out, with the bacon fat mixture. Season with salt and pepper on both sides, too.

Broil the potato skins for 2 to 3 minutes on each side, watching carefully so as not to let them burn. You do want the skins to get a bit crispy.

Now, make sure all the potato skins are skin side down on the pan, scooped-out side facing up. Sprinkle the cheese evenly into the bacon skins, then scatter with the chopped bacon. Place back under the broiler and broil just until the cheese is melted and bubbly.

Remove from the broiler, immediately dollop sour cream on each potato skin (about 1 table-spoon per skin, unless serving with Blue Cheese Dressing or Ranch Dressing, in which case it is optional), and sprinkle with the chives and scallion greens. Serve immediately as is or offer with one of the suggested dipping sauces. Are you salivating yet?

Grilled Swordfish with Pineapple Salsa

   MAKES 4 SERVINGS

Don't let the title turn you away if it is midwinter! We cook this fish on a grill pan indoors all the time, or even just in a heavy cast-iron pan. Of course, if you have a hardwood charcoal grill, by all means use it. The smoky flavor will add another dimension to this dish. (We give directions for both.) The Pineapple Salsa (page 81), which is one of our basics, is a great alternative to a tomato-based salsa for tortilla chips, but we think it really shines alongside the swordfish. We like to serve this dish with rice, which you can prepare while the swordfish is marinating and you are prepping the fire.

---

1 batch Pineapple Salsa (page 81) ready to use

FISH:

2 tablespoons Garlic-Infused Oil (page 68) prepared with olive oil, or purchased garlic-infused olive oil

1 tablespoon freshly squeezed lemon juice

¼ teaspoon ground cumin

⅛ teaspoon kosher salt

Freshly ground black pepper

4 (4- to 5-ounce (115 to 140 g) swordfish steaks, ¾ to 1 inch (2 to 2.5 cm) thick

Vegetable oil, for grill or grill pan

Prepare the fish: Whisk the oil, lemon juice, cumin, and salt together in a large, broad-bottomed, nonreactive bowl and season generously with black pepper. Add the fish, turning the pieces over to coat, and allow to marinate for about 10 minutes.

Meanwhile, prepare a hot fire over hardwood charcoal, or set the gas grill to high. Make sure grates are clean and brush them lightly with vegetable oil. Lift the swordfish out of the marinade, allowing any excess to drip away; discard the marinade. Grill the swordfish for 3 to 4 minutes per side. The fish should take on a little color in addition to grill marks and you can check the insides with the tip of a sharp knife; the flesh should be opaque and your knife should meet little resistance. Alternatively, heat a grill pan or cast-iron skillet over high heat and brush lightly with oil. Cook the fish as above. Serve immediately with the salsa spooned over the top.

> **POST-FODMAP CHALLENGE PHASE OPTION**
>
> **Fructan:** If you passed the fructan garlic challenge, you can use half a garlic clove, finely chopped, and use olive oil instead of the garlic oil in the recipe.

Chicken Tostadas

    MAKES 4 TOSTADAS | SERVES 2

If you are working your elimination phase strictly (as we suggest that you do initially), then onions and garlic as ingredients are off the table and that means you might be missing your Mexican-inspired food. (Sigh). What is one to do? Well, while these Chicken Tostadas do not contain refried beans, they are incredibly satisfying with layers of color, flavor, and contrasting textures and temperatures. The corn tortillas provide crunch; the chicken is an easy, accessible protein; the sautéed peppers add color and nutrition; and what isn't improved by melty cheese and a dollop of silken (lactose-free) sour cream? This recipe takes advantage of leftover cooked chicken, perhaps from our Whole Roast Chicken with Lemon & Herbs (page 276), our basic Garlic-Infused Oil (page 68), and Salsa Fresca (page 80).

The recipe doubles easily but you will need to use two baking sheets and to run them under the broiler in quick succession to get all the food on the table at once.

SAUTÉED PEPPERS:

Scant 1 tablespoon Garlic-Infused Oil (page 68) or Onion-Infused Oil (see variation, page 68) made with vegetable oil, purchased versions of these infused oils, or plain vegetable oil

½ medium-size red bell pepper, cored, cut into 2-inch (5 cm)-long, ¼-inch (6 mm)-wide strips

½ medium-size orange bell pepper, cored, cut into 2-inch (5 cm)-long, ¼-inch (6 mm)-wide strips

½ medium-size yellow bell pepper, cored, cut into 2-inch (5 cm)-long, ¼-inch (6 mm)-wide strips

Kosher salt

Freshly ground black pepper

CHICKEN:

1½ cups (360 ml) shredded cooked chicken, at room temperature or warm

2 tablespoons chopped fresh cilantro or flat-leaf parsley

1 tablespoon freshly squeezed lime juice

Kosher salt

Freshly ground black pepper

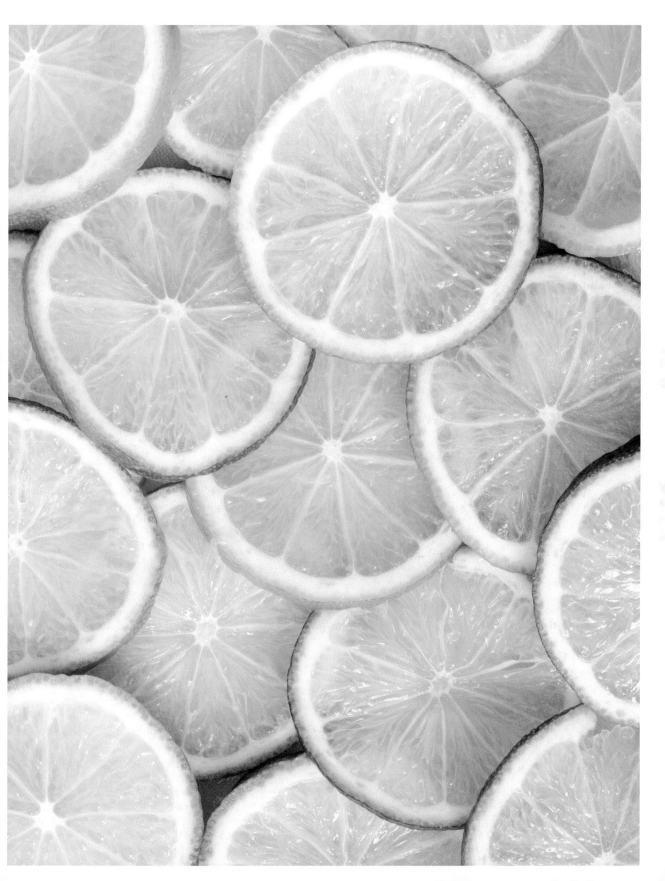

CORN TORTILLAS:

4 white or yellow corn tortillas

Vegetable oil, such as grapeseed or rice bran

TOPPINGS:

3 ounces (85 g) shredded cheese (we recommend half sharp Cheddar and half Monterey Jack)

⅛ head iceberg lettuce, shredded

1 cup (240 ml) Salsa Fresca (page 80)

Lactose-free sour cream, for garnish

Chopped scallions, green parts only, for garnish

Chopped fresh cilantro or flat-leaf parsley, for garnish

Have ready a baking sheet lined with aluminum foil or parchment paper and a triple stack of paper towels to receive the fried corn tortillas.

Prepare the peppers: Heat a 10- to 12-inch (25 to 30.5 cm) skillet over medium heat; add the oil and peppers and sauté over medium heat until the peppers are soft, stirring occasionally, for about 5 minutes. Very lightly season with salt and black pepper and transfer to a heatproof dish; cover with aluminum foil to keep warm.

While the peppers are cooking, prepare the chicken: Toss the chicken together with the cilantro and lime juice and season to taste with salt and black pepper; set aside.

Preheat the broiler to high and arrange a rack 3 to 4 inches from the broiler (top position in most ovens).

When the peppers are done, simply wipe the pan clean with a paper towel and place back on the stove top. Add vegetable oil to a depth of 1 inch (2.5 cm) and heat until the oil begins to shimmer. (If you want to double-check the oil temperature, simply tear an extra tortilla and drop in a piece. The oil should bubble up around the tortilla.) Fry two corn tortillas at a time until just turning light golden brown on the bottom; flip over with tongs, and cook the second side until light golden brown, for about 2 minutes total. Remove with tongs and drain on paper towels; repeat with the remaining tortillas.

Place the tortillas on the prepared sheet pan. Divide the peppers evenly centered on top of the tortillas, followed by the chicken, then the cheese. Place under the broiler and broil until the cheese is melted, for about 1 minute. Remove from the oven and quickly top with the shredded lettuce and salsa, again dividing evenly. Dollop sour cream on top; sprinkle with scallion greens and cilantro. Use a broad spatula to remove from the pan and serve immediately.

KATE'S NOTES

For a bit lighter fare, reduce the fat in the tortillas: try baking them instead. I personally love baked tortillas best. Preheat the oven to 350°F (180°C). Either brush the tortillas lightly with canola oil on both sides or spray with an oil mister. Place on ungreased baking sheets and bake for 8 to 10 minutes, or until crisp.

POST-FODMAP CHALLENGE PHASE OPTION

Fructan: If you passed the fructan onion challenge, you can add half a medium-size white or yellow onion, chopped, to the oil while sautéing the peppers, increasing the oil by 1 teaspoon.

Tofu & Greens

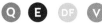 **MAKES 4 SERVINGS**

If you're looking for a lean and clean dinner, this recipe is for you. The tofu and bok choy offer a nice dose of nondairy calcium and vitamins A and C. While the volume of the spinach will seem like a lot at first, rest assured it cooks down to a manageable amount in less than a minute. In fact, if you have already made the rice (we suggest brown rice), this dish will come together in about 20 minutes. Note two things about the tofu: You want to buy extra-firm, and also containers seem to vary by a couple of ounces, depending on the brand. This latter ends up being insignificant, so don't worry. You do need Garlic-Infused Oil (page 68) for this dish.

---

1 (14- to 16-ounce [400 to 455 g]) container extra-firm tofu

3 tablespoons low-sodium soy sauce or tamari (use gluten-free if necessary)

1 tablespoon toasted sesame oil

1 tablespoon rice vinegar

2 tablespoons Garlic-Infused Oil, prepared with vegetable oil or preferably peanut oil, or purchased garlic-infused vegetable oil

3 tablespoons chopped scallion, green parts only

1 tablespoon grated fresh ginger

2½ cups (253 g) chopped bok choy (about 4 large stalks), tough stem ends removed, cut crosswise into ½-inch (12 mm) pieces, including tender stalks and leaves

8 ounces (225 g) baby spinach leaves

Cooked brown rice, to serve

Create a triple layer of paper towels on a cutting board. Slice the block of tofu into ¾-inch (2 cm) slabs and place side by side in one layer on the paper towels. Place a triple layer of towels on top of the tofu and top with another cutting board or a large, flat tray (such as a baking sheet). Weigh down the board or sheet with something heavy, such as canned goods. Allow the tofu to press for 10 minutes while you prep the sauce and vegetables.

Whisk the soy sauce, sesame oil, and vinegar together in a small bowl; set aside and have a pastry brush handy. Cut each slab of tofu into three smaller slabs (each piece will be about 3 x 1½ inches [7.5 x 4 cm]).

Heat a 12-inch (30.5 cm) nonstick skillet over medium-high heat, add 1 tablespoon of the Garlic-Infused Oil, and add the tofu once the oil is sizzling hot. Allow the tofu to cook for several minutes, until golden brown on the bottom. Flip over and cook for a few more minutes, until the second

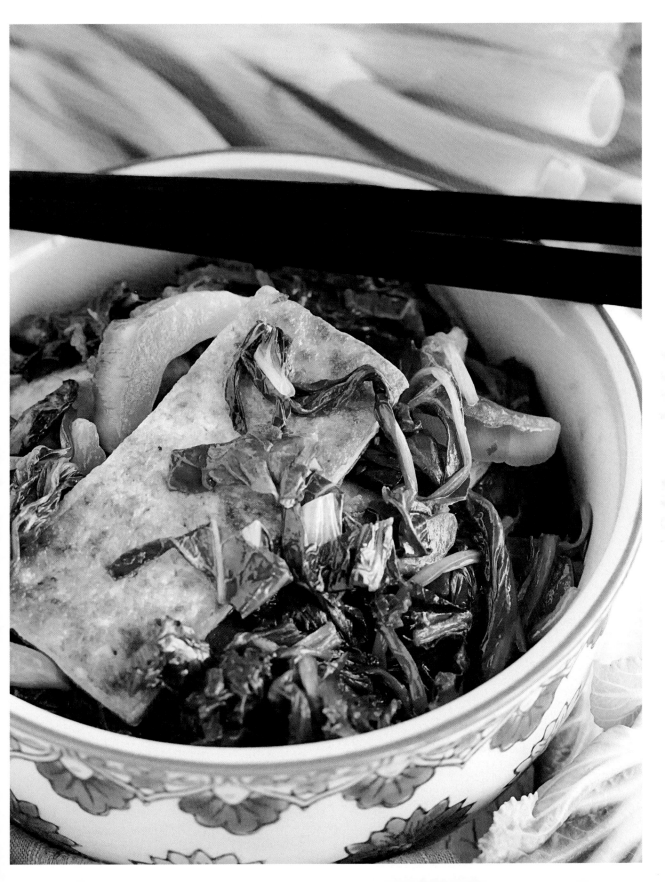

side is golden brown. Transfer the tofu to a cutting board. Brush the tofu with some of the soy sauce mixture; set aside.

Heat the remaining tablespoon of the Garlic-Infused Oil in the pan over medium heat. Add the scallion greens and ginger and sauté for about 1 minute, or until softened and fragrant. Increase the heat to medium high, add the bok choy, and toss around for about 30 seconds to coat, then add the spinach (it will look like a lot) and most of the remainder of the sauce and toss to coat and cook. Keep stirring and the spinach will cook down within a minute. Cook the greens just until the bok choy is crisp-tender, about 1 to 2 minutes more. Add the tofu and any remaining sauce to the pan to reheat, tossing gently with the greens. Serve immediately with brown rice.

DÉDÉ'S TIPS

If you like things spicy, pass FODMAP-approved hot sauce or sambal oelek at the table and add to taste. These are both spicy chile sauces that last for months in the fridge. If you seek out the sambal, read the ingredients label and make sure your version does not contain onion or garlic. It should be easy to find some made with just chiles and salt and sometimes vinegar.

POST-FODMAP CHALLENGE PHASE OPTION

Fructan: If you passed the fructan garlic challenge, you can add one to two garlic cloves, finely chopped, along with the ginger and scallion greens, and use regular vegetable oil in the various steps of the recipe.

Slow-Roasted Pork Tacos with Citrus Slaw & Chipotle Mayo

 MAKES 8 TACOS | SERVING SIZE 2 TACOS

This recipe is built around our Slow-Roasted Shredded Pork (page 297) and our Chipotle Peppers in Adobe Sauce (page 82), which you do have to make first. Here the moist, flavorful pork is nestled within crispy homemade taco shells (baked, not fried), a bright, zingy and crispy citrus-accented coleslaw is piled on top, and the whole shebang is drizzled with a spicy chipotle mayonnaise. Get ready for contrasting textures, temperatures, and flavors that will make your mouth and tummy very happy. There is no getting around the fact that these tacos are a mess to eat. Put out a roll of paper towels and roll up your sleeves.

CHIPOTLE MAYO:

½ cup (113 g) mayonnaise

1½ tablespoons Chipotle Chiles in Adobo Sauce (page 82)

1½ teaspoons freshly squeezed lime juice

CITRUS SLAW:

2 cups (140 g) finely shredded green cabbage (do not use savoy)

2 cups (140 g) finely shredded red cabbage

2 navel oranges

2 tablespoons chopped scallion, green parts only

1 tablespoon freshly squeezed lime juice

1½ teaspoons Garlic-Infused Oil (page 68) made with vegetable oil, or purchased garlic-infused vegetable oil

1 tablespoon chopped fresh cilantro

Kosher salt

Freshly ground black pepper

TACOS:

8 white or yellow corn tortillas

Vegetable oil, nonstick spray, or vegetable oil in an oil mister

2 cups (250 g) shredded pork from the Slow-Roasted Shredded Pork (page 297)

Half a firm, ripe Hass avocado, peeled, pitted, and thinly sliced (optional)

Prepare the chipotle mayo: Simply whisk together the mayonnaise, chopped chipotle chiles, and lime juice in a small bowl. The ingredients should be thoroughly combined and the texture should be thick but fluid; set aside. May be prepared up to 3 days ahead and refrigerated in an airtight container. (Make double and use on sandwiches!)

Prepare the citrus slaw: Toss the green and red cabbage together in a mixing bowl. Section the oranges as follows: use a sharp knife to slice off the stem end and opposite end of one orange. Place the orange, on one cut end, on a cutting board and then use knife to slice down around the sides to cut away all the peel and white pith, reserving as much juicy flesh as possible; save any juice. You should be able to see the membranes that sandwich each segment; they look like white lines. Use the length of the knife to cut into the orange on the left side of a membrane, going all the way to the center. Now go to the left of that segment and cut into the orange on the right side of the next membrane. Wiggle the knife a little and that segment should release. Work your way around the orange, cutting along the membranes, which you will discard, and releasing the tender segments. Chop the segments and add to cabbage along with the scallion greens. Repeat with the second orange. Measure out 2 tablespoons of the reserved orange juice into a small bowl. Whisk the lime juice and oil into the orange juice and pour over the slaw. Stir in the cilantro and season to taste with salt and pepper; set aside. The slaw can be used right away, but it is even better if allowed to sit for about 1 or 2 hours.

Prepare the tacos: Wrap the tortillas in a paper towel and "steam" in a microwave on high for 20 to 30 seconds, or just until warm and pliable. Alternatively, you can wrap in foil and heat on a center rack in a 375°F (190°C) oven for about 5 minutes. The tacos should be heated close to serving time.

If the pork is not hot, reheat as desired. You can place in a pan, sprinkle with a little water, cover with foil, and heat in a 250°F (120°C) oven until hot, or place in a microwave-safe dish, sprinkle with water, cover, and microwave at 50% power until hot.

Place about ½ cup (63 g) of hot shredded pork on each tortilla, top with slaw (drained of any excess liquid), and drizzle with chipotle mayonnaise. Top with a slice or two of avocado, if desired. Serve immediately.

POST-FODMAP CHALLENGE PHASE OPTION

Fructan: If you passed the fructan onion challenge, consider using 2 tablespoons of chopped red onion instead of the scallion greens in the recipe.

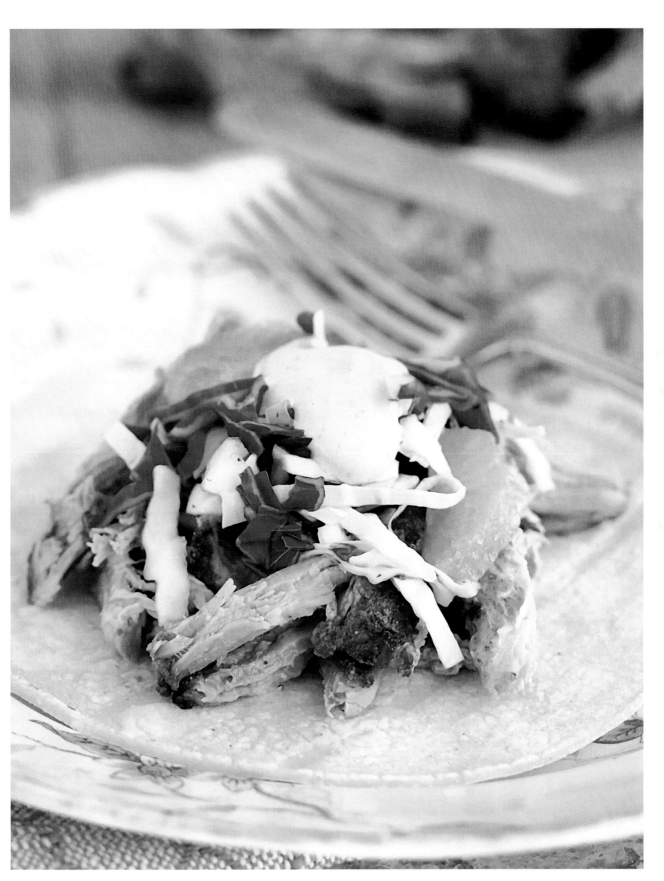

Cheese-Stuffed Turkey Burgers

    MAKES 4 BURGERS | SERVING SIZE 1 BURGER

Beef burgers (page 220) will never completely leave our dinner rotation, but we like these ground turkey–based burgers as a lighter option. Although we like our classic beef burgers a bit pink, you have to cook turkey burgers all the way through, so be patient. Some folks think they don't like turkey burgers, claiming that they are dry and flavorless. Our inclusion of shredded veggies right along with the turkey, and a stuffed center of goat cheese, simply banishes that problem forever.

---

1 pound (455 g) ground turkey

¼ cup (38 g) finely grated zucchini

2 tablespoons grated red bell pepper (yes, use your box grater!)

1 tablespoon finely chopped scallion, green parts only

1 teaspoon Garlic-Infused Oil (page 68) or Onion-Infused Oil (see variation, page 68) made with olive oil, or purchased versions

¼ teaspoon dried thyme

Kosher salt

Freshly ground black pepper

2 ounces (57 g) very cold soft goat cheese, such as Montrachet

4 low FODMAP buns, plain or toasted, or toasted English muffins (use gluten-free if necessary)

Prepared mustard (use gluten-free if necessary)

Ketchup (limit to 1 tablespoon)

Mayonnaise

Sliced tomato

Lettuce

Place the turkey, zucchini, red bell pepper, scallion greens, oil, and thyme in a mixing bowl. Season liberally with salt and black pepper. Use your hands to combine, then form into four equal-size balls. Press a quarter of the cheese into the center of each ball and then form burger patties, about 1 inch (2.5 cm) thick, making sure the cheese is enclosed in the center. The burgers may be refrigerated at this point up to overnight in an airtight container.

Heat a skillet (we like nonstick or cast-iron for these) until very hot. Add the burgers and cook over medium heat until well browned on the bottom, for 4 to 5 minutes. You will be able to see the meat cooking through from along the sides. Flip over and cook the other side for 4 to 5 minutes longer, or until the burgers are cooked through. You can also broil these burgers or grill them outside. Just watch your heat source and cook until the turkey is cooked through.

Serve immediately on buns, if desired, and with low FODMAP condiments and veggies of choice, such as sliced tomato and/or lettuce.

Stuffed Swiss Chard

  MAKES 10 SWISS CHARD BUNDLES | SERVING SIZE 2 TO 3 BUNDLES

This beef and rice–stuffed dish is a takeoff on the classic sweet-and-sour stuffed cabbage. Regular green and red cabbage are low FODMAP approved and could be used, but the Swiss chard is a low FODMAP nutritional powerhouse, a great source of vitamins A, C, and K, and magnesium, too. The chard leaves are softened in boiling water and some of the chopped stems are used in the filling for crunch, also minimizing waste. The rice can be white or brown—we prefer brown—or you could even use quinoa. For that matter, you could use ground turkey or chicken in lieu of the ground beef! You've got flexibility here. The stuffed rolls can even be made up to two days ahead and the flavors improve even more. This dish works well as a plated appetizer or as a main dish for lunch or dinner.

10 large, unblemished Swiss or rainbow chard leaves

1 tablespoon plus 1 teaspoon Garlic-Infused Oil (page 68) prepared with olive oil, or purchased garlic-infused olive oil

1 cup (64 g) finely chopped scallion, green parts only, divided

1 pound (455 g) ground beef, your choice of fat level

¼ teaspoon dried thyme

Kosher salt

Freshly ground black pepper

1¾ cups cooked brown or white rice (298 g), or quinoa (322 g), hot or room temperature

1 (28-ounce [794 g]) can crushed tomatoes (without garlic or onion)

¼ cup (54 g) firmly packed light brown sugar

2 tablespoons red wine vinegar

Wash and dry the Swiss chard. Place each leaf flat on a work surface and remove the stems from the area extending beyond the leaf. If the stem end that is still intact within the leaves is tough and inflexible, remove a few inches (8 cm) of those as well. The leaves must be able to be rolled up without tearing. Finely chop the removed stems to equal ¾ cup (75 g) and set aside; discard the rest.

Bring a large pot of water (large enough to receive the leaves) to a boil. Use tongs to lower the leaves into the boiling water one at a time and blanch for about 5 seconds. Remove with tongs and set aside on a work surface as you continue to blanch the remaining leaves.

Heat a large, deep, nonreactive skillet over medium heat. Add 2 teaspoons of the oil to the pan and swirl to coat. Add ½ cup (32 g) of the scallion greens and sauté until soft, for about 2 minutes.

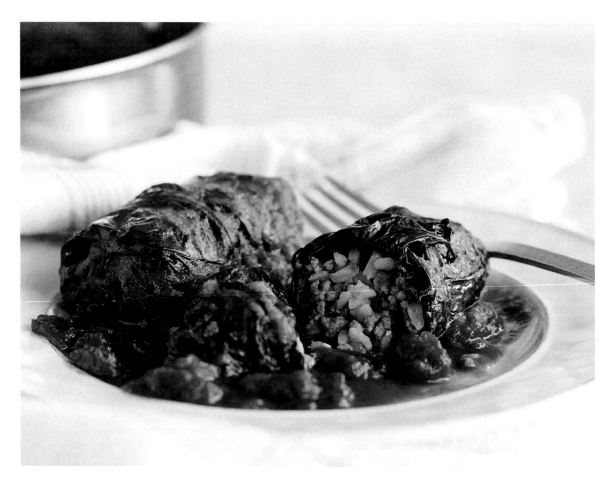

Add the ¾ cup (75 g) of chopped Swiss chard stems and the beef. Use a spatula to chop up the beef. Add the thyme and season well with salt and pepper. Sauté the mixture just until the beef is no longer pink and the chard has softened, for about 3 minutes. Drain the mixture in a colander and place in a mixing bowl. Stir in the cooked rice until combined and set aside.

Wipe out the skillet (no need to wash) and heat over medium heat. Add the remaining 2 teaspoons of oil to the pan and swirl to coat. Add the remaining ½ cup (32 g) of the scallion greens and sauté until soft, for about 2 minutes. Stir in the tomatoes, brown sugar, and vinegar until combined and bring to a simmer. Cover with a splatter guard or partially cover with a lid and simmer for 10 minutes. Season to taste with salt and pepper.

While the sauce is simmering, create the stuffed Swiss chard bundles. Take one blanched chard leaf and place, smooth side down, on a work surface. Place about ⅓ cup (70 g) of the filling just above the broad base of the leaf. Roll the base of the leaf up and over the filling, fold in the sides, and then continue to roll the bundle all the way to the top. Place, seam side down, on another work surface. Repeat with the remaining chard and filling. When the sauce is finished simmering, nestle the chard bundles in the sauce, seam side down, and spoon some of the sauce over the bundles. Cover the skillet and simmer over medium heat for 20 minutes. The stuffed Swiss chard is ready to serve, or allow to cool to room temperature and refrigerate, in a single layer, in their sauce, in an airtight container for up to 2 days. Transfer the bundles carefully to a skillet to be reheated along with the sauce or reheat in the microwave at 50% power (watch for the tomato sauce splashing)!

POST-FODMAP CHALLENGE PHASE OPTIONS

Fructans: If you passed the fructan garlic challenge, sauté one or two garlic cloves, finely chopped, along with the scallion greens.

If you passed the fructan onion challenge, you may substitute 1 cup (142 g) of finely chopped white or yellow onion, or to your tolerance, for the scallion greens.

Vietnamese Summer Rolls with Shrimp or Tofu

 MAKES 12 SUMMER ROLLS | SERVES 6 FOR LIGHT LUNCH

Summer rolls differ from fried spring rolls in that these feature a rice wrapper and they are not fried. Fillings can vary from pork, shrimp, or both, but they always contain fresh herbs, some veggies, and chewy rice noodles. Our version includes avocado and shrimp, with an easy tofu option. (There is enough shrimp and tofu to make a full recipe, so if you make some of each you will have leftover shrimp and tofu.) They make a very satisfying lunch or light meal on a hot summer's day and can even be served as an appetizer. We have given you a choice of two dipping sauces and we recommend that you make both, but feel free to choose one if time is short. Make sure all of your fillings are prepped before you start assembly. Don't be put off by the lengthy directions; they are there to help you have success the first time you make these.

PEANUT DIPPING SAUCE:

½ cup (129 g) natural peanut butter

½ cup (120 ml) 100% canned pure light unsweetened coconut milk, such as Thai Kitchen brand

¼ cup (54 g) firmly packed light brown sugar

2 tablespoons freshly squeezed lime juice

2 teaspoons Asian fish sauce (use gluten-free if necessary)

TANGY LIME DIPPING SAUCE:

¼ cup (54 g) firmly packed light brown sugar

2 tablespoons very hot water

¼ cup (60 ml) Asian fish sauce (use gluten-free if necessary)

¼ cup (60 ml) freshly squeezed lime juice

1 small fresh red Thai bird chile or ½ jalapeño pepper, stem removed, thinly sliced

FOR ASSEMBLY:

2½ ounces (70 g) thin rice vermicelli noodles

12 (8½-inch [22 cm]) rice paper wrappers

18 large shrimp (26/30), cooked, peeled, and deveined, cut in half lengthwise; or 12 ounces (340 g) firm tofu, drained, cut into ¼-inch (6 mm)-thick slabs about 1½ x 4 inches (4 x 10 cm)

12 small to medium-size Bibb or Boston lettuce leaves, washed and dried, large ribs removed

½ ripe but firm Hass avocado, peeled, pitted, and cut into 12 thin slices

1 large carrot, peeled, sliced into 4-inch (10 cm) julienne strips

½ English cucumber, peeled, seeded, and sliced into 4-inch (10 cm) julienne strips

36 medium-size to large fresh mint leaves, stemmed, washed, and dried

Prepare the peanut dipping sauce: Whisk together the peanut butter, coconut milk, and brown sugar in a mixing bowl until smooth. Whisk in the lime juice and fish sauce until combined and smooth. The sauce is ready to use, or you can refrigerate in an airtight container for up to 2 days. Bring to room temperature before serving.

Prepare the tangy lime dipping sauce: Stir together the brown sugar and very hot water in a small mixing bowl until the sugar dissolves. Whisk in the fish sauce, lime juice, and sliced chile. Allow to sit for at least 15 minutes for the flavors to meld. The sauce is ready to use, or you can refrigerate it in an airtight container for up to 2 days. Bring to room temperature before serving.

Prepare the rice noodles: Place the noodles in a large bowl. Pour warm water over them to cover. Allow the noodles to sit for about 30 to 45 minutes or until softened and pliable. Drain well.

To assemble: Have a wide, shallow bowl (we use a large pie plate) filled with room-temperature water next to your work surface, with paper towels handy. Take one wrapper and submerge it flat in the water for about 1 minute, or until very pliable. Remove from the bowl with two hands, taking care not to rip it. Let as much excess water as possible drip back into the bowl. Lay the wrapper flat on your work surface and use a balled-up clean paper towel to gently blot away any excess water but do not blot completely dry; the moisture is going to help the wrap stick to itself in the end.

Add the fillings as follows: If using shrimp, lay three halves, cut side up and slightly overlapping, about 2 inches in from the edge farthest from you, on the center portion of the wrapper. If using tofu, put it in that same place instead of the shrimp. Now, just below your protein (nearer toward you), place a lettuce leaf, folded to fit (it can be a bit larger than the shrimp or tofu), or trimmed if necessary. Place a portion of drained rice noodles (the amount should be a little thicker than a hot dog) along the length of the lettuce. Top the noodles with a slice of avocado, three or four carrot strips, three or four strips of cucumber, and finally, three mint leaves.

Dip the fingertips of both hands in the water, shake dry, and gently bring the left and right sides of the wrapper inward; they probably won't meet and that's okay. Lift the edge of the wrapper closest to you up and over the vegetable filling, keeping the sides tucked in. Now, make one complete rotation of the roll toward the top of the wrapper; this will bring the enclosed vegetables up and over the shrimp or tofu and then adhere any extra wrapper to the roll. You should now be able to see the shrimp or tofu through one layer of wrapper and you can present this side up, as it is the most decorative. Place, seam side down, on a platter. Do not let the finished rolls touch one another as they will stick together. If your fingers stick to the wrappers, redip in water. Repeat with the remaining wrappers and filling—we like to make some rolls with shrimp and some with tofu.

After you make the first one, you will have a sense of whether you were overstuffing or under-stuffing your roll. You will get better at making them with experience. You do want the roll to be taut, but not so tightly rolled so that the fillings tear through the wrapper.

The rolls may be made up to 2 hours ahead and kept at room temperature. Drape a damp paper towel over your finished rolls and cover that with a sheet of plastic wrap.

You can serve whole or slice the rolls in half to expose the colorful filling. Place on a serving platter with the dipping sauce(s), poured into individual bowls, alongside.

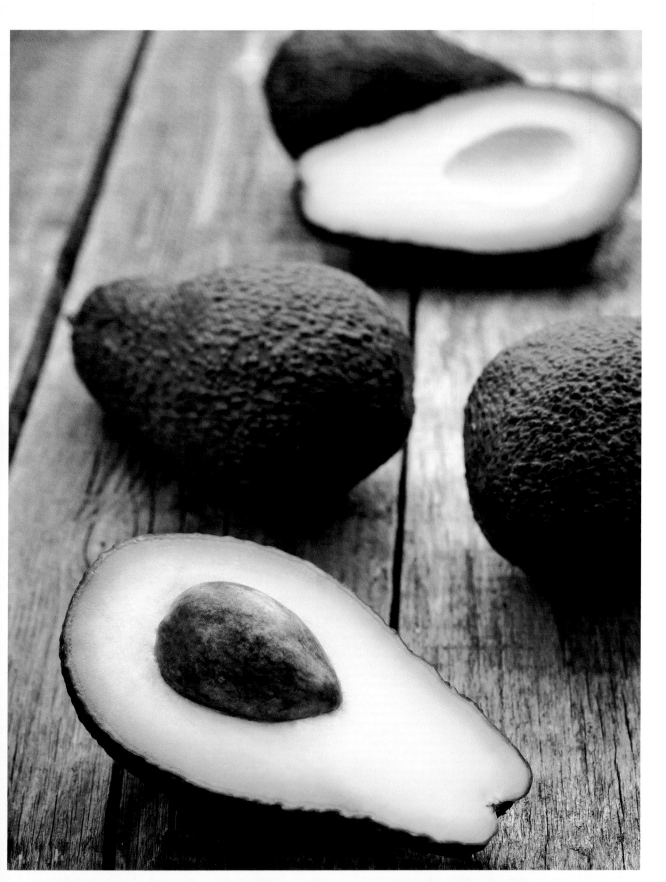

Pan-Seared Salmon & Greens with Balsamic Glaze

   (DF)   **MAKES 2 SERVINGS**

Salmon is easy to prepare as well as packed with anti-inflammation boosting omega-3 fatty acids, which are good for our heart health and may reduce inflammation in the colon, too. Read the recipe through; this is easy to make but the steps should be followed quickly so that it all comes together hot in the end. You can make this dish in fifteen minutes! The recipe may be doubled. Consider offering cooked rice or baked potatoes to round out the meal.

---

2 (5- to 6-ounce (140 to 170 g) center-cut salmon fillets

Kosher salt

Freshly ground black pepper

Scant 3 tablespoons (42 g) balsamic vinegar

2 tablespoons of water

1 teaspoon firmly packed light brown sugar

1 tablespoons vegetable oil or Garlic-Infused Oil (page 68) made with vegetable oil, or purchased garlic-infused vegetable oil, divided

6 ounces (170 g) tender baby spinach, arugula, or kale

Pat the salmon dry with a paper towel and lightly season with salt and pepper. Stir together the vinegar, water, and the brown sugar; set aside.

Warm two dinner plates and set aside. Pour 1 teaspoon of the oil into a large, nonstick skillet, tilting to cover evenly, and heat over medium-high heat until shimmering. Sear the salmon, skin side down, for 2 to 4 minutes, or until the skin is crispy. Carefully turn the fish over and cook for 2 to 4 minutes more. We like to leave the very center of the flesh slightly pink, but you can cook it to your liking. Do not overcook the fish. Leaving the pan over medium-high heat, transfer the fish to the warmed dinner plates and cover loosely with foil while you cook the greens.

Quickly add the remaining 2 teaspoons of oil to the pan, still over medium-high heat. Add the greens and immediately use tongs to coat the greens in the hot oil. Shake the pan occasionally and cook until the greens cook down, for 1 to 2 minutes. Place the greens alongside the salmon on the warmed plates. Pour the vinegar mixture into the pan, still over medium-high heat; it should sizzle immediately. Swirl the pan around or use a silicone spatula to stir and cook for 30 seconds to 1 minute to slightly thicken and reduce the vinegar mixture to a glaze. Immediately pour the glaze over the fish and greens and serve immediately.

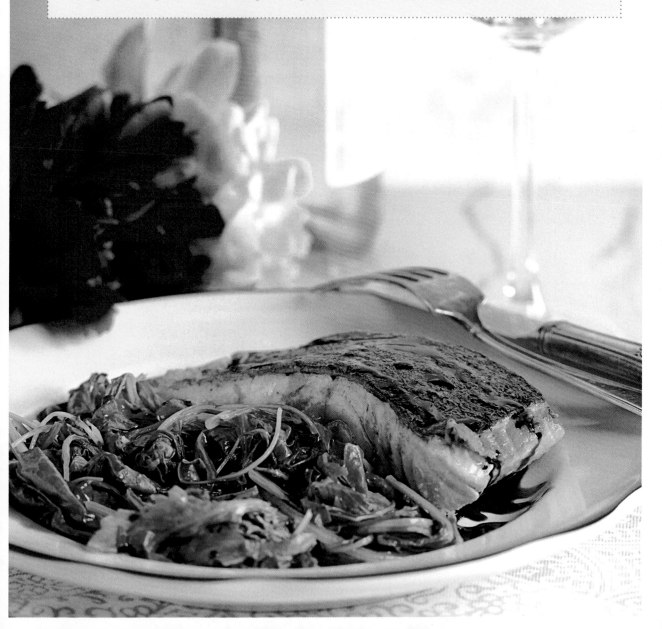

Shrimp & Grits

(E) MAKES 4 TO 6 SERVINGS

This recipe brings together our Cheesy Grits (page 172) and a quick-to-make shrimp dish with bell peppers, scallion greens, and fire-roasted tomatoes. And, by the way, we highly recommend that you keep some cans of fire-roasted tomatoes at hand. They are one of our favorite FODMAP-approved pantry items.

---

1 batch Cheesy Grits (page 172)

2 tablespoons Garlic-Infused Oil (page 68) made with vegetable oil, or purchased garlic-infused vegetable oil

½ cup (32 g) chopped scallion, green parts only

1 medium-size yellow or orange bell pepper, cored and diced

1 medium-size red bell pepper, cored and diced

2 pounds (910 g) large shrimp (26/30), peeled and deveined

1 (14.5-ounce [415 g]) can fire-roasted diced tomatoes (without garlic or onion), such as Muir Glen brand

Freshly ground black pepper

½ to 1 teaspoon hot sauce, such as Texas Pete's (use gluten-free if necessary)

2 tablespoons chopped fresh flat-leaf parsley

Have the grits ready to go, or if you are good at multitasking, make them simultaneously with the shrimp.

Heat the oil in a large sauté pan over medium heat. Add the scallion greens and all the peppers and sauté, stirring frequently, until soft but not browned, for 5 to 7 minutes. Stir in the shrimp and tomatoes. Cook until the shrimp turn opaque and pink all the way through, for 3 to 5 minutes. Taste and season with black pepper and hot sauce. Serve immediately over the hot grits.

POST-FODMAP CHALLENGE PHASE OPTIONS

Fructans: If you passed the fructan garlic challenge, consider adding one to two garlic cloves, finely chopped, along with the scallion greens and peppers and use plain vegetable oil.

If you passed the fructan onion challenge, consider using ½ cup (71 g) of finely chopped white or yellow onion instead of the scallion greens.

Weekday Meat Loaf

E MAKES 8 SERVINGS

We call this Weekday Meat Loaf because it can be mixed together in less time than it takes for the oven to preheat, and while it does have to cook for an hour in the oven, it is completely unattended and gives you time to make the salad or sides, walk the dog, or make tomorrow's lunch—or just relax. Speaking of lunch, when was the last time you had a meat loaf sandwich? With some low FODMAP bread (use gluten-free if necessary) and a schmear of mayo or mustard, plus some lettuce and tomato, this is one satisfying midday meal. You can probably get a couple of meals and a lunch out of this one very simple but tasty dish. The sauce is baked on as well as served alongside; any extra can be used on those sandwiches, too. This main dish will make it into your regular rotation.

SAUCE:

½ cup (120 ml) ketchup (without high-fructose corn syrup, such as Simply Heinz or low FODMAP FODY Food Co.)

¼ cup (54 g) firmly packed light brown sugar

1 tablespoon plus 1 teaspoon balsamic vinegar

MEAT LOAF:

¾ cup (84 g) purchased, dry gluten-free bread crumbs (see Dédé's Tips)

½ cup (120 ml) lactose-free milk (whole, 2%, 1%, or fat-free)

2 pounds (910 g) ground beef, preferably 80%; 1½ pounds (680 g) beef and ½ pound (225 g) ground pork; or part veal and part beef or pork (total should be 2 pounds [910 g])

2 large eggs, at room temperature

⅓ cup (11 g) finely chopped fresh flat-leaf parsley

⅓ cup (22 g) finely chopped scallion, green parts only

2 teaspoons Garlic-Infused Oil (page 68) made with olive oil, or purchased garlic-infused olive oil

1 teaspoon kosher salt

½ teaspoon dried thyme

Freshly ground black pepper

4 slices bacon (use gluten-free, if necessary)

Position a rack in the center of the oven. Preheat the oven to 350°F (180°C).

Prepare the sauce: Whisk all the sauce ingredients together in a small bowl; set aside.

Prepare the meat loaf: Stir together the bread crumbs and milk in a large mixing bowl and allow the bread crumbs to hydrate and soften for 5 minutes. Add the meat, eggs, parsley, scallion greens, olive oil, salt, thyme, and a generous amount of black pepper to the bread crumb mixture and use your hands to mix well. Form into a shallow oval loaf shape about 9 x 6 x 2 inches (23 x 15 x 5 cm) in a roasting pan. Pour about half of the sauce on top and spread around to coat the meat loaf; reserve the remaining sauce to serve alongside the cooked meat loaf. Drape the bacon over the meat loaf on the diagonal and tuck the ends underneath.

Bake for about 1 hour, or until the meat is firm and cooked through and the bacon is crisp. If you have an instant-read thermometer, use it to check the center of the meat, which should register 160°F (72°C). If the bacon isn't as crisp as you would like it, simply run the meat loaf under the broiler for a minute; watch carefully so as not to burn it. The meat loaf is ready to cut into slices and serve with the reserved sauce alongside, which is sort of like gussied-up ketchup. We like it hot, room temperature, or cold in a sandwich.

DÉDÉ'S TIPS

I like Gillian's Foods Original Bread Crumbs for this recipe, which contain only rice flour, water, yeast, salt, and cane sugar. You can use whatever low FODMAP bread crumb you like, but check the texture after sitting for 5 minutes combined with the milk. The mixture should be a somewhat moist paste. If the mixture is dry, add some more milk, a tablespoon at a time, until you have a moist mixture, then proceed as directed.

POST-FODMAP CHALLENGE PHASE OPTION

Fructan: If you passed the fructan onion challenge, consider using ⅓ cup (48 g) of finely chopped white or yellow onion in lieu of the scallion greens.

Meatballs for Spaghetti or Subs

  GF MAKES 20 TO 25 GOLF BALL-SIZE (43 MM) MEATBALLS

Yes, you can have homemade spaghetti & meatballs or a meatball sub on a low FODMAP diet! As with so many of our Italian-inspired dishes, and most dishes requiring garlic, we turn to our trusty Garlic-Infused Oil (page 68) to provide a powerhouse of flavor. Along with suitable gluten-free bread crumbs and a good dose of either Pecorino Romano or Parmigiano-Reggiano, these meatballs have all the taste of the classic rendition but are low FODMAP. For a lower-fat, baked version, see the directions.

⅓ cup (38 g) gluten-free bread crumbs, such as Gillian's Foods Original Bread Crumbs

½ cup (120 ml) warm water

1 large egg

½ cup (50 g) finely grated Pecorino Romano or Parmigiano-Reggiano cheese

1 tablespoon minced fresh flat-leaf parsley

1 pound (455 g) lean ground beef, such as 85% lean; or ½ pound (225 g) lean ground

beef, ¼ pound (115 g) ground veal, and ¼ pound (115 g) ground pork

½ teaspoon kosher salt

⅛ teaspoon freshly ground black pepper

About ⅓ cup (75 ml) Garlic-Infused Oil (page 68) made with olive oil, or purchased garlic-infused olive oil

1 batch Quick Tomato Sauce (page 72)

Combine the bread crumbs and water in a large bowl and allow to sit for about 5 minutes, or until the bread crumbs swell and hydrate. Add the egg, cheese, and parsley and mix thoroughly to combine, then add the meat and mix well (we like to do this with our hands). Season with salt and pepper. Roll into golf ball-size (43 mm) meatballs (see Dédé's Tips) and set aside on a tray until all are rolled. (The meatballs can be shaped and refrigerated 1 day in advance. Simply cover with plastic wrap.)

Heat about a third of the oil in a sauté pan over medium heat until hot but not smoking. Add about a third of the meatballs and fry until the bottoms are golden; flip over and brown the other side. Transfer to a paper towel–lined tray and repeat with two more batches of oil and meatballs.

Alternatively, preheat the oven to 350°F (180°C). Scatter the meatballs, evenly spaced, on a rimmed baking pan. Bake for 30 minutes, shaking the pan gently once or twice during the baking time. Drain on paper towels.

The meatballs are somewhat rare at this point, whether you fried or baked them, and should finish cooking in the tomato sauce.

Heat the tomato sauce in a large, wide saucepan and place the meatballs in the sauce in a single layer. Use two pots if necessary. Bring the sauce to a low simmer, cover, and cook the meatballs for about 10 minutes, or until cooked through and heated. The meatballs are now ready to serve with spaghetti or use for a sub sandwich.

DÉDÉ'S TIPS

To roll the meatballs, you can use a small ice-cream scoop (I like to use my trusty #40 Zeroll scoop). Simply dip the scoop into the meatball mixture to overfill the scoop. Scrape the scoop along the edge of the bowl to create a consistent amount. Pop the meatball out into your hand and round it off with a few quick turns. All your meatballs will be the same size, looking very professional and will cook evenly.

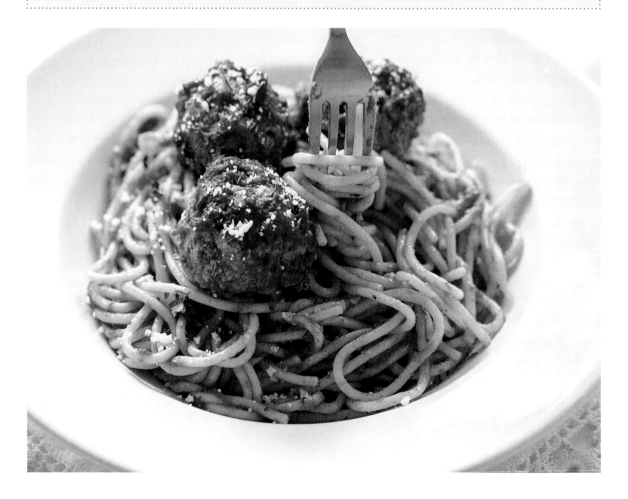

Tomato Basil Pizza

 MAKES TWO 11-INCH PIZZAS (28 CM) PIZZAS | SERVES 3 TO 6

This pizza is a thin-crusted version, crispy and a bit chewy, with a light topping of home-made sauce, sliced fresh tomatoes, mozzarella, and fresh basil. Start the crust about 2½ hours before you want to eat if making start to finish all at once, but we also give you do-ahead tips where you can freeze the partially baked crust. While the crust is rising, you will have plenty of time to make our quick pizza sauce (or you can prepare that way ahead as well). The yeast-raised crust is baked twice at high heat. The first stint sets the crust and provides maximum crispness. The second, shorter baking period is just enough to heat the sauce, melt the cheese, and finish off the crust to a golden brown. In a pinch, consider using a suitable frozen gluten-free crust. We like Udi's Gluten Free Pizza Crust. Follow the directions on the package and feel free to use our Quick Tomato Sauce (page 72). Read the recipe through so you are ready for all of the steps, some of which have to flow pretty quickly in succession.

SAUCE:

1 (28-ounce [794 g]) can crushed or ground peeled tomatoes (without garlic or onion), such as Muir Glen brand

1 tablespoon extra-virgin olive oil

1 teaspoon kosher salt

½ teaspoon dried oregano

Pinch of sugar

CRUST:

Extra-virgin olive oil

2⅔ cups (13.3 ounces; 377 g) gluten-free all-purpose flour, such as Bob's Red Mill Gluten Free 1 to 1 Baking Flour, plus more for dusting

1½ cups (360 ml) warm water (110°F [42°C] is perfect)

⅛ teaspoon sugar

1 tablespoon plus 1 teaspoon active dry yeast

2 teaspoons baking powder (use gluten-free if necessary)

1 teaspoon salt

1 teaspoon xanthan gum

2 teaspoons cider vinegar or white vinegar

FOR ASSEMBLY:

3 plum tomatoes, cored, sliced vertically into ⅛-inch (3 mm) slices, drained lightly on paper towels (optional)

12 ounces (340 g) mozzarella cheese (whole- or skim milk), shredded

15 to 20 fresh basil leaves

Prepare the sauce: Stir together the crushed tomatoes, olive oil, salt, oregano, and sugar in a medium-size nonreactive saucepan and bring to a simmer over medium heat. Cover and simmer, stirring occasionally, for 10 minutes, until slightly thickened. Remove from the heat and allow to cool completely before using. This makes about 2½ cups (600 ml) of sauce. You can make this up to 1 week ahead and refrigerate in an airtight container or freeze for up to 1 month. Bring back to room temperature before using.

Prepare the crust: You can make this by hand or in a stand mixer fitted with a flat paddle attachment. Coat two heavy-duty aluminum rimmed half sheet pans (18 x 13 inches [46 x 33 cm]) and generously coat with olive oil. Line each pan with a piece of parchment paper cut to fit (laying it over the olive oil), lightly flour the top of the parchment, and set aside.

By hand: Measure the warm water in a measuring cup with spout and stir in the sugar. Stir in the yeast and allow to proof for 5 minutes (the yeast will hydrate, become puffy, and expand). Meanwhile whisk together the flour, baking powder, salt, and xanthan gum in a large mixing bowl, to aerate and combine. Once the yeast has proofed, slowly pour the yeast mixture, 2 teaspoons of olive oil, and vinegar over the flour mixture, stirring with a sturdy wooden spoon until absorbed. Now, beat vigorously with a wooden spoon for several minutes, or until the mixture looks like a soft, somewhat wet batter with a little elasticity. It will not form a ball.

In a stand mixer: Measure the water in a measuring cup with spout and stir in the sugar. Stir in the yeast and allow to proof for 5 minutes (the yeast will hydrate, become puffy, and expand). Meanwhile place the flour, baking powder, salt, and xanthan gum in the bowl of a stand mixer fitted with a flat paddle attachment and pulse on and off to combine. Once the yeast has proofed, slowly pour the yeast mixture, 2 teaspoons of olive oil, and vinegar over the dry mixture and beat on medium speed for about 2 minutes, or until the mixture looks like a soft, somewhat wet batter with a little elasticity. It will not form a ball.

For both techniques, proceed as follows: Divide the dough in half and scrape each half onto the center of the parchment paper on a prepared pan, making a round mound. Put a little olive oil on your palms and fingers, and gently coat the balls with oil and coax them into a nice squat ball shape. Cover each dough ball with a piece of plastic wrap pressed right on the surface and place in a warm, draft-free area to rise for 1 hour.

If you haven't made your sauce yet, you can make it now.

After 1 hour, remove the plastic wrap, coat your fingers and palms with a little oil, and press each dough ball into an 11-inch (28 cm) round. Cover with clean plastic wrap and allow the dough to rise for about 20 more minutes while you preheat your oven. (You can hold the dough for up to 45 minutes at this point.)

Position two racks in the hottest areas of the oven. Preheat the oven to 475°F (240°C).

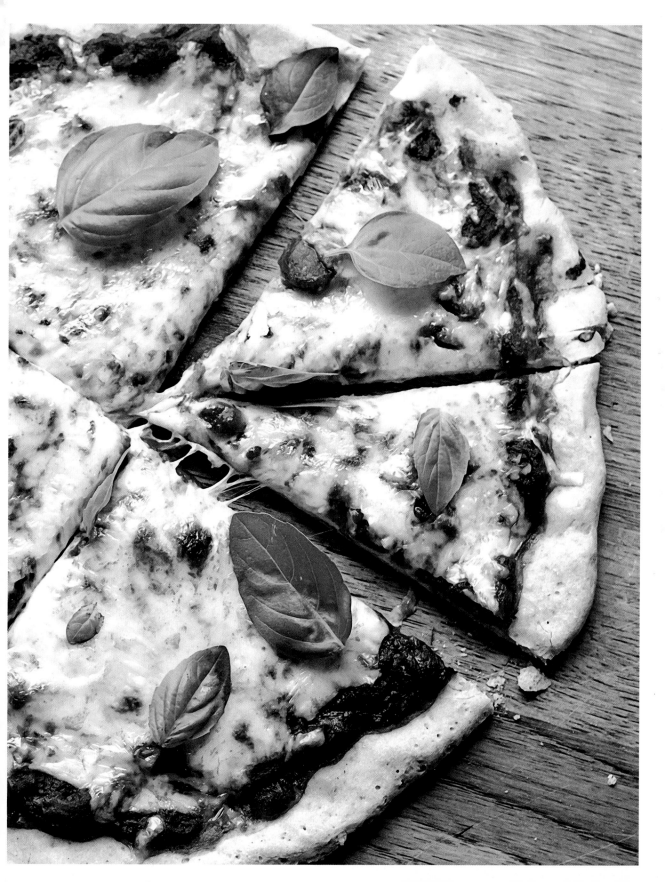

Bake the pizza crusts for 15 to 17 minutes, rotating front to back and from one rack to the other once during baking. The crust should have begun to take on a light golden color and you should be able to lift it from the parchment and feel a dry crust on the bottom that is beginning to crisp up. Go by these visual cues and make sure the crust has begun to "set" and taken on color, regardless of the time.

Taking care not to burn your fingers, quickly lift the crusts off the parchment paper and discard the papers. Place the crusts back on the oiled pans (remember how you oiled the pans under the parchment?) if you are finishing pizzas now. If you want to freeze these pizza crusts, allow them to cool at this point and see the instructions at the end of the recipe.

To assemble: Quickly, so that the pans retain heat, brush the edges of the crust with oil, then spread about ½ cup (120 ml) of the sauce over each crust, leaving about a ½-inch (12 mm) border of unsauced crust. Place the tomatoes here and there over the crusts, dividing equally, if using. Top with the cheese; you might use all of it, or three quarters of it might be enough for you. Bake for 6 to 8 minutes, or until the cheese is melted and beginning to bubble. Transfer the pizzas to a cutting board, scatter with fresh basil, cut into wedges, and serve immediately.

To freeze the crusts: Allow to cool completely, double wrap in plastic wrap, slip into an extra-large resealable plastic bag, and remove the air. Freeze for up to a month, making sure to keep them flat. To bake: Position the oven racks in the two hottest positions. Preheat the oven to 475°F (240°C). Preheat two rimmed baking sheets in the oven until very hot. Quickly brush the pans with some olive oil, then place the still-frozen crusts on the pans. Top with the sauce, tomatoes, if using, and cheese as directed in the main recipe. Bake until the cheese is melted and bubbling, perhaps for 5 minutes longer (maybe 10 to 15 minutes) than stated above. Scatter the basil on top, cut, and serve immediately.

POST-FODMAP CHALLENGE PHASE OPTION

Fructan: If you passed the fructan garlic option, consider adding one or two garlic cloves, finely chopped, to the tomato sauce mixture, if you like.

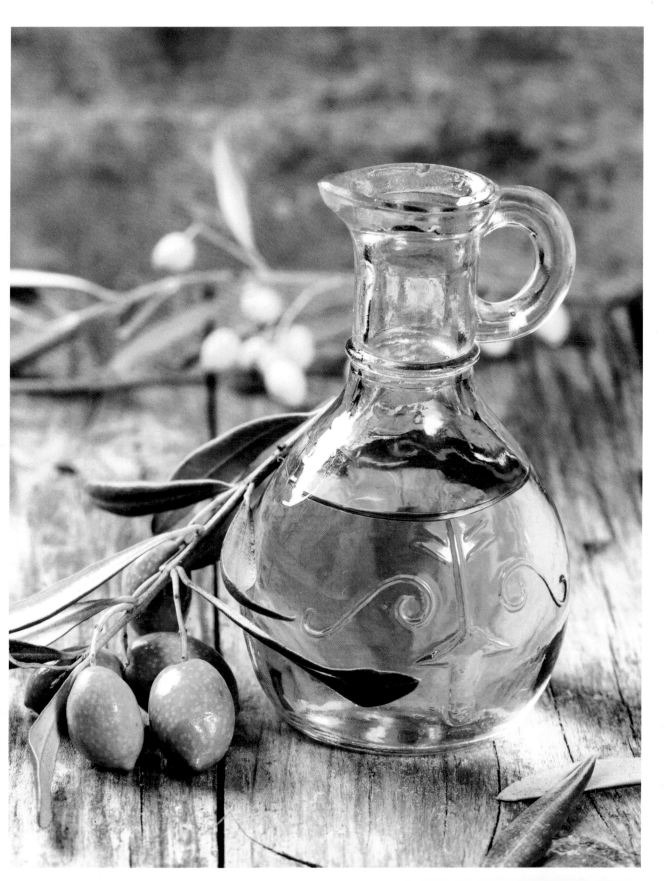

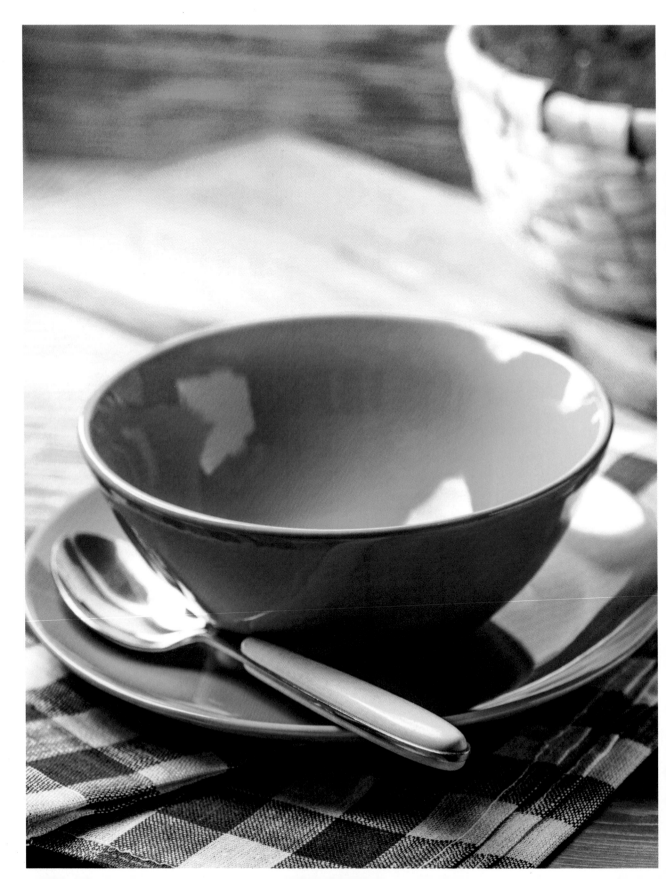

Chapter 11

HEARTY & NOURISHING SOUPS

SOUPS CAN BE THE ULTIMATE comfort food—warmth and sustenance in a bowl. Our low FODMAP choices abound, from Roasted Tomato Soup (page 258), Hearty Vegetable Soup (page 263), and classic Clam Chowder (page 261) to international favorites, such as Egg Drop Soup (page 265) and Tortilla Soup with Chicken & Lime (page 266). And we also have a cool, refreshing Gazpacho (page 272) for you. Looking for something rich and smooth? The Creamy Root Vegetable Soup (page 269) will satisfy your cravings.

Roasted Tomato Soup with Parmesan Crisps

 MAKES ABOUT 1 QUART (960 ML) | 8 SERVINGS

This tomato soup takes advantage of fresh summer plum tomatoes and further develops their flavor by roasting in a hot oven, which caramelizes and concentrates the sugars in the fruit. (Not only are they tasty, but tomatoes are rich in the powerful antioxidant lycopene, which is associated with bone and heart health benefits and linked with lowered cancer risk.) We do like to add a small amount of basil and oregano, but for some this creates a soup that veers flavor-wise into marinara sauce territory. If you want a pure tomato flavor, leave out the herbs. The Vegetable Broth (page 69) keeps this soup vegetarian and vegan (if you don't add the Parmesan crisps, of course). The Chicken Stock (page 70) makes for a slightly richer-flavored and -bodied soup.

The Parmesan Crisps have one ingredient, so you gotta make it good! Start with a hunk of true Parmigiano-Reggiano cheese and grate it yourself, for best results. Purchased pregrated cheese will make rubbery "crisps" and we do not recommend it.

SOUP:

4 pounds (1.8 kg) ripe plum tomatoes (12 to 14 medium-size)

3 tablespoons Garlic-Infused Oil (page 68) or Onion-Infused Oil (see variation, page 68), made with olive oil, or their purchased equivalents

2 teaspoons kosher salt

Freshly ground black pepper

1 to 2 teaspoons dried basil (optional)

1 to 2 teaspoons dried oregano (optional)

2 cups (480 ml) Vegetable Broth (page 69) or Chicken Stock (page 70), or prepared low FODMAP vegetable broth or chicken stock

PARMESAN CRISPS:

Nonstick spray (optional)

1 (2¼-ounce [65 g]) hunk Parmigiano-Reggiano cheese (¾ cup when grated)

Prepare the soup: Position a rack in the upper third of the oven. Preheat the oven to 400°F (200°C). Core the tomatoes and cut in half lengthwise. Place, cut side down, on a rimmed baking pan or large roasting pan. Drizzle with the olive oil and sprinkle with salt and generously with pepper. Sprinkle with the herbs, if using. Roast in the oven for 45 minutes; they should be

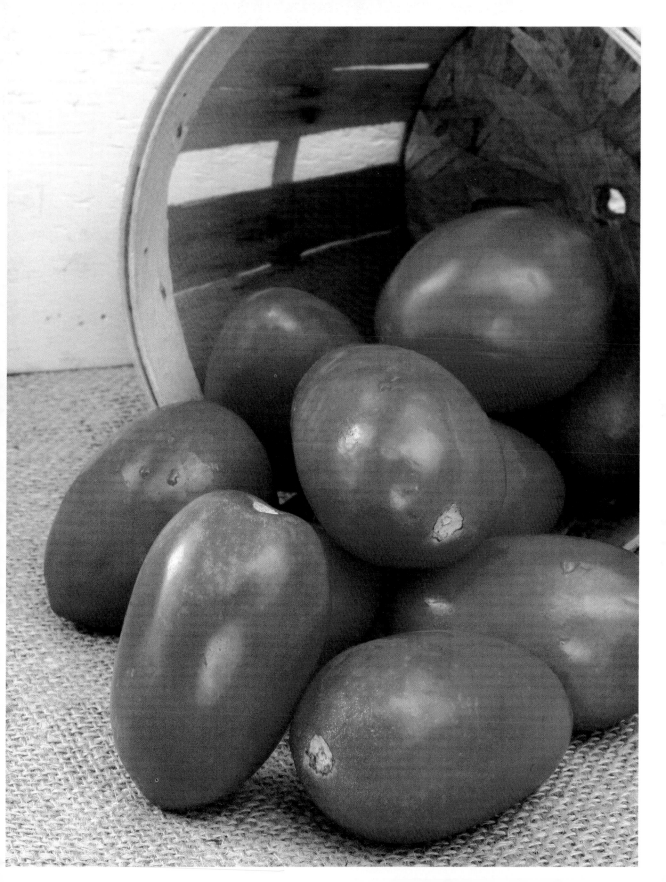

blackening in spots and exuding juice. Roast for 15 minutes more for a total of about 1 hour, or until the tomatoes are very soft and sport black spots here and there.

While the tomatoes are roasting, prepare the crisps: Line a baking sheet with parchment paper and coat with nonstick spray, or line with a silicone baking mat, which will not need to be sprayed. Space twelve equal-size mounds of cheese evenly apart on the prepared pan. Flatten each mound slightly.

As soon as the tomatoes come out of the oven, place the pan of cheese on the upper rack and bake for 3 to 6 minutes, or until the cheese has melted and become lacy and the crisps have turned light golden brown. Remove from the oven. Allow the crisps to cool for a minute or two, then use a sharp metal spatula to remove them from the pan. Stack carefully and set aside to serve with the soup.

Meanwhile, place a food mill fitted with medium blade over a deep, nonreactive saucepan. Scrape the tomatoes and all their juice into the food mill and press through the mill into the pot. Discard the seeds and skin left behind in the food mill. Alternatively, scrape the tomatoes and their juice into a deep, nonreactive saucepan and use an immersion blender to puree; or scrape into a blender and puree, then pour into the pot. Any which way, do not overprocess, or the soup will lighten in color and become aerated and frothy.

Taste the tomatoes and adjust the seasoning. Add stock to taste, about ¼ cup (60 ml) at a time, if you want a thinner texture. Heat over medium heat until almost boiling hot, stirring occasionally. Serve immediately with the crisps.

The soup may be refrigerated in an airtight container for up to 3 days and reheated. The crisps should be served soon after they are prepared.

Clam Chowder

 MAKES ABOUT 1 QUART (960 ML) | SERVES 2

We both live in New England, so having a creamy low FODMAP clam chowder was high on our list. Lactose-free milk allows us to create this most traditional of soups. Buying and cooking with whole clams in the shell might seem daunting, but our technique allows you to make your own clam broth and the entire soup from scratch in less than thirty minutes if you are very organized. We prefer using cherrystones or the larger quahogs or chowder clams; just don't mix them, as they will steam open at different rates. This recipe may be doubled; just make sure you have a large enough stockpot to hold the clams.

BROTH:

4 pounds (1.8 kg) cherrystone clams

1 cup (240 ml) water

6 sprigs flat-leaf parsley

1 sprig thyme

¼ medium-size dried bay leaf

CHOWDER:

1 piece thinly cut smoked bacon, chopped (use gluten-free if necessary)

¼ cup (23 g) finely chopped leek, green parts only

1 pound (455 g) Yukon gold potatoes, peeled and diced

1 cup (240 ml) water

1 cup (240 ml) lactose-free milk (whole, 2%, 1%, or fat-free), at room temperature

1 tablespoon finely chopped fresh flat-leaf parsley

1 tablespoon finely chopped fresh chives

Prepare the broth: Wash the clams well to remove any surface grit. Place in a 5- to 6-quart (1.2 to 1.4 L) stockpot along with the water, parsley, thyme, and bay leaf. Cover and bring to a simmer over medium heat; after 5 minutes, stir the clams with a sturdy wooden spoon to get the ones on top down to the bottom, quickly replace the cover, and cook for about 5 minutes more, or just until the clams open. The timing will vary, depending on the size of the clams: some will open fully, while others will only open a tiny bit, which is fine. Remove from the heat. Remove and discard any clams that do not open. Use tongs to pick remaining clams up one by one, tipping any broth captured in the shells back into the pot. Place the clamshells in a strainer. Some clams will have fallen out of their shells into the broth, which is okay. Pick the clams out of the shells in the strainer and place on a cutting board; use tongs to remove any loose clams from the broth and place them on the cutting board, too. Discard the shells. The clams can cool briefly before chopping, while you strain the broth.

Using a triple-fine meshed strainer or a mesh strainer lined with cheesecloth, strain the broth into a clean container. There might be some grit, which you are trying to capture and leave behind. Set broth aside momentarily.

Chop the clams on the cutting board and then refrigerate until needed.

Prepare the chowder: Wipe out the original stockpot and add the bacon. Cook over medium-low heat to render the fat and cook until the bacon is crisp. Remove the bacon bits and drain on paper towels, reserving the bacon fat in the pot. Add the leek greens to the bacon fat and cook gently over medium-low heat for about 5 minutes, or until the leek is soft but not browned.

Add 1 cup (240 ml) of the strained broth to the pot along with the potatoes and the water. The liquid should just cover the potatoes; add additional broth or water only if necessary. Cover and bring to a low boil over medium-high heat and cook until the potatoes are soft, for 10 to 15 minutes. Use the back of a wooden spoon or a potato masher to mash some of the potatoes right in the pot. This step adds body to the soup.

Add the milk and chopped clams and heat over low heat until very hot (do not allow to boil). If you are not serving right away, but will be doing so within an hour or two, simply stop at this point, keep covered off the heat, then reheat right before serving. Serve with parsley and chives sprinkled on top. You can also sprinkle with the reserved bacon, if you desire. The chowder can be refrigerated overnight without the garnishes and reheated very gently without simmering or boiling; be aware that if reheated, the flavors (particularly the saltiness and clam essence) might intensify.

POST-FODMAP CHALLENGE PHASE OPTIONS

Fructan: If you passed the fructan onion challenge, sub in ¼ cup (36 g) of finely chopped white or yellow onion for the leek greens.

Lactose: If you passed the lactose challenge, feel free to sub in dairy milk (whole milk for the creamiest texture) for the lactose-free version or even up to ¼ cup (60 ml) of heavy cream to make the chowder a little more decadent (keep the serving size of heavy cream to 2 tablespoons).

Hearty Vegetable Soup

  MAKES 5 TO 6 QUARTS (1.2 TO 1.4 L) | 10 TO 12 SERVINGS

If there is one thing all of us battling IBS symptoms need to feel, it is comfort, especially with food, which up till now has felt like the enemy. This hearty vegetable soup is the best kind of comfort food: it is very minestrone-like, but uses all healthy low FODMAP ingredients. It tastes great, nourishes us body and mind, and literally warms us from the inside out. This makes a big batch as it freezes well. Freeze it in single-size servings and microwave at the office for a satisfying winter lunch. Note that you will need Vegetable Broth (page 69). The cheese rind might seem odd, but it adds richness and umami and most cheese stores will sell you a piece; just ask if you don't see it displayed. If you want to shorten the prep time even more, sauté the leeks and then just add everything at once.

3 tablespoons Garlic-Infused Oil (page 68) made with olive oil, or purchased garlic-infused olive oil

1 cup (90 g) finely chopped leek, green parts only

1 pound (455 g) Yukon gold potatoes (2 to 3 medium-size), scrubbed and diced

2 medium-size carrots, scrubbed and cut into ¼-inch (6 mm)-thick rounds

2 medium-size parsnips, peeled, sliced lengthwise and cut into ¼ inch (6 mm)-thick half-moons

2 medium-size turnips, peeled, stem and root end trimmed away, and diced

1 medium-size or large fennel bulb, root and stalk ends trimmed away, bulb halved, then thinly sliced

6 black peppercorns

6 sprigs flat-leaf parsley

2 sprigs thyme

1 bay leaf

10 cups (2.4 L) Vegetable Broth (page 69)

1 (28-ounce [829 g]) can diced tomatoes, preferably fire-roasted (without garlic or onion), such as Muir Glen brand

1 (4-ounce [115 g]) piece Parmigiano-Reggiano rind

1 teaspoon kosher salt, or to taste

Freshly ground black pepper

1 large bunch Swiss or rainbow chard, stems discarded, leaves finely chopped

2 medium-size yellow summer squash, ends trimmed, halved lengthwise, and cut into ½-inch (12 mm) thick half-moons

2 medium-size zucchini, ends trimmed, halved lengthwise, and cut into ½-inch (12 mm) thick half-moons

Chunk of Parmigiano-Reggiano cheese, for garnish (optional but highly recommended)

Heat the oil in an 8- to 10-quart (7.5 to 9.5 L) stockpot over medium heat. Add the leek greens and sauté until soft but not browned, for about 5 minutes. Add the potatoes, carrots, parsnips, turnips, sliced fennel, peppercorns, parsley, thyme, bay leaf, vegetable broth, diced tomatoes, Parmigiano-Reggiano rind, and ½ teaspoon of the salt. Cover and bring to a boil over medium-high heat, then lower the heat to a simmer. Simmer, stirring occasionally, for 30 to 40 minutes, or until the vegetables are cooked. Taste for seasoning; add the remaining salt (and more, if desired) as well as a generous amount of pepper. Add the Swiss chard, yellow summer squash, and zucchini and simmer for about 20 minutes more, or until those vegetables are softened. The soup is ready to serve with optional shavings of Parmigiano-Reggiano (we like a generous amount)—just fish out the bay leaf and the herb stalks and leave the peppercorns behind. To store, allow to cool to room temperature, then divide into more manageable amounts in airtight containers and either refrigerate for up to 4 days or freeze for up to 1 month. Defrost in the refrigerator overnight and reheat as needed.

POST-FODMAP CHALLENGE PHASE OPTION

Fructan: If you passed the fructan onion challenge, consider adding 1 cup (142 g) of finely chopped white or yellow onion, or to your tolerance, in lieu of the leek greens.

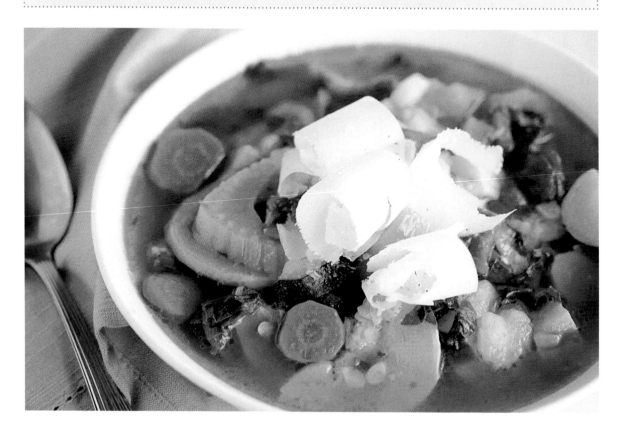

Egg Drop Soup

   MAKES 4 SERVINGS

A good chicken stock, such as the one on page 70, will provide you with the basis for some very easy soups, including our Egg Drop Soup. After simmering with fresh ginger, our stock is ready to receive those lovely threads of egg, which are easier to create than you might think. If you want to increase the protein, add some cubed firm tofu or shredded chicken at the very end.

---

1 quart (960 ml) Chicken Stock (page 70), or prepared low FODMAP chicken stock (use gluten-free if following a gluten-free diet)

1 (½-inch [12 mm]) piece fresh ginger, peeled and cut into a few pieces

1 tablespoon low-sodium soy sauce or tamari (use gluten-free if necessary)

1 tablespoon cornstarch

2 scallions, green parts only, sliced very thinly at a steep oblique angle

2 large eggs, at room temperature, well beaten in pitcher or measuring cup with a spout

Place the chicken stock and the ginger in a medium-size saucepan and bring to a simmer over medium heat. Simmer for 20 minutes to infuse the stock with ginger flavor. Remove and discard the ginger pieces. Set aside 3 tablespoons of the stock in a small bowl. Stir the soy sauce into the stock in the pot, which should remain over medium heat.

Stir together the reserved 3 tablespoons of stock and the cornstarch in a small bowl to create a smooth paste, then whisk the paste into the hot stock. Simmer for 1 minute to thicken the soup, then stir in the scallion greens.

Make sure the soup is simmering. Using a wooden spoon, stir the soup to create a vortex within the liquid, then remove the spoon from the soup. Slowly drizzle the beaten egg into the center of the swirling soup (the pour spout makes this easy). Allow the soup to stop moving on its own; this brief time will allow the egg to cook. Once the egg has set, about 45 seconds, break up the egg into threads, using a fork. Serve immediately in hot bowls.

KATE'S NOTES

Ginger offers many therapeutic properties, especially for those troubled with digestive distress. Active chemicals in the ginger help contract the stomach and aid emptying. Numerous studies have shown its effect on minimizing nausea and more recent research is revealing its anti-inflammatory effects in the colon.

Tortilla Soup with Chicken & Lime

   MAKES 4 SERVINGS

This soup is all about assembly and then balancing the flavors. You will need cooked chicken; we like to use leftovers from our Whole Roast Chicken with Lemon & Herbs (page 276). You can use regular diced tomatoes, but the fire-roasted really add a smoky complexity. Note that most chili powders that you find in the spice aisle are blends that are not low FODMAP approved due to the inclusion of fructan-rich garlic and/or onion. We use pure chipotle chile powder, but be warned, it does pack a wallop of heat; use sparingly and adjust to taste. For a huge time-saver, use purchased tortilla chips to garnish the soup, instead of frying the corn tortillas.

---

1 (15-ounce [430 g]) can fire-roasted, diced tomatoes (without garlic or onion), such as Muir Glen brand

4 cups (960 ml) Chicken Stock (page 70), or prepared low FODMAP chicken stock

¼ to ½ teaspoon chipotle chile powder

Kosher salt

4 cups (500 g) shredded cooked chicken, from the Whole Roast Chicken with Lemon & Herbs (page 276)

Vegetable oil

4 white or yellow corn tortillas

2 limes, quartered

¼ cup (8 g) chopped fresh cilantro

Puree the tomatoes in a blender until smooth; do not overprocess, or they will become frothy. Scrape into a medium-size to large saucepan. If you have an immersion blender, you can puree the tomatoes right in your pot. Add the chicken stock to the tomato puree, whisk to combine, and heat over medium heat until hot. Season to taste with chipotle chile powder and salt. (The flavor balance might not seem quite right yet as the lime juice hasn't been added. Don't worry. Give it your best shot and have extra salt handy to add later, if needed.) Add the cooked chicken and heat until the chicken is warmed through.

Meanwhile heat about ¼ inch (6 mm) of vegetable oil in a skillet (we use a cast-iron) over medium heat until it shimmers. Add one tortilla at a time; the oil should bubble along the edges. Cook the tortilla for about 1 minute, or until beginning to take on some color on the bottom, flip with tongs, and cook the second side for about 1 minute more, or until lightly crisp. Drain on paper towels and repeat with the remaining tortillas.

Ladle the hot soup into bowls. Break or cut the tortillas into pieces and scatter over the soup. If using purchased tortilla chips, grab a handful and crush them by hand over the bowls. Add two lime quarters to each bowl and evenly divide the cilantro over the top. Serve immediately, encouraging diners to squeeze the lime juice into their soup (the acidity is needed to finish off the dish).

POST-FODMAP CHALLENGE PHASE OPTIONS

Fructans: If you passed both the fructan garlic and onion challenges, feel free to use a commercially prepared chicken stock (most prepared chicken broths contain both garlic and onion). We do suggest you use a low-sodium style.

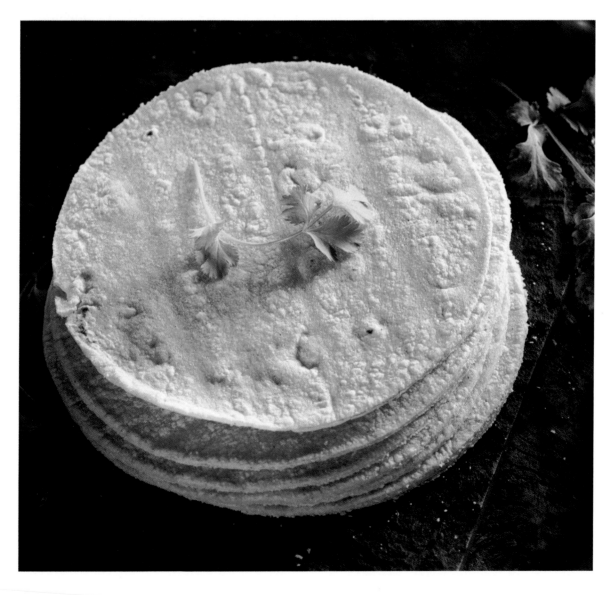

Miso Soup with Tofu & Scallions

    MAKES 4 SERVINGS

Miso soup, unlike so many other soups, is made right before consuming, so we make only what we need at the time. It is slightly salty, slightly sweet, delicate, and incredibly warming and comforting. Think of it as a vegetarian alternative to chicken soup when you are feeling under the weather or anytime you want a light, hot, clear, nourishing soup. Miso is fermented soybean paste; it has been approved for the low FODMAP diet in small amounts. As with any prepared food, read labels and look for naturally fermented and organic miso, such as South River brand Sweet Tasting Brown Rice Miso. You will need to source the miso as well as the bonito (fish) flakes, so plan accordingly. Note that the bonito flakes are shelf stable for a very long time and the miso can be refrigerated for years!

DASHI (FISH BROTH):

4 cups (960 ml) water

1 ounce (30 g) dried bonito flakes (the label might say katsuobushi)

MISO SOUP:

3 tablespoons miso of choice (see headnote)

⅓ pound (152 g) firm tofu, cut into ¼-inch (6 mm) cubes

¼ cup (16 g) finely sliced scallion, green parts only

Prepare the dashi: Bring the water to a boil in a large saucepan, then remove from the heat. Quickly stir in the bonito flakes. Let sit for about 1 minute, or just until the flakes settle to the bottom. Strain the stock through a cheesecloth-lined strainer. The dashi is ready to use, or refrigerate in an airtight storage container for up to 4 days. If refrigerated, return to a very hot temperature before proceeding.

Prepare the miso soup: Place the miso in a small, heatproof bowl. Add about ½ cup (120 ml) of the dashi and whisk until smooth; it should be thick and creamy, but flowable in texture. Stir the miso mixture into the hot dashi in the pot, then add the tofu cubes and heat until they are hot (do not allow to boil).

Remove from the heat, divide the soup among bowls, sprinkle with the scallion greens, and serve immediately.

Creamy Root Vegetable Soup with Gruyère Croutons

MAKES ABOUT 7 CUPS (1.7 L) | **SERVES 4 AS A FIRST COURSE**

This velvety-smooth soup has a rich, creamy texture yet is completely dairy-free. The combination of celery root, potatoes, carrots, and parsnips comes together to create a luxurious thick texture after being roasted in a hot oven with olive oil and then pureed with the addition of liquid. We like to use the peelings from the root vegetables to make a simple stock while the veggies roast. If you add this liquid to the vegetables, the soup will have an exceptional earthy flavor that we just love. You could use water for a milder flavor, or even chicken stock, which adds a sweetness and another layer of flavor. The Gruyère croutons are optional, but folks love them. The recipe may be doubled, in which case you will need two roasting pans. It is also easily adaptable to become dairy-free, vegan, or gluten-free; see ingredient notes.

SOUP:

4 medium-size carrots, washed

3 medium-size Yukon gold potatoes, washed

2 medium-size parsnips, washed

1 (14- to 16-ounce [400 to 455 g]) celery root (a.k.a. celeriac), scrubbed free of dirt

2 tablespoons plus 2 teaspoons Garlic-Infused Oil (page 68) made with olive oil, purchased garlic-infused olive oil, or plain olive oil, divided

Kosher salt

Freshly ground black pepper

6 cups (1.4 L) water

½ cup (32 g) chopped scallion, green parts only

5 cups (1.2 L) water or Chicken Stock (page 70) (optional; use water if following a vegetarian diet)

GRUYÈRE CROUTONS
(OMIT IF FOLLOWING A DAIRY-FREE OR VEGAN DIET):

1 tablespoon unsalted butter, melted, or Garlic-Infused Oil (page 68) made with olive oil, purchased garlic-infused olive oil, or olive oil

8 (¼-inch [6 mm]) slices low FODMAP French bread or similar bread (use gluten-free if following a gluten-free diet)

1 cup (115 g) grated Gruyère cheese

Prepare the soup: Position a rack in the hottest zone of the oven. Preheat the oven to 400°F (200°C).

Peel the carrots and remove the stem ends. Place the peelings and ends in a medium-size saucepan. Chop the carrots into ½-inch (12 mm) rounds and toss into a roasting pan. Peel the potatoes, adding the peelings to the saucepan. Chop the potatoes into 2-inch (5 cm) chunks and add to the roasting pan. Peel the parsnips and remove the stem ends. Place the peelings and ends in the saucepan. Chop the parsnips into ½-inch (12 mm) rounds and add to the roasting pan. Peel the celery root, adding the peelings to the saucepan. Chop the celery root into 1-inch (2.5 cm) chunks and add to the roasting pan.

Drizzle the vegetables in the roasting pan with 2 tablespoons of the oil and toss well to coat. Season with salt and pepper. Spread out the veggies in a single layer and roast for 40 to 50 minutes, or until tender when pierced with a knife.

Meanwhile, add the 6 cups (1.4 L) of water to the pot of peelings and bring to a boil over high heat. Lower the heat and simmer, uncovered, for 40 minutes while the vegetables roast. Strain, reserving the broth and discarding the solids.

While the veggies roast and the broth simmers, heat the remaining 2 teaspoons of oil in a deep saucepan over medium heat. Add the scallion greens and sauté, stirring often, until soft, about 2 minutes. Add the roasted vegetables when they are done. Add about 3 cups (720 ml) of the broth (or use water or chicken stock instead) and puree, using an immersion blender, right in the pot. Or you can puree the vegetables and broth in a blender and return them to the pot. Add enough liquid (use the broth, water, or chicken stock, or a combination) to make a creamy soup; you might not need all the liquid. Taste and adjust the seasoning as desired. Keep the soup hot while you make the croutons, if using. Alternatively, allow to cool to room temperature, then refrigerate in an airtight container for up to 4 days. Reheat as needed.

Prepare the croutons: When you are ready to serve the soup, adjust an oven rack to 3 to 4 inches (7.5 to 10 cm) from the broiler and preheat the broiler on high. Lightly brush one side of each bread slice with butter or oil and place, oiled side up, on a foil- or parchment-lined baking sheet. Broil until lightly toasted, flip the croutons over, divide the cheese evenly on top of the bread, then broil again until the cheese melts. Ladle the soup into bowls; top each with croutons and serve immediately.

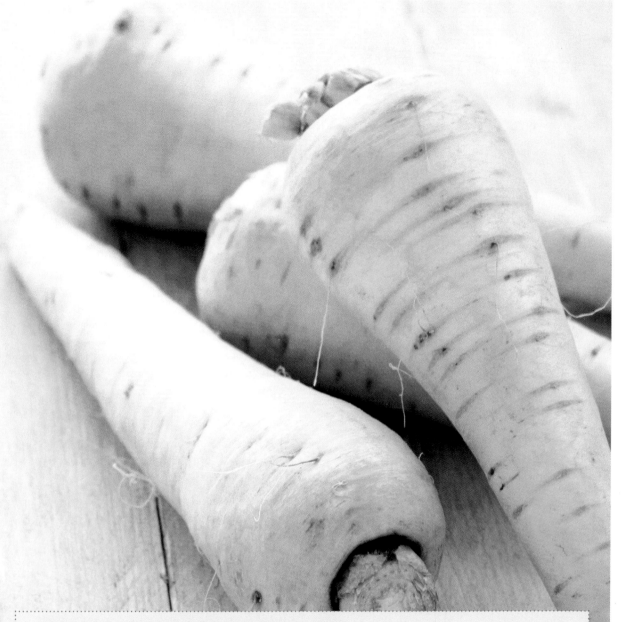

POST-FODMAP CHALLENGE PHASE OPTIONS

Polyols: If you passed the mannitol challenge, sub in one medium-size peeled and diced sweet potato for one regular potato among the vegetables to be roasted. Note that this will make the soup much sweeter.

Polyols and GOS: If you passed both the mannitol and GOS challenge, you may add 1 cup (120 g) of peeled, seeded, and diced butternut squash to the vegetables to be roasted, in which case you will need more liquid for pureeing. The soup will also be much sweeter.

Note: These versions will be a more vivid orange color and have a sweeter flavor.

Gazpacho

  MAKES 8 SERVINGS

Gazpacho is a chilled summer soup, best made when tomatoes are at their ultimate peak of ripeness. Although you could chop the veggies in a food processor, the results will be far less elegant and visually pleasing than if you chop by hand. Yes, this is going to give you and your chef's knife a workout, but on a blistering hot and humid summer day, you won't want to eat anything else. The classic version contains garlic and onions; let's agree to recognize this version as a refreshing low FODMAP alternative. The soup is best if served the day it is made, and it can be served right after preparation, but the flavors improve and meld after a few hours, so plan accordingly. And make another recipe if all you can find are lackluster tomatoes. This is all about the vegetables and their bright freshness.

---

8 large, ripe beefsteak tomatoes

1 English cucumber

2 cups (128 g) finely chopped scallion, green parts only

1 medium-size green bell pepper, stemmed, cored, and finely chopped

1 medium-size yellow or orange bell pepper, stemmed, cored, and finely chopped

2 small or 1 medium-large jalapeño pepper, stemmed, seeded, and finely chopped

3 tablespoons sherry vinegar

Kosher salt

Freshly ground black pepper

Garlic-Infused Oil (page 68) made with olive oil, or purchased garlic-infused olive oil

Hot sauce, such as Texas Pete's (use gluten-free if following a gluten-free diet)

Bring a large pot of water to a boil. Drop two or three tomatoes in at a time and blanch for about 1 minute, or until the skins slip off easily. Transfer to a colander and rinse under cold water to stop the cooking, then slip off the skins and discard. Repeat with the remaining tomatoes. Once cooled, cut in half, squeeze and/or scoop out and discard all the seeds, and finely chop the flesh into very tiny dice, catching all the juice. Place the tomatoes and juice in a large, nonreactive mixing bowl.

Peel the cucumber; remove and discard the ends. Slice the cucumber in half lengthwise. Use a small spoon to scoop out and discard the seeds. Very finely dice the cucumber and add to the tomatoes. Stir in the scallion greens, bell peppers, and jalapeño. Stir in the vinegar, then season to taste with salt and black pepper. Cover with plastic wrap and refrigerate for at least an hour or up to 8 hours.

Taste after chilling and correct the seasoning, if necessary. Serve with a drizzle of garlic-infused oil and pass the hot sauce at the table.

POST-FODMAP CHALLENGE PHASE OPTIONS

Fructans: If you passed the fructan onion challenge, use 1¼ cups (178 g) of finely chopped white or yellow onion, or to your tolerance, instead of the scallion greens.

If you passed the fructan garlic challenge, add two cloves of garlic, finely chopped, along with the scallion to the soup mixture and use plain extra-virgin olive oil instead of the garlic-infused oil to drizzle on top.

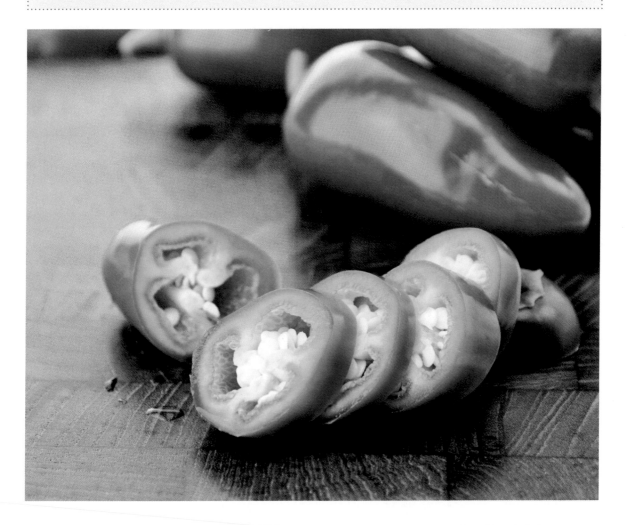

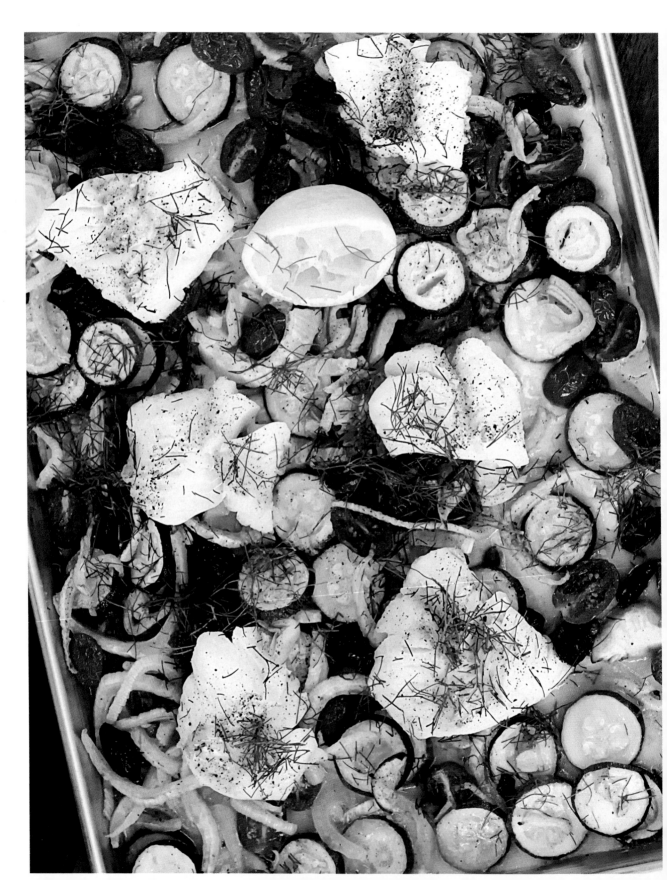

Chapter 12

ONE-POT, ONE-DISH MEALS

WE KNOW WHAT IT IS LIKE TO BE BUSY and have the need to eat healthily within our low FODMAP lifestyle. That's why we love one-dish dinners. These are perfect for a work night or those cooking for one, who want ease and built-in leftovers. Here you will find Perfect Pot Roast (page 292), Mediterranean Fish with Fennel, Tomatoes & Zucchini (page 284), and All-Beef Chili (page 294), among other choices. Don't overlook the Citrus Sage Turkey Breast (page 282). We make it year-round and use leftovers for sandwiches, tacos, chicken salad, and handy high-protein noshing.

Whole Roast Chicken with Lemon & Herbs

 SERVES ABOUT 6

A whole roast chicken is a thing of beauty. It makes a great family meal, and if you are lucky enough to have leftovers, you could be set with low FODMAP meals for days—Chicken Tostadas (page 226), Tarragon Chicken Salad with Grapes and Pecans (page 118), and Mason Jar Salads (page 124) are just a few of our favorites. This chicken also makes a great filler-free, lower-salt, and tasty protein-rich topping for salads and filling for a hearty sandwich.

Roasting a chicken is easy, but the details make a difference, so be sure to follow them closely for best results; they will create a juicy, tender chicken with a crackling crust. The herbs are truly optional. Sometimes it is nice to let a chicken taste like chicken. If you don't have them or forgot to shop for them, don't worry. We make this dish without them all the time.

---

1 (4-pound [1.8 kg]) whole chicken, preferably air chilled and organic

Kosher salt

Freshly cracked black pepper

1 lemon

Sprigs of thyme or rosemary (optional)

EQUIPMENT:
Butcher's twine

Position a rack in the middle of the oven. Preheat the oven to 450°F (230°C).

Meanwhile, remove the chicken from the refrigerator, unwrap, and place on a paper towel–lined tray. Pat dry inside and out with paper towels and bring to room temperature.

Remove the neck and any giblets or innards from the bird's cavity (they might be in a bag or loose; discard or use for stock). Season the bird liberally with salt and pepper inside and out. Place the chicken, breast side up, in a roasting pan. Roll the lemon around on a countertop, applying pressure to loosen the juices within. Prick several times with a fork and stuff the whole lemon into the cavity of the chicken. If you are using the herbs, stuff them into the cavity as well. Cross the legs right at the end of the drumsticks and tie with butcher's twine. Place in the oven, close the door, and lower the temperature to 400°F (200°C).

Roast the chicken for about 50 minutes undisturbed—do not open the oven door. The chicken is done when it registers 165°F (74°C) on an instant-read thermometer inserted into the thickest part of the thigh but not touching bone. You can also jiggle the wings and legs—they should feel loose in their sockets, or prick in one spot on the thigh with the tip of a knife and the juices should run clear. The total roasting time will be between 50 minutes and 1 hour 10 minutes, depending on the size of the chicken and what temperature it was when it went into the oven.

Remove the chicken from the oven, tent loosely with foil, and let the bird rest for 10 or 15 minutes, which will allow the juices to redistribute. This is a very important step to ensure maximum juiciness. Use this time to dress your salad and prepare your side dishes. Carve the chicken into the breasts, thighs, and legs, and serve immediately. Pick any remaining meat off the bones and save it for other meals. The leftovers will keep for about 5 days, refrigerated in airtight containers, or can be frozen for up to 3 months.

DÉDÉ'S TIPS

For an effortless accompaniment, make Schmaltz Croutons. Schmaltz is the rendered chicken fat and there will be some in the bottom of the pan. Remove the chicken from the roasting pan when done and allow it to rest on a cutting board, draping it with aluminum foil. Tear up hunks of a good low FODMAP bread (you want a country-style, baguette-type bread here; use gluten-free and/or dairy-free if necessary) and throw it in the bottom of the pan in the chicken fat. Toss the hunks around to coat, season with a little salt, if desired, and roast in the 400°F (200°C) oven until they get a bit crispy and crunchy. You want them to have some crunch and some chew, so don't overroast them. By the time the chicken is done resting, you will have the most incredible oven croutons to serve alongside.

Roast Chicken Thighs with Smoked Paprika, Lemon & Herbs, Carrots & Potatoes

 SERVES 4 TO 6

This might be the one dinner that makes a weekly appearance in Dédé's kitchen, year-round. She loves this recipe not only for its ease (you can get it ready all in one pan while the oven preheats) and flavor, but also because there was really only one tweak that was needed to make it low FODMAP. By using garlic oil in lieu of the garlic powder, Dédé was able to continue to serve a family favorite while keeping her IBS symptoms at bay. We recommend doubling this recipe if you have a large family, as the leftovers are great even at room temperature or the chicken can be repurposed for tacos, salad, or sandwiches. The smoked paprika lends a fabulous rich and deep smoky flavor to the dish and is worth seeking out.

---

8 chicken thighs, bone-in, skin on

1 pound (455 g) red, fingerling, or Yukon gold potatoes, quartered or sliced into large bite-size pieces

½ pound (225 g) "baby" carrots

2 tablespoons Garlic-Infused Oil (page 68) made with olive oil, or purchased garlic-infused olive oil

2 tablespoons freshly squeezed lemon juice

2 tablespoons fresh thyme, chopped, or 1 tablespoon dried

1 tablespoon plus 1 teaspoon smoked paprika

Salt

Freshly ground black pepper

Position a rack in the center of the oven. Preheat the oven to 375°F (190°C).

Pat the chicken thighs dry with paper towels and place in a large roasting pan. There should be room around the thighs; use two pans, if necessary. Scatter the potatoes and carrots over and around the chicken. Drizzle with the garlic oil and lemon juice. Sprinkle the thyme and paprika evenly over all, then season very generously with salt and pepper.

Roast the chicken for 45 to 60 minutes, or until an instant-read thermometer registers 165°F (74°C). The roasting time will depend on the size of the chicken parts and what temperature they were when it went into the oven. Remove from the oven and allow the chicken to rest for at least 5 minutes before serving. Store leftovers in airtight containers in the refrigerator for up to 4 days.

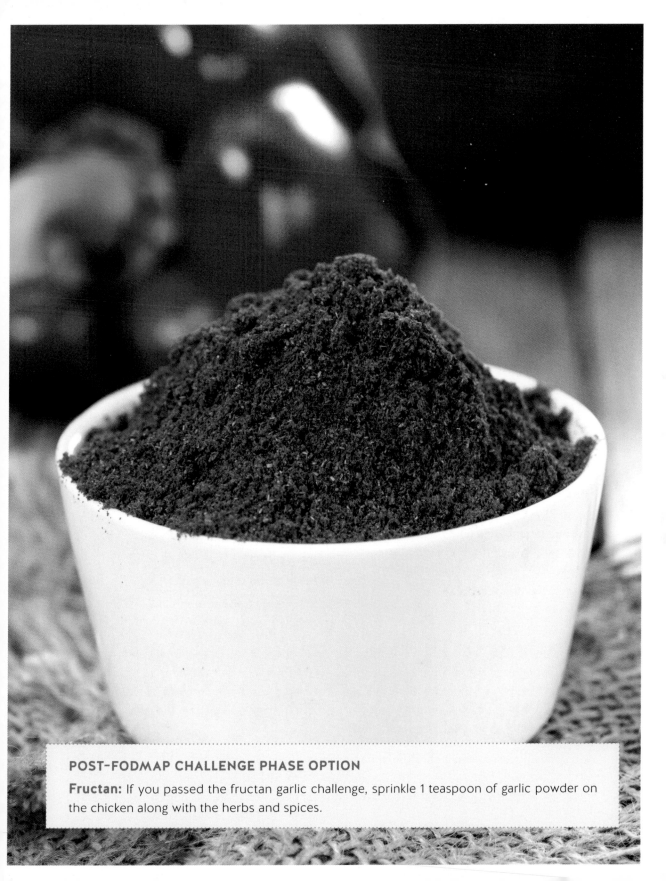

POST-FODMAP CHALLENGE PHASE OPTION

Fructan: If you passed the fructan garlic challenge, sprinkle 1 teaspoon of garlic powder on the chicken along with the herbs and spices.

Chicken and Rice (Arroz con Pollo)

   MAKES 4 TO 8 SERVINGS | SERVING SIZE 1 OR 2 CHICKEN PIECES

Dédé grew up with Spanish and Basque heritage and this chicken and rice dish made regular appearances. This recipe uses eight chicken thighs, and as you will cook the rice in the same pot, make sure you have a large enough pan. We use a 12-inch (32 cm)-wide, 2½-inch (6.5 cm)-deep straight-sided, lidded skillet. This dish even improves on days two and three, so feel free to make ahead and reheat. You do need Chicken Stock (page 70), but if you are making this last minute, you can use water; just adjust the seasonings as you go: you will need more salt and pepper or might consider some of the more highly seasoned variations in the Tips.

---

8 chicken thighs, or 4 thighs and 4 legs

Kosher salt

Freshly ground black pepper

1 tablespoon Garlic-Infused Oil (page 68) made with olive oil, or purchased garlic-infused olive oil

2 ounces (55 g) smoked ham, cut into ¼-inch (6 mm) dice (see Dédé's Tips) (use gluten-free if necessary, and without other FODMAP ingredients)

½ cup (32 g) chopped scallion, green parts only

1 green bell pepper, cored and diced

1½ cups (150 g) long-grain white rice

3 cups (720 ml) Chicken Stock (page 70), or prepared low FODMAP chicken stock

2 cups (400 g) canned diced tomatoes, preferably fire-roasted

¾ cup (107 g) pimiento-stuffed green olives, chopped

½ cup (85 g) chopped, canned roasted red peppers

1 tablespoon tomato paste

¼ cup (8 g) chopped fresh flat-leaf parsley

Pat the chicken pieces dry with paper towels and season both sides liberally with salt and black pepper. Heat the oil in a large, deep skillet over medium heat. Place the chicken in the pan, skin side down, and cook until well browned, for about 5 minutes. Flip the pieces over and cook for 3 or 4 minutes more to brown. Remove from the pan. Drain the excess fat from the pan, leaving about 2 tablespoons (just do this by eye).

Add the ham and scallion greens to the pan, scrape up any browned bits, and sauté for about 1 minute. Add the green pepper and sauté for about 4 minutes more, or until the pepper begins to soften. Add the rice and toss to coat and cook for about 1 minute, stirring constantly. Stir in the chicken stock, tomatoes, olives, roasted red peppers, and tomato paste until combined. Season with more salt and pepper. Nestle the chicken pieces in a single layer in the rice. Cover, bring to a simmer, and cook at a low simmer over low heat until the liquid is absorbed and the rice is cooked, for about 25 minutes. The dish is ready to serve with a sprinkling of parsley. Alternatively, allow to cool to room temperature, refrigerate in an airtight container for up to 4 days, and reheat in the microwave on 50% power or, moistened with some stock or water, in a skillet over low heat.

POST-FODMAP CHALLENGE PHASE OPTIONS

Fructans: If you passed the fructan garlic challenge, add two garlic cloves, finely chopped, along with the ham, and/or substitute chorizo, a garlic-infused sausage, for the ham.

If you passed the fructan onion challenge, substitute ½ cup (121 g) of chopped white or yellow onion for the scallion greens.

GOS: If you pass the GOS challenge, add ½ cup (36 g) of frozen peas along with the chicken stock, for some added color and flavor.

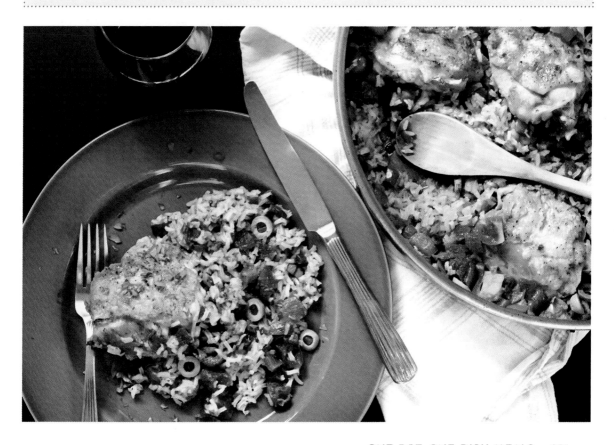

Citrus Sage Turkey Breast

  MAKES 10 TO 12 DINNER-SIZE SERVINGS

We like a whole turkey on our Thanksgiving table, but in our opinion, turkey is a versatile protein year-round that gets overlooked. Cooking a turkey breast couldn't be easier and you will have leftovers for amazing sandwiches and salads in addition to a fabulous dinner when it first comes out of the oven. We chose to season it with the classic Turkey Day herb—sage—but also incorporated the bright flavor of citrus, making this recipe perfect for a holiday event or even midsummer when you want lots of turkey on hand for a quick protein-rich salad topper or sandwich.

---

1 (7-pound [3.2 kg]) turkey breast, at room temperature

½ cup (1 stick; 113 g) unsalted butter, at room temperature

2 tablespoons grated orange zest (use a Microplane or rasp-style zester)

1 tablespoon Garlic-Infused Oil (page 68) or Onion-Infused Oil (see variation, page 68) made with olive oil or vegetable oil, or a purchased equivalent

1 tablespoon freshly squeezed lemon juice

2 teaspoons kosher salt

1 teaspoon dried sage

1 teaspoon freshly ground black pepper

1 cup (240 ml) water

Position a rack in the center of the oven. Preheat the oven to 325°F (165°C). Place a flat roasting rack in a roasting pan and set aside.

Trim the turkey of any excess fat and pat dry all over with paper towels; set aside.

Combine the butter, orange zest, oil, lemon juice, salt, sage, and pepper in a small bowl. Rub the turkey all over with the mixture. We use our hands! It's messy, but the best way. Gently slide your hand between the skin and the flesh, starting at the broad end of the breast, and rub the mixture under the skin as well, over the top and sides of the flesh to coat evenly. Pat the skin back into place.

Place the turkey breast on the rack. Add the water to the pan (the rack should sit above the water). Roast the turkey, adding more water if it evaporates during roasting, rotating the pan from front to back once during roasting and basting once or twice, and tenting with foil at any time if the turkey is browning too quickly. The total roasting time should be 1 hour 30 minutes to 2 hours, or until an instant-read thermometer inserted in the thickest part, without touching bone, registers 165°F (74°C). Remove from the oven, tent with foil, and allow to rest for 15 minutes, for the juices to redistribute. To serve, slice across the grain into ¼-inch (6 mm)-thick slices, pouring any pan juices on top. The turkey breast may also be served chilled or at room temperature. Refrigerate, wrapped airtight, for up to 4 days.

KATE'S NOTES

Food safety first! Remember to wash your counters and hands thoroughly with soap and warm water after handling raw meats, fish, or poultry to avoid food-borne illness.

Mediterranean Fish with Fennel, Tomatoes & Zucchini

    MAKES 4 SERVINGS

The mild flavor of cod loins, flounder, or similar white fish get the big flavor treatment in this supereasy and quick-to-make one-pan meal: shaved fennel, tomatoes, zucchini, black olives, capers, garlicky olive oil, and a bright squeeze of lemon juice make for satisfying low FODMAP eating. Plan ahead; with all the ingredients at hand, you can get this ready in the time it takes for the oven to preheat. Serve with rice, steamed or baked potatoes, or suitable low FODMAP crusty bread (use gluten-free and/or dairy-free if necessary).

---

2 tablespoons plus 2 teaspoons Garlic-Infused Oil (page 68) made with olive oil, or purchased garlic-infused olive oil, divided

2 medium-size zucchini (280 g), ends discarded, sliced into ¼-inch (6 mm) rounds

1 small fennel bulb, leafy fronds (leaves) reserved, stalks and root end discarded, bulb cut in half vertically, then cut into ¼-inch (6 mm) slices to equal 1 cup (98 g) of thin slices

1 dry pint (284 g) cherry or grape tomatoes, halved

½ cup (71 g) pitted kalamata olives, drained and halved

2 tablespoons brine-packed capers, drained

Kosher salt

Freshly ground black pepper

1½ pounds (680 g) cod loins or other mild white fish, such as flounder fillets, grouper, catfish, halibut steaks, or bass, cut into 4 to 6 pieces for even cooking

1 lemon, halved

Position a rack in the center of the oven. Preheat the oven to 450°F (230°C).

Coat the bottom of a large rimmed roasting pan or a heavy-duty half sheet pan with 2 tablespoons of the oil. Add the zucchini, fennel, tomatoes, olives, and capers, and toss in the oil to coat. Season with salt and pepper. Cover the pan tightly with foil.

Roast the veggies for 15 minutes, then remove the foil, stir, and continue to roast for about 15 minutes more, or until all the vegetables are tender.

Meanwhile, chop and reserve ¼ cup (3 g) of the fennel fronds (discard the rest or use for vegetable stock).

Place the fish pieces on top of the vegetables, drizzle with the remaining 2 teaspoons of the oil, sprinkle with the chopped fronds, season with salt and pepper, and bake until the fish is just cooked through and opaque, for 5 to 10 minutes (depending on the thickness of the fish). Squeeze the lemon juice over all and serve immediately.

POST-FODMAP CHALLENGE PHASE OPTION

Fructan: If you passed the fructan onion challenge, add half a medium-size white or yellow onion, very thinly sliced, to the zucchini, fennel, olives, and capers.

(Recipe photo on page 274)

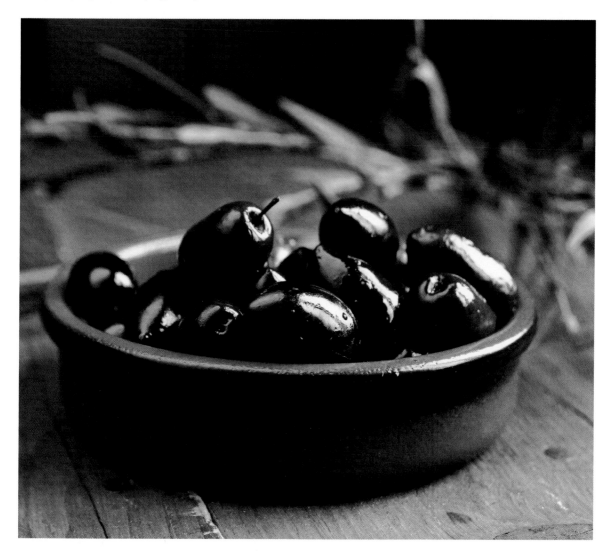

Cod with Roasted Potatoes, Garlic & Parsley

  SERVES 4

This is a simple one-dish dinner. It does take time; however, it is largely unattended time while the potatoes roast in the oven. The patience will reward you with crispy, luscious, crusty potatoes slathered with butter and garlicky olive oil. The thinness of the potato slices is key. You can cut them by hand, but slicing them on a mandoline or in a food processor will make the prep superquick and give you consistently sized slices, which in turn will roast up more uniformly crispy. Although you can make this with cod fillets, we prefer the thicker cod loins as they retain their delicate moisture. If using fillets, cut down the fish-roasting time to about 4 minutes, at which point check for doneness.

---

4 tablespoons (½ stick; 57 g) unsalted butter, melted, divided

2 tablespoons Garlic-Infused Oil (page 68) made with olive oil, or purchased garlic-infused olive oil

1½ pounds waxy potatoes, either red, white, or Yukon gold, peeled and cut into ⅛-inch (3.5 mm) slices

Kosher salt

Freshly ground black pepper

1½ pounds (680 g) cod loins

Zest of 1 lemon

¼ cup (8 g) finely chopped fresh flat-leaf parsley

1 tablespoon freshly squeezed lemon juice

Position a rack in the middle of the oven. Preheat the oven to 450°F (230°C). Use 1 tablespoon of the melted butter to coat the insides of a 13 x 9-inch (33 x 23 cm) casserole dish or similarly sized roasting pan; set aside.

Combine the remaining melted butter with the garlic-infused olive oil. Using some of the potatoes, overlap slightly to create a single layer of potatoes in the prepared dish, filling the pan. Brush with the butter mixture and season with salt and pepper. Add another layer of potatoes arranged similarly, brushing with the butter mixture and seasoning as you go, until you use up all the potatoes. Brush the tops of the potatoes with the butter mixture, reserving some for the fish. Season with salt and pepper and cover the pan tightly with foil. Roast for 15 minutes, then remove the foil and continue to roast until the potatoes are golden and crusty, for 15 to 20 more minutes.

Meanwhile, season the fish with salt and pepper. Toss the lemon zest with the parsley in a small bowl and set aside.

When the potatoes are nice and crispy, top with the cod loins, brush with the remaining butter mixture, and roast for about 10 minutes, or just until the fish is opaque and cooked through. Right before serving, sprinkle with the lemon juice and shower with the parsley mixture. Serve immediately.

KATE'S NOTES

Potatoes have received a bad rap, often thought of as lacking in nutrition and full of calories, but a medium-size spud contains a mere 110 calories as well as potassium, vitamins B6 and C, and even a little iron; eat the skin and you get 3 grams of fiber, too. Potassium plays a role in smooth muscle contraction, aiding digestive muscle function, Vitamin C enhances iron absorption, especially from plant sources of iron; vitamin B6 helps your body metabolize protein and carbs; and the fiber helps with laxation.

POST-FODMAP CHALLENGE PHASE OPTION

Fructan: If you passed the fructan garlic challenge, sauté two garlic cloves, finely chopped, in olive oil over medium heat until softened, in lieu of the garlic-infused oil.

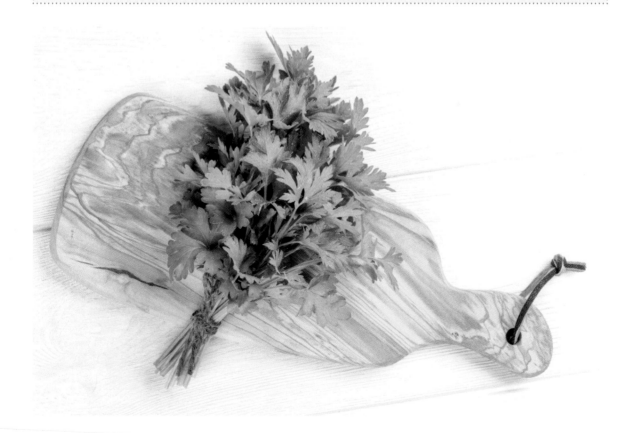

Shrimp & Broccoli Stir-Fry

     MAKES 6 SERVINGS

No need to order Chinese takeout, this stir-fry comes together very quickly and packs a punch with ginger, the crisp crunch of broccoli, and tender, sweet shrimp. Have rice already cooked, if using (we recommend generous mounds), as you will be getting dinner on the table in less than ten minutes. (Before you panic when you see the words "shrimp stock," read Dédé's Tips for a simple method to make your own.)

½ cup (120 ml) shrimp stock, Chicken Stock (page 70), or water (see Dédé's Tips)

2 tablespoons low-sodium soy sauce or tamari (use gluten-free if necessary)

1 teaspoon cornstarch

1 teaspoon crushed red pepper flakes

1 teaspoon sugar

2 tablespoons Garlic-Infused Oil (page 68) made with vegetable oil, or purchased garlic-infused vegetable oil

2 tablespoons peeled and finely julienned fresh ginger

2 cups (144 g) small broccoli florets (or combination of florets and stems)

1 pound (455 g) large shrimp (26/30), peeled and deveined

2 teaspoons toasted sesame oil (optional)

¼ cup (16 g) chopped scallion, green parts only

Whisk your choice of the stock or water (our order of preference is: shrimp stock, then chicken stock, then water), soy sauce, cornstarch, red pepper flakes, and sugar together in a small bowl until combined; set aside.

In a wok or large skillet, heat the vegetable oil over medium heat. Add the ginger and stir-fry for about 1 minute. Increase the heat to high, add the broccoli, and stir-fry for about 2 minutes, or until the broccoli begins to soften but is still crisp and bright green. Add the shrimp to the skillet and stir-fry for about 30 seconds, or until they just begin to turn pink. Add the stock mixture and keep tossing and stir-frying until the shrimp are just opaque and the sauce has coated the shrimp and broccoli and has thickened, for about 1 minute more. Drizzle with the sesame oil, if using, sprinkle with the scallion greens, and serve immediately.

DÉDÉ'S TIPS

To make your own shrimp stock, buy your shrimp with the shells on, peel the shrimp, and place the shells in a small saucepan along with ¾ cup (180 ml) of water. Bring to a boil and simmer for 5 minutes. Drain out ½ cup (120 ml) of the stock and use in the recipe.

When you see a number associated with shrimp, such as "26/30," it means there are 26 to 30 shrimp of that size per pound. The terms large or extra-large are less accurate. Best to buy shrimp by the number recommended in a recipe.

I use frozen shrimp for this dish all the time. Best-case scenario would be shrimp that aren't treated with preservatives, such as sodium sulfite. Defrost in the refrigerator overnight. If you must defrost at the last minute, do so in the bag with the bag submerged in cool water, not the shrimp directly in water, which will waterlog them.

POST-FODMAP CHALLENGE PHASE OPTION

Fructan: If you passed the fructan garlic challenge, sauté two garlic cloves, finely chopped, along with the ginger in the vegetable oil over medium heat until softened, in lieu of the garlic-infused oil.

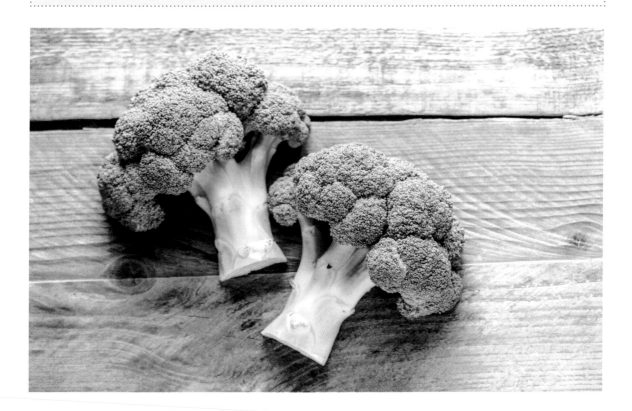

Mussels with Coconut Milk, Basil & Lime

   MAKES 6 SERVINGS

Mussels are on many restaurant menus and appear to be a fancy dish. Once you make them at home and see how quick and easy they are to prepare, you will be making them often. This is a one-pot dish that comes together in less than thirty minutes (twenty if you are really organized). We like to serve these with steamed white rice or FODMAP-approved crusty bread (use gluten-free and/or dairy-free if necessary) as a main dish to make a heartier meal, but they are also good on their own, as a starter or main attraction.

---

1 tablespoon Garlic-Infused Oil (page 68) made with vegetable oil, or purchased garlic-infused vegetable oil

1 cup (92 g) chopped leek, green parts only

2 cups (120 ml) 100% pure canned light unsweetened coconut milk, such as Thai Kitchen brand

2 cups (120 ml) water

3 to 4 tablespoons Asian fish sauce (use gluten-free if necessary)

2 tablespoons freshly squeezed lime juice

1 tablespoon firmly packed light brown sugar

¼ to ½ teaspoon hot sauce, such as Texas Pete's (use gluten-free if following a gluten-free diet)

½ cup (8 g) torn fresh basil leaves, divided

4½ pounds (2 kg) fresh mussels, scrubbed clean

Heat the oil over medium heat in a large, heavy-bottomed pot or Dutch oven. Sauté the leek greens until soft but not brown, for 3 to 5 minutes. Whisk in the coconut milk, water, 3 tablespoons of the fish sauce, the lime juice, brown sugar, ¼ teaspoon of the hot sauce, and ¼ cup (4 g) of the basil leaves. Heat until warm; taste and adjust the seasoning as needed. Add the mussels, cover the pot, and bring to a simmer over medium-high heat. Cook until the mussels open, for 8 to 10 minutes. Serve immediately, dividing into bowls and garnishing with the reserved basil. Place an empty bowl on the table to receive the shells and serve with big soup spoons.

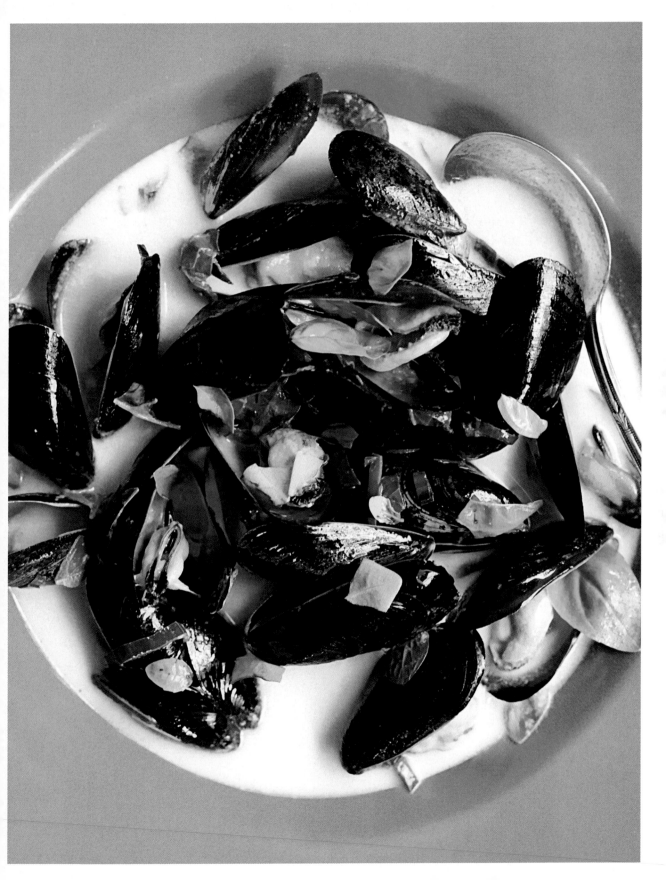

Perfect Pot Roast

  MAKES 6 TO 8 SERVINGS

This one-pot dish serves a big family and has that old-fashioned comfort food appeal that we all crave, especially when we are following a "diet." Well, you will be thrilled to know that this pot roast is made with all low FODMAP-approved ingredients and tastes like Grandma's. Note that some of the vegetables are cooked with the meat and later pureed to make the sauce; more vegetables are added toward the end of cooking to enjoy eating along with the beef. Serve with steamed potatoes, mashed potatoes, grits, Cheesy Grits (page 172), hunks of low FODMAP-approved bread (use gluten-free and/or dairy-free if necessary), or gluten-free pasta.

---

4 pounds (1.8 kg) (or as close to it as you can get) beef chuck roast, rump, or bottom round

3 tablespoons gluten-free all-purpose flour, such as Bob's Red Mill Gluten Free 1 to 1 Baking Flour

2 teaspoons kosher salt, plus more as needed

½ teaspoon freshly ground black pepper, plus more as needed

3 tablespoons Garlic-Infused Oil (page 68) made with vegetable oil, or purchased garlic-infused vegetable oil, divided

1 medium-size white or yellow onion, peeled and halved (make sure to follow the directions)

1 medium-size garlic clove (make sure to follow the directions)

2 cups (184 g) finely chopped leek, green parts only

2 cups (480 ml) dry red wine

1 cup (240 g) canned crushed tomatoes (without garlic or onion)

2 tablespoons tomato paste

1 teaspoon dried thyme, plus more as needed

5 medium-size carrots, scrubbed (peeled if desired), and cut into 1-inch (2.5 cm) chunks, divided

3 medium-size parsnips, peeled and cut into 1-inch (2.5 cm) chunks, divided

Bring the meat to room temperature for best browning. Meanwhile, stir together the flour, salt, and black pepper in a mixing bowl. Place the meat in the bowl and use your hands to thoroughly coat every surface of the meat with the seasoned flour, patting it in well.

Heat 2 tablespoons of the oil in a 5 quart (4.75 L) Dutch oven over medium heat and brown the meat well on all sides, for 6 to 8 minutes total, using sturdy tongs to move the meat around to make sure every side has an opportunity to brown. Transfer the meat to a plate or cutting board. Wipe the pot clean. Add the remaining tablespoon of oil to the pot along with the onion halves, cut side down, and sauté until the onion is soft, for 3 to 5 minutes, stirring the onion occasionally so as not to burn. Remove and discard all the onion pieces. Repeat with garlic clove, sautéeing until soft, then remove all garlic pieces. This is very important to stay within low FODMAP guidelines. Add the leek and sauté over medium-low heat, stirring frequently, until soft but not browned, for about 8 minutes.

Add the red wine and scrape up any browned bits, cooking over medium heat. Whisk in the crushed tomatoes, 1 tablespoon of the tomato paste, and the thyme. Add the meat back to the pot along with two of the chopped carrots and one of the chopped parsnips. Cover the pot, bring to a boil, then lower the heat to a low simmer and cook for about 3 hours, or until the meat is very tender but not quite fall-apart tender.

Remove the meat from the pot and set aside. Use an immersion blender to puree the cooked vegetables in the cooking liquid to make a sauce. Alternatively, allow to cool briefly, puree in a blender, and return the mixture to the pot. Taste and adjust the seasoning as desired with salt, pepper, thyme, and/or the reserved tablespoon of tomato paste.

Return the meat to the pot along with the three reserved chopped carrots and two reserved chopped parsnips and cook for another 30 minutes, or until the meat is completely tender and vegetables are as well. The pot roast is ready to serve, but much improves upon refrigerating for a day or two or three! Take advantage of this for parties. Refrigerate right in the pot and reheat as needed.

POST-FODMAP CHALLENGE PHASE OPTIONS

Fructans: If you passed the fructan onion challenge, finely chop the onion and leave in the pot as you proceed with the recipe.

If you passed the fructan garlic challenge, finely chop the garlic clove and leave in the pot as you proceed with the recipe.

All-Beef Chili

 GF MAKES 6 TO 8 SERVINGS

Did you know that chili does not contain beans? Well, at least according to the Chili Appreciation Society International, referred to as CASI. This one-pot all-beef chili is rich and spicy. It freezes well, you can easily adjust the heat level, and there is something here for everyone. Dédé traditionally thickened her chili with masa flour, which is not an easy-to-find ingredient. She found that finely ground yellow cornmeal worked just as well. Serve the chili with white (or brown) rice, Corn Bread (page 337), and as many bowls of low FODMAP add-ins as you are up to prepping.

CHILI:

4 pounds (1.8 kg) boneless chuck roast, cut into chunks

2 tablespoons Garlic-Infused Oil (page 68) made with vegetable oil, or purchased garlic-infused vegetable oil

2 medium-size white or yellow onions, peeled and halved (make sure to follow the directions)

1 to 2 tablespoons chipotle chile powder

2 tablespoons ground cumin

2 teaspoons paprika

2 teaspoons smoked paprika

1 teaspoon dried oregano

1 teaspoon kosher salt

½ teaspoon freshly ground black pepper

2 cups (470 ml) tomato sauce (without garlic or onion)

3 to 4 cups (720 to 960 ml) water

Cayenne pepper

¼ cup (35 g) finely ground yellow cornmeal

ADD-INS:

Shredded sharp Cheddar or Monterey Jack cheese (omit if following a dairy-free diet)

Shredded green cabbage (do not use Savoy) or lettuce

Diced bell pepper

Chopped scallion greens (green part only)

Lactose-free sour cream or yogurt (omit if following a dairy-free diet)

Salsa Fresca (page 80)

Fit a food processor with a metal blade. Add a handful of the meat and pulse on and off until coarsely ground. Scrape into a bowl and set aside; repeat until all the meat is ground.

Heat the oil in a heavy-bottomed 5-quart (4.75 L) Dutch oven over medium heat and add the onions, cut side down. Sauté for 3 to 5 minutes, or until the onions begin to soften, but do not

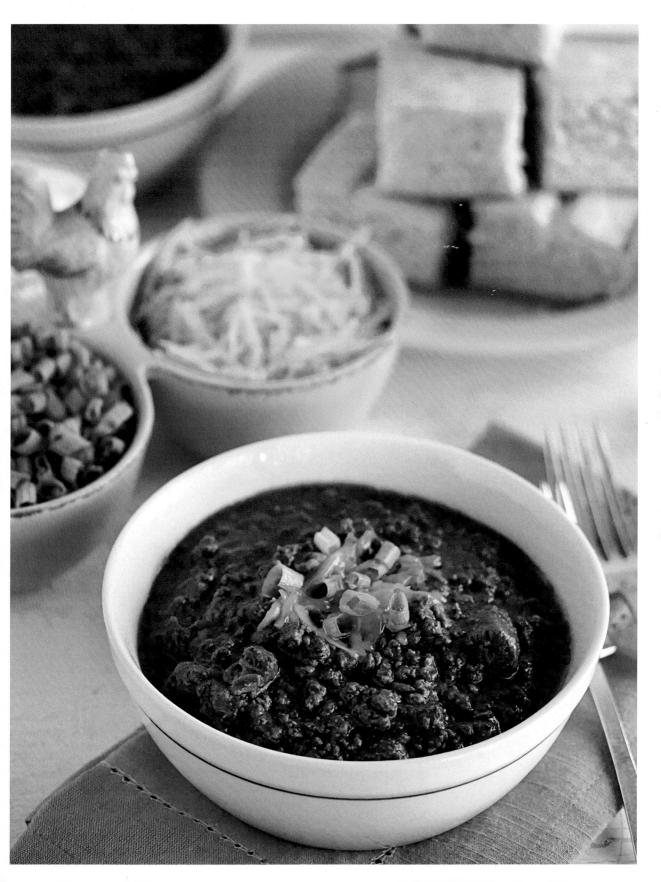

brown. Remove and discard all the onion pieces from the oil and discard. This is very important to stay within low FODMAP guidelines.

Add the meat, stir to combine with the oil, and cook for several minutes until browned, stirring often.

Add 1 to 2 tablespoons of the chipotle chile powder (depending on the level of heat desired) and the cumin, paprika, smoked paprika, oregano, salt, and black pepper and stir to coat the meat. Stir in the tomato sauce and 3 cups (720 ml) of the water to combine. Cover, lower the heat to a low simmer, and cook, stirring occasionally and making sure it does not burn, adding additional water if necessary, for 1 hour to 1 hour 15 minutes. Check the liquid level and meat doneness. The meat should be tender and there should be some liquid, but it should not be soupy. Simmer for a bit more if needed. Taste the chili, adjust the salt and pepper if desired, and add cayenne if you want more heat.

Place the cornmeal in a small bowl. Use a ladle to remove some of the cooking liquid and add it to the cornmeal, stirring to make a paste. Add this to the chili and stir in to distribute. Simmer, covered, for 10 more minutes to thicken the chili. The chili is ready to serve, but we think it is even better on day two or three. Allow to cool to room temperature and either refrigerate in airtight containers for up to a week or freeze for up to a month. (Defrost in the refrigerator overnight.) Reheat on the stove top over low heat. Serve with your choice of add-ins and encourage diners to add as they like.

POST-FODMAP CHALLENGE PHASE OPTIONS

Polyol: If you passed the sorbitol challenge, garnish the top of your chili with one quarter diced Hass avocado (smaller amounts, such as ⅛ avocado, is an acceptable low FODMAP portion even during your elimination phase).

Fructan: If you passed the fructan onion challenge, you can add 1 to 2 tablespoons of chopped red, yellow, or white onion as a garnish.

Slow-Roasted Shredded Pork

   MAKES ABOUT 9 CUPS SHREDDED PORK | UP TO 18 SERVINGS

This recipe takes hours to cook, but only 5 minutes to prep—and the time in the oven can be unattended, so it couldn't be easier. A flavorful dry rub is massaged into the meat, and after slow roasting in the oven, this pork is so tender you can shred it with a fork, yet the dry-roast method also provides some crispy outer bits that, when combined with the tender, juicy shreds from the interior, make for some quality eating. This recipe provides enough meat for days of succulent feasting. Use it for sandwiches, nachos, or our Slow-Roasted Pork Tacos with Citrus Slaw & Chipotle Mayo (page 233).

You will need a "butt" or "Boston butt," which is actually cut from the top of the pig's shoulder, forming a somewhat rectangular hunk of well-marbled meat. You can use bone-in, which we like for added flavor, or boned. If you can only find a cut labeled "picnic shoulder," you can use it but it will not be quite as tender.

Note that the roasting time is about an hour per pound; adjust accordingly, as your piece of meat might vary in weight.

---

2 tablespoons kosher salt

1 tablespoon firmly packed light brown sugar

1 tablespoon dry mustard

1 tablespoon paprika

1 tablespoon smoked paprika

1 teaspoon chipotle chile powder

1 teaspoon ground cumin

1 (5- to 6-pound [2.3 to 2.7 kg]) bone-in Boston butt, at room temperature

Position a rack in the center of the oven. Preheat the oven to 300°F (150°C). Have ready a large roasting pan.

Stir together the salt, brown sugar, mustard, paprika, smoked paprika, chipotle chile powder, and cumin in a small bowl. Use your hands to thoroughly rub the mixture into the pork, covering every surface, including over any fat cap and under any flaps of meat or fat.

Place the meat in the roasting pan, fat cap (fatty layer) down, and roast for about 6 hours. Check with an instant-read thermometer, cooking the meat until it reaches 150°F (65°C). This will take about an hour per pound, give or take a little, depending on how cold the meat was when you placed it in the oven. Allow the meat to rest for at least 20 minutes, for the juices to redistribute. Simply shred the meat, using two forks, pull apart with your fingers, or chop into hunks with a knife.

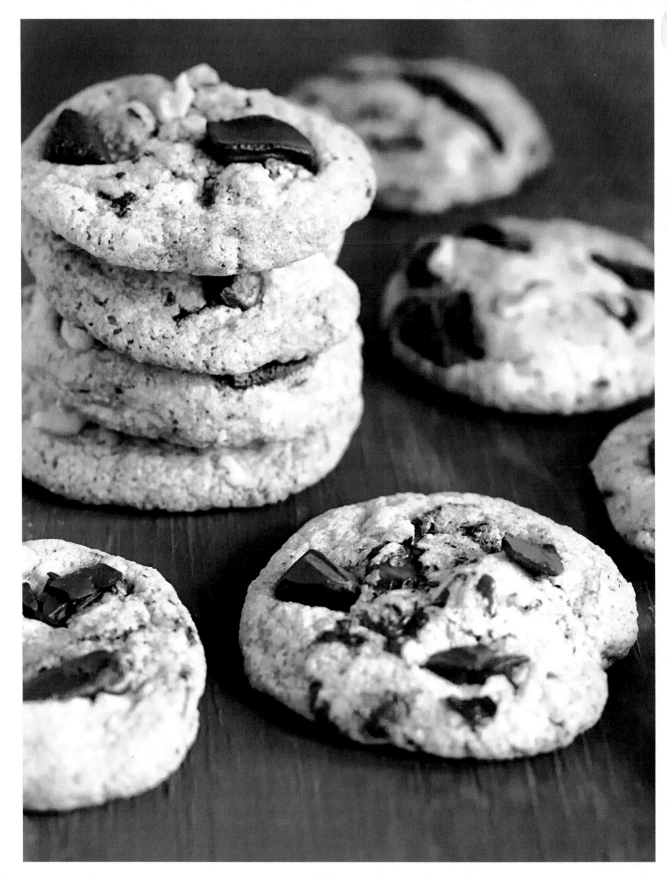

Chapter 13

DESSERTS & BAKED GOODS: SIMPLE & SPECTACULAR

YOU MIGHT BE WONDERING whether you are still allowed baked goods and treats now and then. The answer is yes! Of course, even if you fall in love with the Chocolate Chunk Cookies (page 319) or Carrot Cake with Cream Cheese Frosting (page 310), use your best judgment. These aren't for every day, but when the hankering does strike, or it's a birthday or pot-luck or other special event where you need a low FODMAP sweet, this chapter will be your guide. We have also included more everyday baked goods, such as Corn Bread (page 337) and Banana Bread (page 303), so you don't have to wait for a special occasion.

Blueberry Muffins

   MAKES 12 STANDARD-SIZE MUFFINS | SERVING SIZE 1 MUFFIN

These muffins freeze well—you can remove one muffin at a time from the freezer for quick weekday breakfasts or to pack as a snack. Crushing some of the blueberries adds to the moistness, so don't skip that step. The sprinkling of sugar on top of the muffins creates a bakery-worthy finish but is not necessary.

Nonstick spray (optional)

2 cups (290 g) gluten-free all-purpose flour, such as Bob's Red Mill Gluten-Free 1 to 1 Baking Flour

2 teaspoons gluten-free baking powder

½ teaspoon salt

½ cup (1 stick; 226 g) unsalted butter, at room temperature, cut into pieces

1 cup (198 g) sugar, plus 2 tablespoons for sprinkling (optional), divided

2 teaspoons pure vanilla extract

2 large eggs, at room temperature

½ cup (120 ml) lactose-free milk (whole, 2%, 1%, or fat-free), at room temperature

2¼ cups (383 g) fresh blueberries

Position a rack in the middle of the oven. Preheat the oven to 400°F (200°C). Coat twelve standard-size muffin wells with nonstick spray, or line with fluted paper cups; set aside.

Whisk together the flour, baking powder, and salt in a medium-size bowl, to aerate and combine; set aside.

Beat the butter in a separate bowl, using an electric mixer on medium-high speed, until creamy, for about 3 minutes. Add the sugar and beat until lightened, for about 2 minutes, scraping down the bowl once or twice. Beat in the vanilla, then the eggs, one at a time, scraping down after each addition, and allowing each egg to be absorbed before continuing.

Add the flour mixture in three additions, alternately with the milk. Do not combine completely; there should be streaks of flour left.

Place ⅔ cup (113 g) of the blueberries in a bowl and crush with a potato masher. Fold these crushed blueberries, along with any juice, and the whole blueberries into the muffin batter.

Divide the batter evenly among the prepared muffin wells. Sprinkle the tops with the 2 table-spoons of sugar, if using.

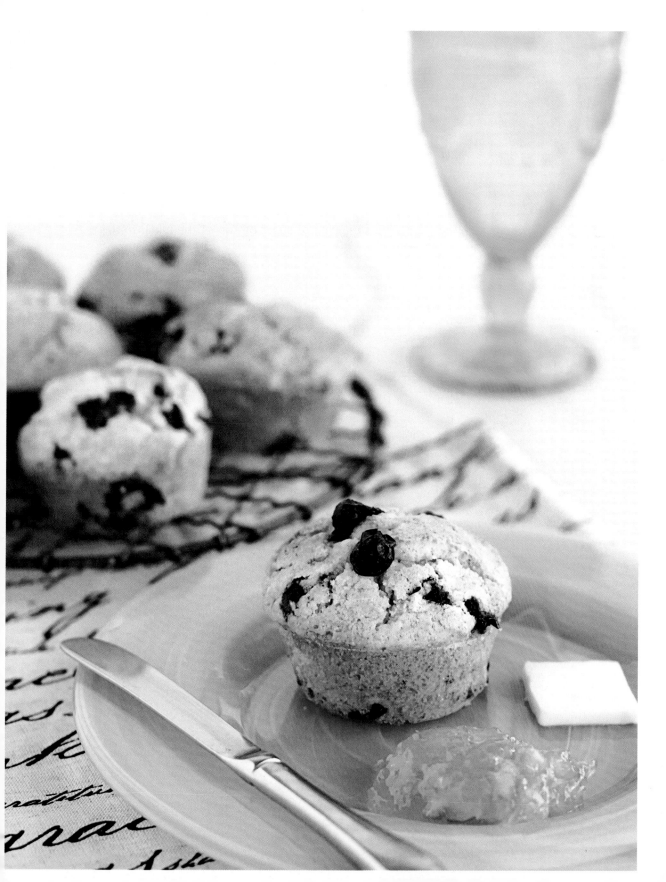

Place in the oven and immediately lower the oven temperature to 375°F (190°C). Bake for 20 to 25 minutes, or until a toothpick inserted into the center shows a few moist crumbs. Allow the pan to cool on a wire rack for 5 minutes, then remove the muffins from the pan and place them directly on the rack to cool. Serve as soon as possible, either warm or at room temperature. Store at room temperature in an airtight container for up to 1 day or freeze for up to 1 month.

DÉDÉ'S TIPS

You can make these with frozen blueberries. Do not defrost before folding in. The baking time might be a bit longer.

You can make these vegan by using ½ cup (120 ml) of solid coconut oil instead of the butter (creaming it like butter) and using unsweetened almond milk in lieu of the milk.

POST-FODMAP CHALLENGE PHASE OPTION

Fructan: If you passed the fructan wheat challenge, you can sub in all-purpose unbleached flour for the gluten-free flour (do not use this substitution if following a gluten-free diet). Use weight equivalents for the most accurate results with this substitution.

Banana Bread

   MAKES ONE 8-INCH (20 CM) LOAF | 9 SLICES | SERVING SIZE 1 SLICE

Dédé's work in the world of baking means she has made hundreds of versions of banana bread and this one is one of her friend's and family's favorites! It is incredibly moist, supereasy to prep, lasts for days, and even freezes well. The addition of light brown sugar, with its slightly caramel-like flavors, actually enhances the tropical banana taste. Feel free to use the walnuts and/or chocolate morsels if you like—or go for straight banana bread flavor and texture and leave them out.

Nonstick spray

1½ cups (218 g) gluten-free all-purpose flour, such as Bob's Red Mill Gluten Free 1 to 1 Baking Flour

1 teaspoon baking soda

½ teaspoon salt

½ cup (120 ml) vegetable oil

½ cup (99 g) granulated sugar

½ cup (107 g) firmly packed light brown sugar

2 large eggs, at room temperature

1½ cups (360 ml) fork-mashed banana (about 3 medium-size just ripe bananas)

1 teaspoon pure vanilla extract

1 cup (99 g) toasted walnut halves, finely chopped (optional)

½ cup (85 g) miniature semisweet chocolate morsels (optional)

Position a rack in the center of the oven. Preheat the oven to 350°F (180°C). Coat an 8½ x 4¼-inch (21.5 x 10.5 cm) loaf pan with nonstick spray (see Dédé's Tips).

Whisk together the flour, baking soda, and salt in a large bowl and set aside.

Whisk the oil, granulated sugar, and brown sugar together in a medium-size bowl until thoroughly combined. Whisk in the eggs, one at a time, until incorporated. Whisk in the banana and vanilla.

Pour the wet ingredients over the dry ingredients and whisk gently just until combined, finishing with a rubber spatula. Gently fold in the walnuts and/or chocolate morsels at this time, if using.

Scrape the batter into the loaf pan and bake for 1 hour to 1 hour 10 minutes. A toothpick should test clean when inserted into the center of the bread, the top will be golden and risen, and the edges will just be pulling away from the sides of the pan.

Allow the pan to cool on a wire rack for 10 minutes, then turn the bread out onto the rack and allow to cool completely. The bread is ready to eat immediately; however, it slices best after being wrapped in plastic wrap and allowed to sit at room temperature overnight. The bread will keep for about 4 days (but you can never keep it around that long); you can also freeze it for up to 1 month. Defrost in the fridge overnight.

Try it toasted for breakfast.

DÉDÉ'S TIPS

You can make this banana bread recipe in a standard 9 x 5-inch (23 x 12 cm) loaf pan or the smaller size indicated. Check for doneness about 5 minutes earlier than suggested if baking in the larger pan.

POST-FODMAP CHALLENGE PHASE OPTION

Fructan: If you passed the fructan wheat challenge, you can sub in all-purpose unbleached flour for the gluten-free flour, or try whole wheat pastry flour (do not use these substitutions if following a gluten-free diet). A whole wheat version will be heavier; we recommend using half whole wheat pastry flour and half all-purpose flour at first and adjust to your taste from there. Use weight equivalents for most accurate results with these substitutions.

Cinnamon Pecan Streusel Coffee Cake

   MAKES 14 TO 16 SERVINGS

This big, impressive, ring-shaped coffee cake is packed with all of the classic coffee cake flavors and textures: a rich sour cream batter, a cinnamon pecan streusel ribboned inside and crowning the top, and a white glaze drizzled over all. The lactose-free sour cream and gluten free-flour makes this all possible to enjoy even during your elimination phase.

Nonstick spray

Gluten-free all-purpose flour, such as Bob's Red Mill Gluten Free
    1 to 1 Baking Flour, for pan

CINNAMON PECAN STREUSEL:

½ cup (1 stick; 113 g) unsalted butter, cut into pieces

¾ cup (160 g) firmly packed light brown sugar

1 tablespoon ground cinnamon

½ teaspoon salt

1 cup (145 g) gluten-free all-purpose flour, such as Bob's Red Mill Gluten Free 1 to 1 Baking Flour

½ cup (50 g) lightly toasted pecan or walnut halves, finely chopped

CAKE:

3 cups (435 g) gluten-free all-purpose flour, such as Bob's Red Mill Gluten Free 1 to 1 Baking Flour

1½ teaspoons gluten-free baking powder

1½ teaspoons baking soda

½ teaspoon salt

1½ cups (3 sticks; 339 g) unsalted butter, at room temperature, cut into pieces

1½ cups (297 g) granulated sugar

2¼ teaspoons pure vanilla extract

3 large eggs, at room temperature

1½ cups (341 g) lactose-free sour cream, at room temperature

GLAZE:

1 cup (90 g) sifted confectioners' sugar

1 tablespoon water

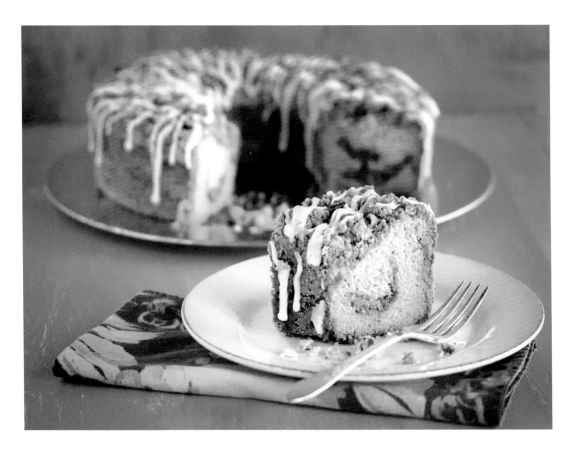

Position a rack in the center of the oven. Preheat the oven to 325°F (165°C). Coat a 12-cup (2.9 L) ring pan with nonstick spray, then dust with the flour, tapping out any excess.

Prepare the streusel: Melt the butter in a medium-size microwave-safe mixing bowl in the microwave on low. (Or melt the butter in a small saucepan on your stove top, if you like, then transfer to a medium-size mixing bowl.) Whisk in the brown sugar, cinnamon, and salt, then stir in the flour and nuts. Create texture by squeezing the mixture together with your fingers. Set aside.

Prepare the cake: Whisk together the flour, baking powder, baking, soda, and salt in a medium-size bowl, to aerate and combine; set aside.

Beat the butter until creamy with the flat paddle attachment of a stand mixer on medium-high speed until creamy, for about 2 minutes. If using a handheld electric mixer, the beating times could be twice as long or longer; use visual cues. Add the granulated sugar gradually and continue to beat for about 3 minutes at medium-high speed, until very light and fluffy. Beat in the vanilla. Add the eggs, one at a time, beating well after each addition, scraping down the bowl as needed. The mixture might look curdled; that's okay. Add the flour mixture in three additions, alternately with the sour cream. Begin and end with the flour mixture and beat briefly until smooth.

Scrape a little over half of the thick batter (you can do this by eye) into the prepared pan and smooth the top with a small offset spatula. Sprinkle a scant half of the streusel evenly over the batter, covering it completely. Top with the remaining batter, spreading carefully with an offset spatula to cover the streusel, then top with the remaining streusel, covering the entire surface. Press the streusel topping gently so that it adheres to the batter.

Bake for 55 to 65 minutes, or until a bamboo skewer inserted into the center of the cake shows a few moist crumbs. The streusel will be golden brown and the cake will crown a bit. Allow the pan to cool on a wire rack for at least 20 minutes; the pan should be barely warm. Invert to unmold the cake onto a plate, then invert again to place it right side up on the rack. Once cooled, transfer to a display platter.

Prepare the glaze: Place the confectioners' sugar in a saucepan. Whisk in water until beginning to combine; it will be thick before you heat it. Cook over medium heat, whisking often, until it liquefies and becomes completely smooth and very warm to the touch. Do not let it get too hot or simmer. This cooking time will be brief—for about 15 seconds, give or take. Whisk until completely smooth and use immediately.

Drizzle the glaze over the cake, using a spoon or fork. It will set almost instantly.

The cake is now ready to serve. Store at room temperature in an airtight container for up to 3 days.

POST-FODMAP CHALLENGE PHASE OPTION

Fructan: If you passed the fructan wheat challenge, you can sub in all-purpose unbleached flour for the gluten-free flour (do not use this substitution if following a gluten-free diet). Use weight equivalents for most accurate results with this substitution.

Lemon Ginger Scones

  MAKES 8 SCONES | SERVING SIZE 1 SCONE

Scones are a perfect breakfast or coffee break treat for weekdays or special brunches. They are rich, and as such we consider them an occasional indulgence. In the regular baking world, some scones contain eggs and some do not. We found that eggs were really necessary for the gluten-free approach, to create a desirable texture—and these are crave worthy! The double hit of ginger via the crystalized ginger and the grated fresh ginger really boosts that flavor profile. Look for bulk crystallized ginger in natural food stores, where it will be most economical. The scones are delicious as is, but you have three options, which we detail below: plain, with a crunchy sugar topping, or lemon glazed.

SCONES:

1¾ cups (254 g) gluten-free all-purpose flour, such as Bob's Red Mill 1 to 1 Gluten Free Baking Flour, plus more for hands and knife, if needed

⅓ cup (66 g) granulated sugar

2 teaspoons gluten-free baking powder

1 teaspoon ground ginger

½ teaspoon salt

½ cup (1 stick; 113 g) unsalted butter, cold, cut into pieces

⅓ cup (64 g) finely chopped crystallized ginger

1 tablespoon freshly grated lemon zest (use a Microplane or rasp-style zester)

⅓ cup (75 ml) lactose-free milk (whole, 2%, 1%, or fat-free), cold

2 large eggs, cold

OPTIONAL TOPPING:

2 tablespoons coarse decorating sugar or 1 cup (90 g) sifted confectioners' sugar

1¼ tablespoons freshly squeezed lemon juice

Prepare the scones: Position a rack in the center of the oven. Preheat the oven to 400°F (200°C). Line a baking sheet with parchment paper; set aside.

Whisk the flour, sugar, baking powder, ground ginger, and salt in a medium-size mixing bowl, to aerate and combine. Using a handheld pastry blender, two butter knives, or your fingertips, work in the butter until the mixture resembles a very coarse, crumbly meal, with larger pockets of butter left here and there. Toss in the crystallized ginger and the lemon zest.

Measure the milk in a liquid measuring cup, then whisk the eggs into the milk. Pour the wet mixture over the dry and mix just until combined. Scrape out onto the prepared pan and use very lightly floured hands to pat the dough into an 8-inch (20 cm) round about ½ inch thick (12 mm). Use a sharp knife to cut into eight equal wedges. (Dip the knife into extra flour if it is sticking, wiping clean between cuts.) Separate the wedges so that they are evenly spaced on the pan. The scones can be left plain or sprinkle some with the coarse sugar, if desired. (If you wish to glaze instead, that will happen after cooling.)

Bake for 15 to 20 minutes, or until lightly browned top and bottom. Allow the pan to cool on a wire rack for 5 minutes. The warm scones are ready to serve. Transfer the scones to the wire rack to cool completely if you want to glaze them.

Prepare a glaze, if using: Place the confectioners' sugar in a small saucepan. Whisk in the lemon juice until beginning to combine; it will be thick. Cook over low-medium heat, whisking often, until it liquefies and becomes completely smooth and just warm to the touch. Do not let it get too hot or simmer. This cooking time will be brief—for about 15 seconds, give or take. Whisk until completely smooth, then use a spoon or fork to drizzle over the cooled scones. The glaze will harden almost immediately. The glazed scones are ready to serve and are best enjoyed as soon as possible; certainly the same day.

POST-FODMAP CHALLENGE PHASE OPTIONS

Lactose: If you passed the lactose challenge, you can use regular dairy milk (whole milk) instead of the lactose-free milk.

Fructan: If you passed the fructan wheat challenge, you can sub in all-purpose unbleached flour for the gluten-free flour (do not use this substitution if following a gluten-free diet). Use weight equivalents for most accurate results with this substitution.

Carrot Cake with Cream Cheese Frosting

  MAKES ONE 13 X 9-INCH CAKE (33 X 23 CM) | 24 SERVINGS

Carrot cake is one of those classic recipes that lends itself quite easily to a low FODMAP makeover. We have made it gluten-free and added just the right amount of raisins and nuts to keep it low FODMAP approved. Lactose-free cream cheese allows us to have the expected cream cheese frosting; however, this type of cream cheese has to be handled a bit differently from regular cream cheese, so make sure to follow the frosting preparation carefully. The 13 x 9-inch (33 x 23 cm) size makes this a perfect cake for a school birthday, a bake sale, or for an office party. And you can prep this cake in the time it takes for the oven to preheat.

Nonstick spray

CARROT CAKE:

2 cups (290 g) gluten-free all-purpose flour, such as Bob's Red Mill Gluten Free 1 to 1 Baking Flour

2 teaspoons gluten-free baking powder

2 teaspoons ground cinnamon

1 teaspoon baking soda

1 teaspoon salt

1 cup (240 ml) vegetable oil

¾ cup (149 g) granulated sugar

½ cup (107 g) firmly packed light brown sugar

4 large eggs, at room temperature

1 pound (455 g) carrots, finely grated

1 cup (99 g) toasted and chopped pecans or walnuts

1 cup (160 g) raisins

CREAM CHEESE FROSTING:

6 tablespoons (¾ stick; 85 g) unsalted butter, at room temperature, cut into pieces

3 cups (270 g) sifted confectioners' sugar

1½ teaspoons freshly squeezed lemon juice

½ cup (113 g) lactose-free cream cheese, cold, such as 1 (8 ounce [225 g]) tub Green Valley Organics brand

Prepare the cake: Position a rack in the middle of the oven. Preheat the oven to 350°F (180°C). Coat a 13 x 9-inch (33 x 23 cm) cake pan with nonstick spray. Line the bottom with parchment paper, then spray the parchment, if you want to unmold it before frosting.

Whisk together the flour, baking powder, cinnamon, baking soda, and salt in a large bowl, to aerate and combine; set aside.

Whisk together the oil, granulated sugar, and brown sugar in a medium bowl until well blended. Whisk in the eggs, one at a time, until combined. Stir in the grated carrot, nuts, and raisins.

Pour the wet ingredients over the dry and stir until just combined. The batter will be heavy; make sure you mix well and that there are no pockets of flour left, particularly on the bottom of the bowl. Scrape the batter into the prepared pan and smooth the top with an offset spatula.

Bake for 35 to 40 minutes, or until a toothpick inserted into the center shows a few moist crumbs. Allow the pan to cool on a wire rack for 15 minutes. If desired, unmold the cake right onto the rack, peel off the parchment, and allow to cool completely. Alternatively, allow to cool completely in the pan. The cake is ready to frost, or wrap in plastic wrap and store at room temperature and frost within 24 hours.

Make the frosting: Beat the butter in a large bowl, using an electric mixer on medium-high speed, until very creamy and smooth, for about 2 minutes. Add half of the sugar (just eyeball it), beating on low speed, until it is absorbed and the mixture is creamy. Add the lemon juice and about half of what is left of the sugar and beat until smooth, scraping down the bowl as needed. Add the cream cheese and remaining sugar and beat until completely smooth. The frosting is ready to use and best if used immediately.

If the cake has cooled in the pan, simply spread the frosting on top in attractive swirls, using a spoon, butter knife, or small offset icing spatula. The cake can be transported easily and served directly out of the pan.

If the cake is unmolded, place on a serving platter and spread the frosting on top (and on the sides, if desired) as described above.

The cake may be served immediately, or refrigerated for up to 2 days under a cake dome. Bring to room temperature before serving.

DÉDÉ'S TIPS

I am thrilled to have access to lactose-free dairy products, such as Green Valley Organics Lactose Free Cream Cheese, but do not try to approach it as you would regular cream cheese. Upon agitation this product liquefies, so you cannot simply substitute it in your own traditional cream cheese frosting recipe. It will not work.

POST-FODMAP CHALLENGE PHASE OPTION

Fructan: If you passed the fructan wheat challenge, you could use unbleached all-purpose flour instead of the gluten-free flour (do not use this substitution if following a gluten-free diet). Use weight equivalents for the most accurate results with this substitution.

Birthday & Celebration Cake for Everyone (Yellow Cake & Chocolate Frosting)

  ONE 8- OR 9-INCH (20 OR 23 CM), THREE LAYER CAKE | SERVES 16. ALTERNATIVELY, MAKES ONE DEEP 13 X 9-INCH (33 X 23 CM) RECTANGLE OR ABOUT 36 CUPCAKES

We all have birthdays, kids and adults, and celebratory events arise from office parties to school functions and bake sales where a classic American layer cake is needed. What is a FODMAPer to do? This recipe is the answer: a tender, buttery three-layer yellow cake with old-fashioned creamy, swirly chocolate frosting that looks and tastes just like the nostalgic cakes of our childhood. Like many baked goods, this cake is best enjoyed as fresh as possible. Dédé likes to make the cake the day before the event and then either frosts it the day before or the day of. Whatever you do, do not refrigerate, as that will dry out the cake. Alternatively, this recipe makes one 13 x 9-inch (33 x 23 cm) rectangle or about three dozen cupcakes (see Dédé's Tips).

Nonstick spray

CAKE:

4 scant cups (575 g) gluten-free flour, such as Bob's Red Mill 1 to 1 Gluten Free Baking Flour

1 tablespoon plus ¼ teaspoon gluten-free baking powder

¾ teaspoon salt

1½ cups (3 sticks; 339 g) unsalted butter, at room temperature, cut into small pieces

2½ cups (495) granulated sugar

1 tablespoon pure vanilla extract

6 large eggs, at room temperature

1½ cups (360 ml) lactose-free milk (whole, 2%, 1%, or fat-free), at room temperature

FROSTING:

7½ ounces (215 g) semisweet or bittersweet chocolate (50% to 60% cacao), finely chopped

¾ cup (1½ sticks; 170 g) unsalted butter, at room temperature, cut into pieces

6¾ to 8¼ cups (608 to 743 g) sifted confectioners' sugar

1 tablespoon pure vanilla extract

½ to ¾ cup (120 to 180 ml) lactose-free milk (whole, 2%, 1%, or fat-free), at room temperature

Gluten-free nonpareils or sprinkles (optional)

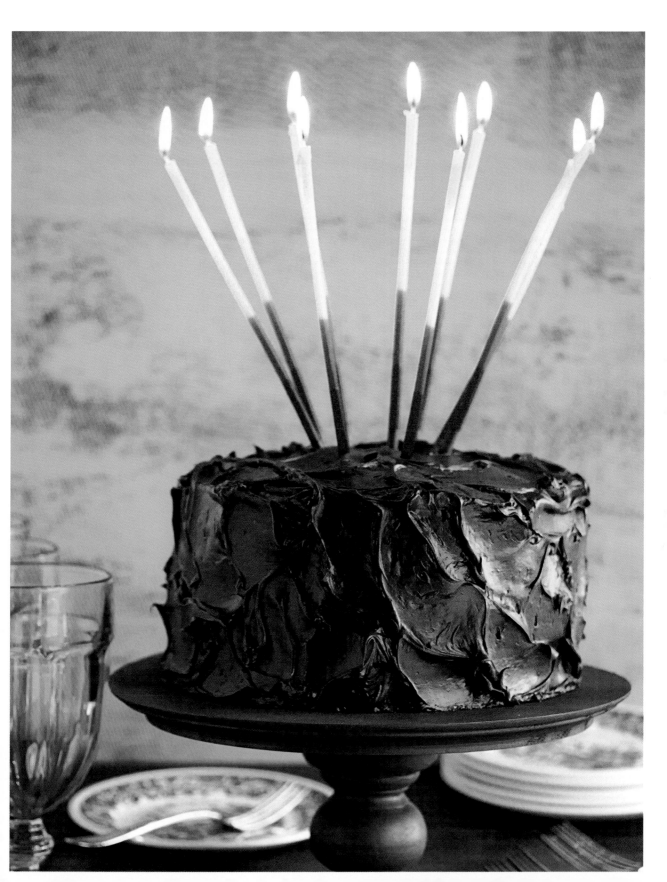

Prepare the cake: Position a rack in the center of your oven. Preheat the oven to 350°F (180°C). Coat three 8- or 9-inch (20 or 23 cm) round cake pans with nonstick spray, line the bottoms with parchment rounds, then spray the parchment (see Dédé's Tips if using the suggested alternative pans).

Whisk together the flour, baking powder, and salt in a medium-size bowl, to aerate and combine; set aside.

Beat the butter in a large bowl, with an electric mixer on medium-high speed, until creamy, for 2 to 3 minutes. Add the granulated sugar gradually and beat until very light and fluffy, for about 3 minutes, scraping down the bowl once or twice. Beat in the vanilla.

Beat in the eggs, one at a time, scraping down after each addition, and allowing each egg to be absorbed before continuing. Add the flour mixture in four additions, alternating with the milk. Begin and end with the flour mixture and beat briefly until smooth. Divide the batter equally among the prepared round pans (see Dédé's Tips if using the suggested alternative pans).

Bake for 25 to 35 minutes, or until a toothpick inserted into the center of the cake shows a few moist crumbs. The cake will have begun to come away from the sides of the pan. Allow the pans to cool on wire racks for 10 minutes. Unmold directly onto the wire racks, peel off the parchment, and allow to cool completely. The cake is now ready to fill and frost. Alternatively, place the layers on clean cardboard and double wrap in plastic wrap; store at room temperature if assembling within 24 hours.

Prepare the frosting: Partially melt the chocolate either in a small, microwave-safe bowl in the microwave on low or in the top of a double boiler. Remove from the microwave or the heat and stir until completely melted; set aside to cool briefly until just warm.

Meanwhile, beat the butter in a large bowl, using an electric mixer on medium-high speed, until creamy, for 2 to 3 minutes. Add about half of the confectioners' sugar (eyeball it), the melted chocolate, the vanilla, and ⅓ cup of the milk and beat until combined and very creamy and smooth, for at least 2 to 3 minutes more, or as long as it takes to achieve a thick, creamy, and smooth consistency. Add additional confectioners' sugar only if necessary. This frosting's texture is a balance between the confectioners' sugar and the milk: add more sugar for a thicker frosting, more milk to thin it out. You want the texture to at least be thick enough to hold swirls when you apply it to your cake. If the frosting looks spongy or coarse, simply keep beating.

To assemble: Trim the tops of the cake layers if they are excessively domed. Place one cake layer, top side down, on a display plate. Apply a thick layer of frosting to the up-turned bottom, using a small offset spatula to spread it all the way to the edges. Add a second layer of cake, top side down, and add a layer of frosting. Place the third layer on top (bottom side up if you want it perfectly flat, or top side up for a more rounded appearance). Apply the frosting thickly to the final cake layer, spreading out toward the edges, then frost the sides. If the frosting becomes stiff while using, simply rebeat it. You can use the icing spatula or even a dessert spoon to create swirls in the frosting. Scatter the top with nonpareils or sprinkles, if desired. Get the candles ready for a delicious low FODMAP birthday celebration! The cake is ready to serve, or may be stored at room temperature under a cake dome for up to 24 hours.

DÉDÉ'S TIPS

If using a 13 x 9-inch (33 cm x 23 cm) pan, coat with nonstick spray and line the bottom with parchment (if unmolding after); bake for 30 to 35 minutes and allow to cool in the pan on a wire rack, then unmold if desired. If making cupcakes, line three dozen cupcake wells with fluted paper liners and fill each two-thirds full with the batter, then bake for about 20 minutes. Allow the pan to cool on a wire rack for 5 minutes, then unmold the cupcakes directly onto the rack to cool. The frosting can be used to frost all of these as well.

POST-FODMAP CHALLENGE PHASE OPTIONS

Lactose: If you passed the lactose challenge, you can use regular dairy milk (whole milk) instead of the lactose-free milk for the cake and frosting.

Fructan: If you passed the fructan wheat challenge, you could use unbleached all-purpose flour instead of the gluten-free flour (do not use this substitution if following a gluten-free diet). Use weight equivalents for the most accurate results with this substitution.

NY-Style Cheesecake with Glazed Strawberries

 MAKES ONE 9-INCH (2CM) CHEESECAKE | 12 TO 24 SERVINGS

This is a New York–style cheesecake, based on cream cheese and enhanced with sour cream—all lactose-free, of course. Any low FODMAP cookie crumb can be used to make the crust; we used Pamela's Pecan Shortbread. The strawberry topping is optional but highly recommended. This cheesecake is not only gorgeous, but the freshness of the fruit is the perfect complement to the rich creamy cheesecake. The cheesecake is baked in a water bath; to protect the cake from any water leaking into the pan, we use extra-wide, heavy-duty aluminum foil wrapped around the outside of the pan. As with any cheesecake, this keeps well (without topping) and should be refrigerated at least overnight for the neatest slicing, so plan ahead.

Nonstick spray

CRUST:

1 (7.25 ounce [210 g]) box Pamela's Pecan Shortbread, or enough low FODMAP cookie crumbs of choice to measure 1¼ cups (300 ml) (use gluten-free, if necessary)

1 to 6 tablespoons (1 tablespoon to 85 g) unsalted butter

FILLING:

4 (8-ounce [227 g]) containers lactose-free cream cheese, such as Green Valley Organics brand, at room temperature

¾ cups (149 g) sugar

1 teaspoon freshly squeezed lemon juice

1 teaspoon pure vanilla extract

5 large eggs, at room temperature, whisked very well in a bowl

1 cup (227 g) lactose-free sour cream, such as Green Valley Organics brand, at room temperature

TOPPING:

1 pound (455 g) strawberries, preferably all medium-size and deep red in color

¼ cup (50 g) sugar

1 tablespoon freshly squeezed lemon juice

1 tablespoon cold water

1½ teaspoons cornstarch

Prepare the crust: Position a rack in the center of the oven. Preheat the oven to 375°F (190°C). Coat the inside of a 9-inch (23 cm) springform pan with nonstick spray. Double wrap the outside of the pan with 18-inch (46 cm)-wide (extra-wide) aluminum foil, bringing the foil all the way up and around the sides of the pan to the top edge; set aside.

Grind the cookies to a fine crumb in a food processor fitted with a metal blade. Alternatively, place in a heavy resealable plastic bag and crush well with a rolling pin, using a rolling and smashing action to get the job done. Measure out 1¼ cups (300 ml) of crumbs and place in a medium-size bowl. Stir in just enough melted butter to moisten the crumbs enough so that they stick together when pressed against the sides of the bowl. (Pamela's Pecan Shortbread is very buttery on its own and might only need 1 tablespoon of butter. Classic graham-type crumbs might need the largest amount.) Press the crust mixture firmly into an even layer in the prepared pan.

Bake for 10 to 12 minutes, or until light golden brown. You want the crust to dry out a bit. Remove the crust from the oven and set aside on a wire rack. Lower the oven temperature to 325°F (165°C).

Meanwhile, prepare the filling: Lactose-free cream cheese acts differently from regular cream cheese, so please follow our technique: place one (8-ounce [225 g]) container's worth of the cream cheese in a large mixing bowl and blend, with an electric mixer on low speed, until creamy and smooth. Add the sugar, lemon juice, and vanilla and blend very briefly on low speed. Pour in the eggs a little bit at a time, mixing just enough to incorporate and no more. The mixture might be very liquid at this point; that's okay. Add the remaining three containers' worth of cream cheese and sour cream and beat just until combined, for 30 seconds to 1 minute. If the mixture is not blending, use a large balloon whisk to whisk by hand, using a folding action. Make sure the mixture is well combined but do not overmix. Scrape the filling into the crust and smooth the top with a small offset spatula.

Place the foil-wrapped pan in a large roasting pan. Add very hot tap water to the roasting pan to come up the sides of the wrapped pan by about 1 inch (2.5 cm). Bake for 1 hour. The cake should be set along the edges and slightly jiggly in the center. Turn off the oven and leave the cake in the oven for 20 minutes more. While the cake is still on its oven rack, dip the tip of a small paring knife in warm water and use it to run around the top edge of the cake (going down about ½ inch [12 mm]) to loosen it from the pan; this will prevent the sides from pulling away from the pan as it cools, then remove the cake from the oven. Remove the cake pan from the roasting pan and remove the foil. Refrigerate the cake in its springform pan overnight or up to 48 hours. Dip a small icing spatula in warm water, shake dry, and run all the way around the outer edge of the cake, going all the way down to the bottom. Release the springform rim, and remove and place the cake on a display plate.

Prepare the topping: Wash and dry the berries and hull. Divide the whole berries into two portions (by eye), reserving the best-looking berries for the top of the cake. Finely chop the rest and place them, along with the sugar and lemon juice, in a saucepan and stir to combine. Cook over medium heat, crushing the berries with a potato masher or fork, until they become juicy and break down into a thick sauce, for about 3 minutes. Combine the cold water and cornstarch in a small bowl and stir into the sauce. Continue to cook, stirring frequently, until the sauce thickens, for about 1 minute. Scrape into a fine-mesh strainer set over a bowl and press the sauce through, using a rubber or silicone spatula. Place the reserved whole berries, stemmed side down, in the center of the cake in an attractive circular grouping. Use a pastry brush to coat with the strained sauce. If the sauce thickens too much, simply thin with a little bit of water. The cake is ready to serve, or may be refrigerated until serving time, preferably within the day. The cheesecake is best served cold. Use a long, thin-bladed knife dipped in hot water to slice, wiping clean between cuts.

Chocolate Chunk Cookies

   MAKES ABOUT 2 DOZEN COOKIES | SERVING SIZE 1 TO 2 COOKIES

Everyone needs a recipe for chocolate chip or chocolate chunk cookies in their repertoire, and that includes FODMAPers. We prefer chunks because then we can choose a really high-quality chocolate, but feel free to use morsels. In any event, read labels to check for acceptable low FODMAP ingredients in whatever chocolate you choose. As with any classic-style chocolate chip cookie recipe, this is very easy to make. The resting and chilling time allows the dry ingredients to become hydrated by the eggs and creates the chewy texture we love. We aim for crisp edges and chewy centers, which is accomplished with our choice of ingredients, preparation technique, and also baking time. Even thirty seconds too long in the oven and you can end up with crisp cookies. Just be aware that you can control the outcome of the finished cookie's texture by playing with the baking time. We have provided visual cues as well as time cues to help you along.

2⅓ (338 g) cups gluten-free all-purpose flour, such as Bob's Red Mill 1 to 1 Gluten Free Baking Flour

1 teaspoon baking soda

1 teaspoon salt

1 cup (2 sticks; 226 g) unsalted butter, at room temperature, cut into pieces

1 cup (213 g) firmly packed light brown sugar

½ cup granulated sugar

2 teaspoons vanilla extract

2 large eggs, at room temperature

12 ounces (340 g; about 2 cups) semisweet or bittersweet chocolate chunks, cut into ½-inch (12 mm) pieces (we like 60% to 70% cacao)

1⅓ cups (132 g) toasted walnut or pecan halves, chopped (optional)

Whisk together the flour, baking soda, and salt in a medium-size bowl to aerate and combine; set aside.

Beat the butter in a large bowl, with electric mixer on medium-high speed, until creamy. Add the brown sugar and granulated sugar and beat until lightened, for about 3 minutes, scraping down the bowl as needed. Beat in the vanilla, then the eggs, one at a time, allowing each one to be incorporated before adding the next. Beat in the dry mixture until a few streaks of flour remain. Add the chocolate and nuts, if using, and beat just until combined. Cover the bowl and chill for at least 4 hours, preferably overnight.

Position racks in the upper and lower thirds of the oven. Preheat the oven to 375°F (190°C). Line two baking sheets with parchment paper.

Form golf ball–size balls and place eight on each pan, spaced evenly apart. No need to press them down.

Bake for 9 to 12 minutes, or until lightly browned with the edges firmer than the centers, which should be soft. The cookies firm up tremendously upon cooling. Allow the cookies to cool completely on the pans set on wire racks. (Bake the remaining batter on cooled pans.) The cookies are best served the same day, but may be stored at room temperature in an airtight container for up to 3 days.

KATE'S NOTES

Let's talk a bit about one of my favorite subjects: chocolate! Semisweet or bittersweet chocolate is low FODMAP in a small portion, one about the equivalent of a scant 3 tablespoons of semisweet chocolate chip morsels or 30 grams, but do avoid white and milk chocolate if you are sensitive to lactose in portions greater than 15 grams.

POST-FODMAP CHALLENGE PHASE OPTION

Fructan: If you passed the fructan wheat challenge, you could use unbleached all-purpose flour instead of the gluten-free flour (do not use this substitution if following a gluten-free diet). Use weight equivalents for the most accurate results with this substitution.

(Recipe photo on page 298)

3-Ingredient, 17-Second Peanut Butter Cookies

    MAKES 15 COOKIES | SERVING SIZE 1 COOKIE

Did the title get you? These cookies do indeed have only three ingredients and are naturally gluten-free and FODMAP-friendly, as there is no flour whatsoever. After tasting these, you will never make traditional peanut butter cookies again. As for the seventeen-second declaration, Dédé once made these live on TV and was timed to see how fast the dough could be put together. There was a stopwatch, countdown, and everything, and indeed, it took a mere seventeen seconds. Of course, you have to measure out the peanut butter first and then dole out the dough onto the prepared cookie sheets, but you can easily make these in less time than it takes for the oven to preheat. These are a classic cookie jar treat—and they are perfect for the low FODMAP diet.

1 cup (270 g) smooth, lightly salted natural peanut butter

1 cup (198 g) sugar

1 large egg, at room temperature

Preheat the oven to 350°F (180°C). Line a baking sheet with parchment paper.

Combine the peanut butter, sugar, and egg in a medium-size bowl and mix until smooth, using an electric mixer on high speed or beat vigorously with a wooden spoon.

Drop golf ball–size balls of dough, spaced evenly apart, onto the prepared baking sheet. Make a crisscross impression into the dough with a fork. Bake for 10 to 12 minutes. Do not overbake! These cookies are best when they are still a bit soft in the center and just barely brown on the bottom. They firm up upon cooling. Allow the cookies to cool on the pan on a wire rack.

Store the cookies in an airtight container at room temperature for up to 4 days.

VARIATIONS:

Peanut Butter Cookies with Chocolate Chips: Stir in ½ cup (85 g) miniature or standard-size semisweet chocolate morsels (use dairy-free if necessary) into the batter after it is all mixed. Form, bake, and cool as directed.

Sunflower Seed Butter Cookies: Use 1 cup (270 g) of sunflower seed butter (make sure the ingredients are just sunflower seeds and oil) instead of peanut butter. Mix, form, bake, and cool as directed. Not recommended for the elimination phase; see Kate's Notes.

KATE'S NOTES

For those with peanut and tree nut allergies, substituting sunflower seed butter can work in this recipe (see Dede's Tips above); however sunflower seeds do contain fructans (oligosaccharides) in large servings, per the Monash University app, and sunflower seed butter has yet to be tested. The amount included in this recipe per cookie should still be suitable for those following a low FODMAP diet. We included this version as many suffer with allergies that preclude them from enjoying typical nut butter cookies. Perhaps start with a one-cookie serving to assess your tolerance. Remember the low FODMAP diet is not a FODMAP-free diet and you will find that some experimentation is in order so that you can enjoy the most liberal diet your body tolerates.

Chocolate Walnut Brownies

   MAKES 16 BROWNIES | SERVING SIZE 1 BROWNIE

A life without brownies? No way! We wouldn't hear of it. That said, these are an occasional treat and given the amount of cocoa, please do pay attention to portion size. Cut them as suggested, eat one per serving, and then step away from the pan. We know, it's hard, but knowing you can have treats like this will not only keep you from feeling deprived but your inner chocoholic will be thoroughly satisfied. Perfect for bake sales, potlucks, work parties, and packing for picnics. These freeze well, too. And don't miss the variations at the end of the recipe, including the Double Chocolate Brownies.

Nonstick spray

10 tablespoons (1¼ sticks; 142 g) unsalted butter, cut into 1-inch (2.5 cm) pieces

¾ cup (149 g) granulated sugar

½ cup (107 g) firmly packed light brown sugar

2 large eggs, at room temperature

1 teaspoon pure vanilla extract

⅛ teaspoon salt

¾ cup (64 g) sifted unsweetened natural cocoa powder

⅓ cup (48 g) gluten-free all-purpose flour, such as Bob's Red Mill Gluten Free 1 to 1 Baking Flour

¾ cup (75 g) lightly toasted chopped walnuts

Position a rack in the center of the oven. Preheat the oven to 325°F (165°C). Line an 8-inch (20 cm) square baking pan with parchment paper, leaving an overhang by a few inches on two opposite sides of the paper, for easy removal after baking. Coat the parchment paper with nonstick spray.

Melt the butter in a medium-size saucepan over medium heat, then transfer to a mixing bowl, or melt in the microwave on low in a large enough microwave-safe bowl that you will be able to continue to make the brownies in the same bowl for easy cleanup.

Whisk the granulated sugar and brown sugar into the melted butter until well blended. Then, whisk in the eggs, one at a time, allowing each to become incorporated before adding the next. Whisk in the vanilla and salt. Stir in the cocoa powder and flour just until some floury streaks remain, then fold in the walnuts. Scrape into the prepared pan and smooth the top with a small offset spatula.

Bake for 22 to 27 minutes, or just until a toothpick inserted into the center comes out with a few moist crumbs clinging. Allow the pan to cool on a wire rack. Use the paper overhang to remove the brownies from the pan, place on a cutting board, peel the paper down and away, and place the brownies directly on the cutting board. Cut into a 4 x 4 grid, yielding sixteen square brownies. The brownies are ready to eat, and may be stored in an airtight container for up to 3 days.

VARIATION:

Double Chocolate Brownies: Add 1 cup (170 g) of miniature or standard-size semisweet chocolate morsels to the batter along with the nuts. Or leave out the nuts, add the morsels, and go for pure chocolate decadence.

POST-FODMAP CHALLENGE PHASE OPTION

Fructan: If you passed the fructan wheat challenge, you could use unbleached all-purpose flour instead of the gluten-free flour (do not use this substitution if following a gluten-free diet). Use weight equivalents for the most accurate results with this substitution.

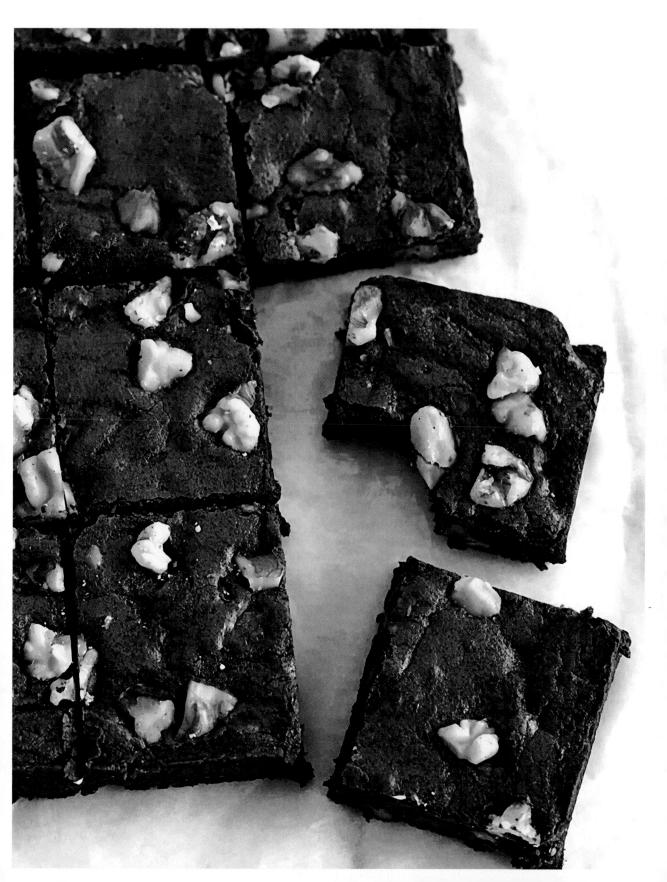

Lemon Bars

  MAKES 16 BARS | SERVING SIZE 1 BAR

The most common question we get about low FODMAP living is "What about baked goods"? People do not want to be without their treats. Lemon bars are a beloved classic and we were thrilled with this low FODMAP version and know you will be, too. These are all about the fresh, clean, tangy lemon flavor, which can truly only come from freshly squeezed lemon juice, so we encourage you to go that route. Check out the poppy seed variation at the end.

Nonstick spray

CRUST:

½ cup (1 stick; 113 g) unsalted butter, melted

3 tablespoons sugar

¼ teaspoon salt

1 cup plus 1 tablespoon (145 g plus 1 tablespoon) gluten-free all-purpose flour, such as Bob's Red Mill Gluten Free 1 to 1 Baking Flour

LEMON FILLING:

1¼ cups (248 g) sugar

3 tablespoons gluten-free all-purpose flour, such as Bob's Red Mill Gluten Free 1 to 1 Baking Flour

⅔ cup (165 ml) freshly squeezed lemon juice

3 large eggs, at room temperature

Position a rack in the center of the oven. Preheat the oven to 350°F (180°C). Line an 8-inch (23 cm) square pan with parchment paper, leaving an overhang by a few inches on two opposite sides of the paper, for easy removal after baking. Coat the paper with nonstick spray; set aside.

Prepare the crust: Whisk together the melted butter, sugar, and salt in a medium-size bowl. Stir in the flour just until combined. Pat into the prepared pan in an even layer.

Bake for 20 to 25 minutes, or until very lightly browned all over the crust.

Prepare the filling: While the crust is baking, whisk together the sugar and flour in a clean bowl, then whisk in the lemon juice. Whisk in the eggs, one at a time, until combined. When the crust is done, lower the oven temperature to 325°F (165°C), pour the filling over the crust, and bake for 18 to 22 minutes, or until the lemon filling is set. Allow the pan to cool on a wire rack. The bars are easier to cut if chilled for at least an hour. Use the paper overhang to remove the bars from the pan, place on a cutting board, peel the paper down and away, and place the bars directly on the cutting board. Cut into a 4 x 4 grid, yielding sixteen square bars. The bars are ready to serve, or store refrigerated in airtight container in single layers for up to 2 days or refrigerated for up to 4 days.

VARIATION:

Lemon Poppy Seed Bars: Simply add 2 teaspoons of poppy seeds to the crust along with the flour. Proceed as directed.

DÉDÉ'S TIPS

Lemon zest will add even more lemon flavor to your bars—but it will also add a slightly chewy texture to the filling. If you want to max out with lemon flavor, add 1 to 2 teaspoons of very light and fluffy lemon zest (created with a Microplane or rasp-style zester) to the filling. Just whisk it in and proceed as directed.

POST-FODMAP CHALLENGE PHASE OPTION

Fructan: If you passed the fructan wheat challenge, you could use unbleached all-purpose flour instead of the gluten-free flour (do not use this substitution if following a gluten-free diet). Use weight equivalents for the most accurate results with this substitution.

Blondies with Chocolate Chunks & Pecans

     MAKES 25 BARS | SERVING SIZE 1 TO 2 BARS

Blondies are all about that rich brown sugar and butter flavor, which we accentuate by browning the butter. The only trick with this recipe is to let that mixture cool before proceeding so that the chocolate chunks do not melt (see Dédé's Tips). These blondies pack well for an on-the-go treat.

Nonstick spray

1¼ cups (182 g) gluten-free all-purpose flour, such as Bob's Red Mill Gluten Free 1 to 1 Baking Flour

Heaping ½ teaspoon gluten-free baking powder

¼ teaspoon salt

6 ounces (170 g) semisweet or bittersweet chocolate, cut into ½-inch (12 mm) chunks, or 1 cup (170 g) bittersweet or semisweet morsels

⅓ cup (33 g) pecan halves, lightly toasted and chopped

½ cup (1 stick; 113 g) unsalted butter, cut into pieces

1 cup (213 g) firmly packed light brown sugar

1½ teaspoons pure vanilla extract

1 large egg, at room temperature

Position a rack in the middle of the oven. Preheat the oven to 350°F (180°C). Coat an 8-inch (20 cm) square pan with nonstick spray.

Whisk together the flour, baking powder, and salt in a small bowl, to aerate and combine; toss in the chocolate and nuts and set aside.

Melt the butter over medium heat in a medium-size saucepan. Once melted, continue to simmer over medium-low heat for a couple of minutes, or until the melted butter is golden brown. The milk solids on the bottom will also turn golden brown, but take care to not allow them to burn. There will be an irresistible toasty, buttery aroma. Remove from the heat and pour into a large mixing bowl. Allow to cool until just barely warm to the touch. Whisk in the brown sugar and vanilla until combined, then whisk in the egg. Stir in the flour mixture just until blended. Spread evenly in the prepared pan.

Bake for 20 to 25 minutes, or until a toothpick inserted in the center shows a few moist crumbs clinging when removed. The bars should be light golden brown, slightly puffed, and the edges will have just begun to come away from the sides of the pan. Allow the blondies to cool in the pan set on a wire rack.

Cut into a 5 x 5 grid, yielding twenty-five square bars. Store at room temperature for up to 3 days in an airtight container in single layers separated by parchment paper.

DÉDÉ'S TIPS

We like using heavy-duty aluminum baking pans with square edges; this way all the blondies will have nice sharp edges once cut, just as they are in a professional bakery. If you use an ovenproof glass dish, lower the oven temperature by 25°F (–4°C) and watch the baking times and visual cues for doneness, as they may vary.

POST-FODMAP CHALLENGE PHASE OPTION

Fructan: If you passed the fructan wheat challenge, you could use unbleached all-purpose flour instead of the gluten-free flour (do not use this substitution if following a gluten-free diet). Use weight equivalents for the most accurate results with this substitution.

Strawberry Shortcakes

  MAKES 6 SHORTCAKES | 1 PER SERVING

In summer we like to make shortcakes often, as the crumbly biscuits showcase so many different fruits so well, but a strawberry version is still the most requested. Luckily for us FODMAPers, we can indulge in this timeless American classic. We begin with a flaky, rich biscuit that we like to separate in half with a fork, as opposed to a knife, all the better to create more texture within the cut surfaces to catch the juices of the strawberries. To make the filling, the berries are divided in half with a portion cooked with sugar and the other half folded in fresh for maximum fruitiness. A topping of lightly whipped cream finishes off this time honored dessert. The components should be made the same day they are to be eaten, for best results.

BISCUITS:

½ cup (120 ml) lactose-free milk (whole, 2%, 1%, or fat-free), chilled

1½ teaspoons freshly squeezed lemon juice

1 large egg, chilled

1½ cups (218 g) gluten-free all-purpose flour, such as Bob's Red Mill Gluten Free 1 to 1 Baking Flour, plus more for dusting

3 tablespoons sugar

1 tablespoon gluten-free baking powder

½ teaspoon baking soda

½ teaspoon salt

½ cup (1 stick; 113 g) unsalted butter, chilled, cut into pieces

STRAWBERRY FILLING:

1 quart (590 g) strawberries, preferably small to medium-size

¼ cup (50 g) sugar, divided

1½ teaspoons freshly squeezed lemon juice

TOPPING:

1½ cups (360 ml) heavy cream, chilled

2 tablespoons sugar

Prepare the shortcakes: Position a rack in the center of the oven. Preheat the oven to 425°F (220°C). Line a baking sheet with parchment paper; set aside.

Combine the milk and lemon juice in a small bowl and allow to sit for 5 minutes to thicken, then whisk in the egg; set aside.

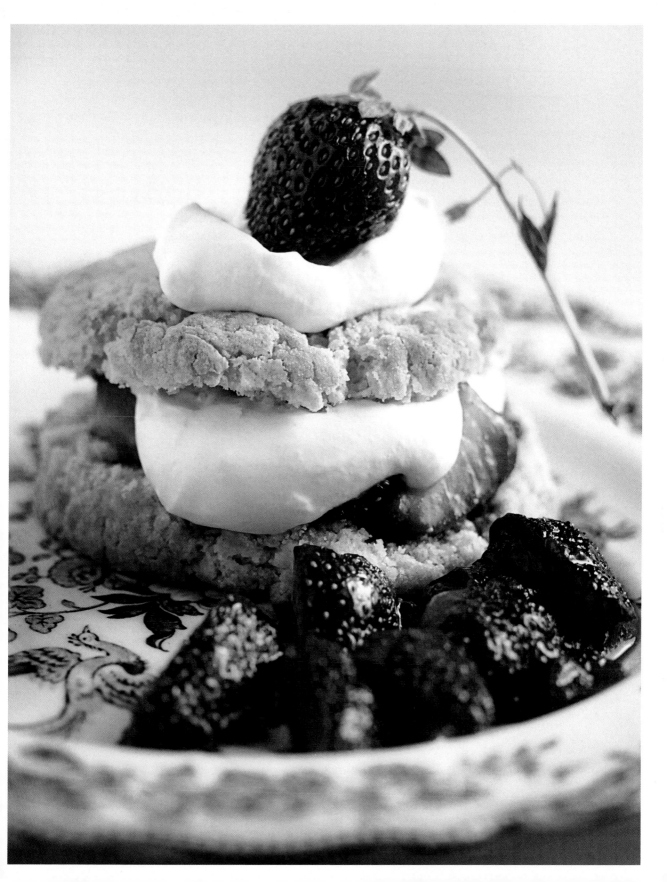

Whisk together the flour, sugar, baking powder, baking soda, and salt in a large mixing bowl, to aerate and combine. Cut in the butter with a pastry blender or two knives until the butter is the size of flat raisins. (Alternatively, you can do this in a stand mixer fitted with the flat paddle attachment, pulsing on and off.)

Add the wet mixture to the dry ingredients and gently bring together by stirring with a wooden spoon just until combined. Gently pat out the dough on a very lightly floured surface to a 6 x 4-inch (15 x 10 cm) rectangle. Cut into six equal pieces, then gently use your hands to shape each piece into a round biscuit about 1 inch (2.5 cm) thick. Arrange the biscuits, spaced equally apart, on the prepared pan.

Bake for 10 to 15 minutes, or until the tops and bottoms are just tinged with color and the biscuits are baked all the way through. Allow to cool on the pan set on a wire rack, at which point they are ready to use. Alternatively, store at room temperature for up to 8 hours, loosely wrapped in foil.

Prepare the filling: Hull the strawberries. Roughly chop half of them and combine with 3 tablespoons of the sugar in a saucepan. Cook over medium heat, stirring frequently, until the fruit is bubbling and juicy, for about 5 minutes. The juices should darken and concentrate. Remove from the heat and allow to cool completely. Halve or quarter the remaining berries so that they are bite-size. Toss these raw berries with the remaining tablespoon of sugar and the lemon juice in a bowl and allow to sit, stirring occasionally, until the juices exude and the sugar dissolves, for about 15 minutes. Fold the two berry mixtures together. Use immediately, or refrigerate for up to 3 hours in an airtight container.

Right before serving, prepare the topping: Place the cream and sugar in a large bowl, and with an electric mixer on high speed, beat just until the mixture is visibly thickened, then lower the speed and continue to whip just until very soft peaks form. Do not overwhip, or you will lose the silky texture.

Pry the shortcakes in half horizontally with a fork. Place the bottom halves, cut side up, on six dessert plates, or preferably, shallow bowls. Spoon a good quantity of strawberries and juice over the bottom halves, top with a generous dollop of cream, and crown with the top of each biscuit. Allow to sit for about 5 minutes for the juices to penetrate the biscuits. Serve immediately.

KATE'S NOTES

You may be surprised to see heavy cream in this recipe . . . but, good news: When whipped up, the volume of heavy cream nearly doubles and a ½-cup (120 ml) serving of whipped cream is low enough in lactose to be deemed low FODMAP approved. A dollop of whipped cream on these strawberry shortcakes is heavenly! So, have your cake and whipped cream, too!

3-Berry Crisp

    SERVES 16

Fruit crisps are a thing of beauty. They offer the juiciness of a fruit pie with the ease of a one-bowl topping, and preparation time is a mere 10 minutes, max. You can get the crisp ready while the oven preheats. Although our preference is to use fresh fruit, all these low FODMAP berries—blueberries, raspberries, and strawberries—are available frozen. This means you can get your fix even in the dead of winter, if the desire strikes (see Dédé's Tips). This 3-Berry Crisp is great warm, at room temperature, and even for breakfast the next day with a dollop of lactose-free yogurt. Note that there is no sweetener in the filling; we let the lush, fresh fruit flavor shine through.

Nonstick spray

3 cups (300 g) strawberries, hulled and halved

2½ cups (300 g) raspberries

1½ cups (255 g) blueberries

½ cup (1 stick; 113 g) unsalted butter, cut into large pieces

1 cup (213 g) firmly packed light brown sugar

¾ cup (109 g) gluten-free all-purpose flour, such as Bob's Red Mill Gluten Free 1 to 1 Baking Flour

¾ cup (75 g) old-fashioned rolled oats (not quick or instant; use gluten-free if necessary)

½ teaspoon ground cinnamon

¼ teaspoon salt

Position a rack in the middle of the oven. Preheat the oven to 375°F (190°C). Coat a 9-inch (23 cm) ovenproof glass or ceramic pie plate with nonstick spray.

Toss the fruit together in the prepared plate; set aside.

Melt the butter in a medium-size microwave-safe mixing bowl in the microwave on low. (Or melt the butter in a small saucepan on your stove top, if you like, then transfer to a medium-size mixing bowl.) Whisk in the brown sugar, then whisk in the flour, oats, cinnamon, and salt until well combined. Use your hands to help form clumps and scatter them evenly over the fruit. Place the pie plate on a parchment-lined baking sheet to catch any drips.

Bake for 35 to 45 minutes, or until the topping is golden and the fruit is bubbling around the edges. Let sit for 5 minutes before serving, to allow the juices to thicken. The crisp may be served at room temperature, or rewarmed after cooling. Best eaten the day it is made.

DÉDÉ'S TIPS

If you are using frozen fruit, do not defrost before measuring. Just measure straight out of the bag.

KATE'S NOTES

Remember to stick to one fruit serving size per meal—and sometimes that might come packaged up in one of our delicious fruit-based dessert recipes. As you move along the low FODMAP diet after the challenge phase, and perhaps learn you can consume larger serving sizes than we specify in our recipes without any symptoms, then go for it! But in the beginning, try to adhere to the portion sizes we recommend, as they will guide you through successful low FODMAPing.

POST-FODMAP CHALLENGE PHASE OPTION

Fructan: If you passed the fructan wheat challenge, you could use unbleached all-purpose flour or whole wheat pastry flour instead of the gluten-free flour (do not use these substitutions if following a gluten-free diet). Use weight equivalents for the most accurate results with this substitution.

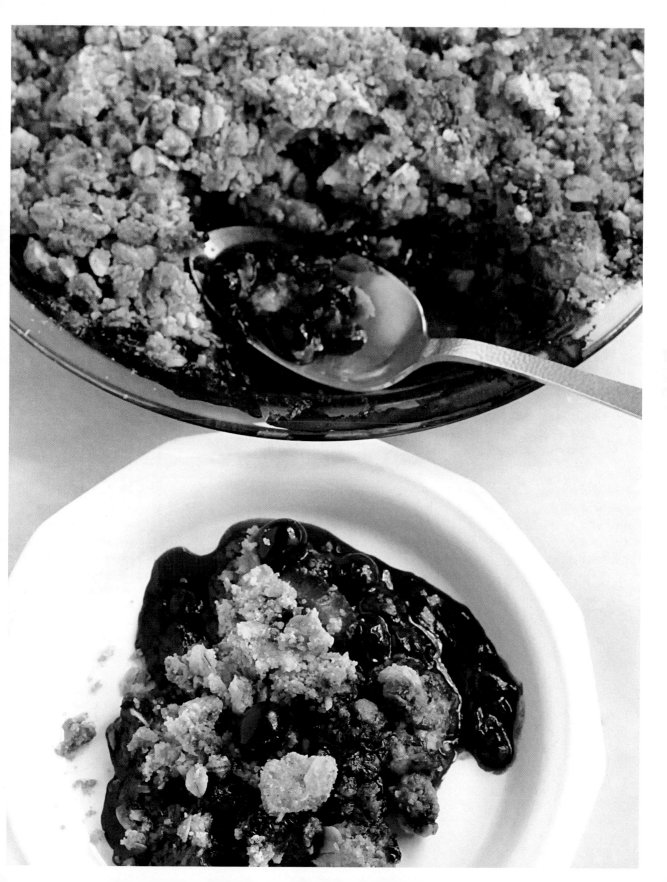

Rich & Creamy Chocolate Pudding

   SERVES 8

This recipe began its life as a classic dairy-packed comfort-food dessert and translated quite nicely to a low FODMAP version using lactose-free milk—if you stick to the portions! While the optional Whipped Cream (page 86) is a nice touch, this pudding is decadent enough without it; your choice.

⅓ cup (29 g) sifted unsweetened natural cocoa powder

⅓ cup (66 g) sugar

2 tablespoons cornstarch

Pinch of salt

2 cups (480 ml) lactose-free milk (whole, 2%, 1%, or fat-free), such as Organic Valley brand, divided

4 ounces (115 g) semisweet or bittersweet chocolate (55% to 61% cacao), finely chopped

1 teaspoon pure vanilla extract

Whipped Cream (page 86; optional)

Have eight ramekins (at least 4 ounces [120 ml] in size), goblets, or glasses ready to receive the pudding.

Whisk together the cocoa powder, sugar, cornstarch, and salt in a medium-size saucepan. Slowly whisk in about 1 cup (240 ml) of the milk until smooth, then whisk in the remaining milk. Bring to a simmer over medium heat (might take about 5 minutes) and simmer for 1 minute, whisking frequently, until thickened. Add the chocolate and whisk frequently for about 1 minute more, or until the chocolate melts and the pudding is thick and smooth. The pudding should be thick enough for the whisk to leave marks in the surface. Remove from the heat, whisk in the vanilla, and then immediately pour into the waiting dishes or goblets.

Allow to cool until almost room temperature, then refrigerate for at least 2 hours or overnight until set. Serve chilled, topped with the whipped cream, if using.

> **POST-FODMAP CHALLENGE PHASE OPTION**
>
> **Lactose:** If you passed the lactose challenge, you can use regular dairy milk (whole milk) instead of the lactose-free milk in this recipe.

Corn Bread

  MAKES ONE 9-INCH (23 CM) PAN | ABOUT 16 SERVINGS

Corn bread can be divisive. It sounds so innocent, and yet there are factions that staunchly believe theirs to be "the best." Broadly speaking, southern style is heartier and drier—a bit more savory. Northern style is more tender, sweeter, and has a lighter texture. Even though Dédé has been developing recipes for thirty years, it is very hard for her to hang her hat on just one corn bread recipe. This version is a fluffier, richer, northern style. We like this because it seems at home next to a bowl of All-Beef Chili (page 294) and works well for breakfast with a dollop of jam. It also lasts a bit longer than the leaner style. We do offer you an option in regard to serving and pan size; see Dédé's Tips.

Nonstick spray

1½ cups (360 ml) lactose-free milk (whole, 2%, 1%, or fat-free), at room temperature

1 tablespoon plus 1 teaspoon freshly squeezed lemon juice

1¾ cups (242 g) fine stone-ground yellow cornmeal

1¼ cups (182 g) gluten-free all-purpose flour, such as Bob's Red Mill Gluten Free 1 to 1 Baking Flour

⅓ cup (66 g) sugar

1 tablespoon plus 1 teaspoon baking powder (use gluten-free if necessary)

1 teaspoon salt

7 tablespoons (99 g) unsalted butter, melted, cooled slightly

2 large eggs, at room temperature

Position a rack in the center of the oven. Preheat the oven to 375°F (190°C). Coat a 9-inch (23 cm) square baking pan with nonstick spray; set aside.

Stir the milk and lemon juice together in a small bowl and allow to sit for 5 minutes to thicken while the oven preheats.

Whisk together the cornmeal, flour, sugar, baking powder, and salt in a large mixing bowl, to aerate and combine. Make a small well in the center and set aside.

Whisk together the thickened milk, melted butter, and eggs until combined. Pour into the well of the dry mixture and whisk together just until combined. Scrape into the prepared pan and spread evenly with a small offset spatula.

Bake for 35 to 40 minutes, or just until a toothpick inserted into the center comes out clean. Allow the pan to cool on a wire rack until just barely warm. The corn bread is ready to cut into squares and serve warm, or allow to cool completely, then wrap with plastic wrap and store at room temperature for up to 2 days. It will become a bit drier upon sitting.

DÉDÉ'S TIPS

When baked in the recommended 9-inch square pan, the resulting corn bread is impressively tall; however, if I want the corn bread to serve a larger group of people, I take a different approach. Crank up the oven to 400°F (200°C) and bake this same batter in a 13 x 9-inch (33 x 23 cm) baking pan for 15 to 20 minutes. The corn bread will not be as tall but is just as delicious. Watch the baking time, as it will be ready much sooner than the square-pan version, so consider this adaptation when time is tight.

You may reduce the sugar to 2 tablespoons, if you want a less sweet version.

POST-FODMAP CHALLENGE PHASE OPTION

Fructan: If you passed the fructan wheat challenge, you could use unbleached all-purpose flour or whole wheat pastry flour instead of the gluten-free flour (do not use these substitutions if following a gluten-free diet), in which case this will be a bit drier. Use weight equivalents for most accurate results with these substitutions.

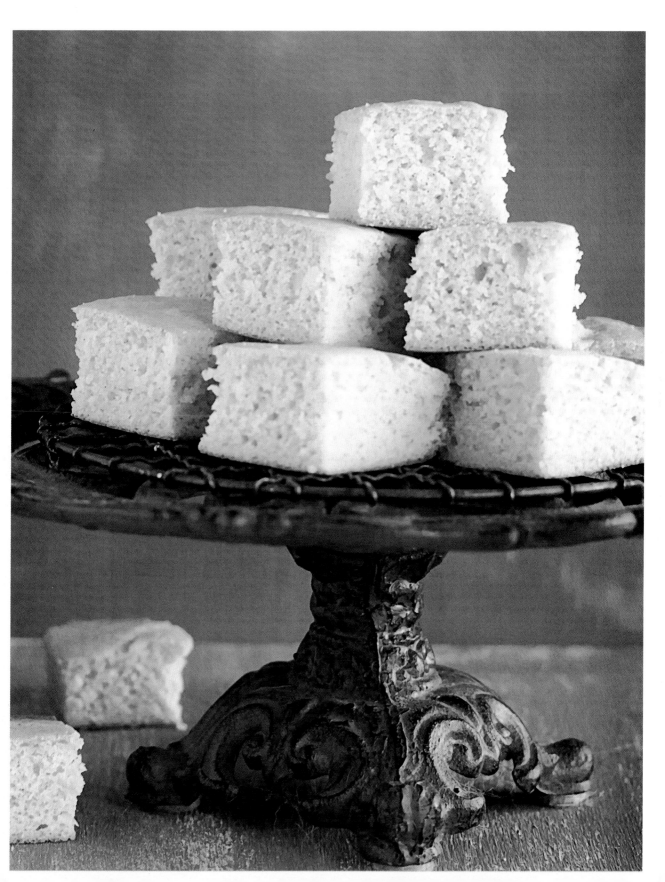

3-Ingredient Coconut Ice Cream

     MAKES ABOUT 1 QUART (960 ML) | SERVING SIZE ⅓ CUP (75 ML)

We debated whether to call this treat ice cream or sorbet. It does not contain dairy (as in milk or cream), so calling it ice cream might be a bit of a misnomer; however, it is so creamy and satisfying in the way that ice cream is, that sorbet didn't seem to fit the bill. Whatever you call it, it couldn't be easier to put together. The three aspects that will affect the final product are your choice of coconut milk, chilling your mixture before freezing, and your ice-cream machine. Thai Kitchen brand coconut milk (the full-fat version) gives great results and we recommend it. This brand contains coconut milk, water, and guar gum. If you are using a different brand, try to find one with the same ingredient list for equivalent results. Make sure to chill your mixture before processing in the ice-cream machine, for best final texture. As far as ice-cream machines go, yes you do need one for this recipe and different machines yield different results, also mostly in the texture of the ice cream. Dédé uses a Cuisinart ICE-100, which makes a very creamy ice cream.

---

2 (13- to 14-ounce [370 to 400 g]) cans pure full-fat unsweetened coconut milk,
   such as Thai Kitchen brand

1 cup (198 g) sugar

1½ teaspoons pure vanilla extract

Whisk together all the ingredients in a medium bowl. Make sure to get all of the thick coconut cream as well as coconut milk out of the cans. Cover the bowl with plastic wrap and refrigerate for at least 6 hours or overnight. Process the mixture in an ice-cream machine according to the manufacturer's instructions. Scrape into an airtight container and freeze until firm. This further develops the ice cream's desirably firm texture. Allow to sit for a minute or two before scooping and serving.

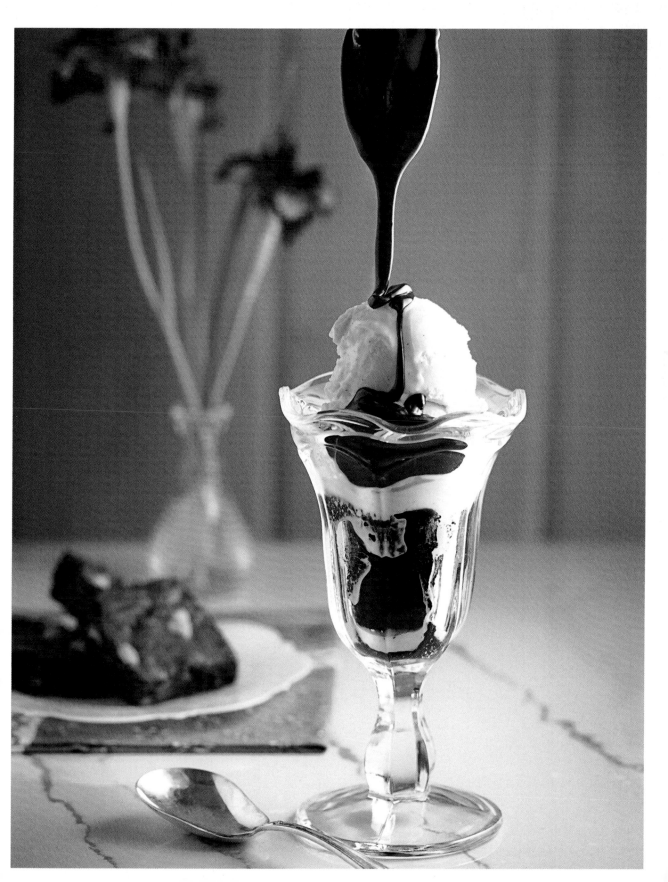

Hot Fudge Sauce

    MAKES ABOUT 2 CUPS (480 ML) | SERVING SIZE 2 TABLESPOONS

This is a classic hot fudge sauce—thick, sticky, and oh, so chocolaty—reimagined for a low FODMAP diet. You might be surprised to see the Lyle's Golden Syrup and light corn syrup. Golden syrup is a liquid sweetener with the incredible flavor of toffee and it is an approved low FODMAP ingredient in 1½-teaspoon servings. It is a refined sugar product, as is the corn syrup (which is not the same as high-fructose corn syrup). If you can find the Lyle's, it adds a complexity to the sauce and is worth the inclusion. Please pay attention to serving size. Whether you are a FODMAPer or not, too much of a good thing is not necessarily better.

---

1 cup (240 ml) canned pure light coconut milk, such as Thai Kitchen brand

1 cup (198 g) sugar

¼ cup (60 ml) Lyle's Golden Syrup or light corn syrup

6 ounces (170 g) semisweet chocolate, finely chopped

4 ounces (115 g) unsweetened chocolate, finely chopped

3 tablespoons unsalted butter, at room temperature, cut into ½-inch (12 mm) pieces

¼ cup (21 g) sifted Dutch-processed cocoa powder

1 teaspoon pure vanilla extract

Pinch of salt

Whisk together the coconut milk, sugar, and golden syrup in a medium-size, heavy-bottomed saucepan.

Cook over medium heat, stirring occasionally, until the sugar dissolves and the mixture comes to a boil, for about 5 minutes total. Lower the heat and simmer for 1 minute. Remove from the heat and stir in the semisweet and unsweetened chocolate and butter. Let sit for 1 to 2 minutes for the residual heat to melt the chocolate and butter. Stir until smooth. Whisk in the cocoa powder slowly to prevent lumping. Whisk in the vanilla and salt. Allow to cool slightly and the hot fudge is ready to use, or scrape into an airtight container and refrigerate for up to 3 weeks. May be reheated on the stove top over low heat or in the microwave on low, which is our preferred method.

KATE'S NOTES

Golden syrup is high FODMAP for 1 tablespoon but low at ½ tablespoon. Stick to the 2-tablespoon serving size for the fudge sauce and you are well within the FODMAP cutoffs.

Dark Caramel Sauce

       MAKES ABOUT 2 CUPS (480 ML) | SERVING SIZE 2 TABLESPOONS

Caramel comes in a range of colors and flavors from light and faint to dark and bold. This is on the bolder end of the spectrum, but you can vary it to your liking by simply going by color (you will see what we mean in the recipe. For a lighter-flavored caramel, simply do not cook the clear caramel as long). No need for a thermometer here! After making a basic caramel with sugar and water, heavy cream is usually added, but for our low FODMAP version we have used canned coconut milk. The only trick here is to use the style of pot as described. Don't miss the variation for Salted Dark Caramel Sauce at the end.

---

2 cups (396 g) sugar

½ cup (120 ml) water

1 cup (240 ml) canned pure full-fat coconut milk, such as Thai Kitchen brand, well shaken, at room temperature

Place the sugar and water in a light-colored, deep, heavy-bottomed saucepan (we use a 4-quart [3.8 L] stainless-steel pot. A dark-colored pot will not allow you to see the color of the caramel). Stir to moisten the sugar and cook over medium-high heat, without stirring, until the syrup begins to color, for 5 to 10 minutes. Wash down the sides of the pot once or twice with a damp pastry brush, if necessary.

When the syrup is a medium amber color, watch closely, as the color will deepen quickly. Within the next minute or so, the caramel will turn a very dark mahogany brown, the bubbles will turn tan in color, and wisps of smoke might appear. Immediately remove from the heat and swirl the pot to dissipate the heat.

Slowly pour in the coconut milk. The mixture may bubble up furiously; the deep pot will protect you from overflow. Just let the bubbling subside and whisk until smooth. If the coconut milk is too cool, it will cause the caramel to seize. Just place the pot back over low heat and stir until the sauce liquefies.

Allow to cool to room temperature. Refrigerate in an airtight container for up to 1 month. Reheat in a double boiler or the microwave on low before using. Perfect over ice cream, cake, or for eating off a spoon.

> **DÉDÉ'S TIPS**
>
> For Salted Dark Caramel Sauce, simply stir in ½ teaspoon of kosher salt or fleur de sel at the end. Taste and add more if you like. I also like to sprinkle some large flake-style salt, such as Maldon or more fleur de sel, on whatever I am serving with this version of the sauce.

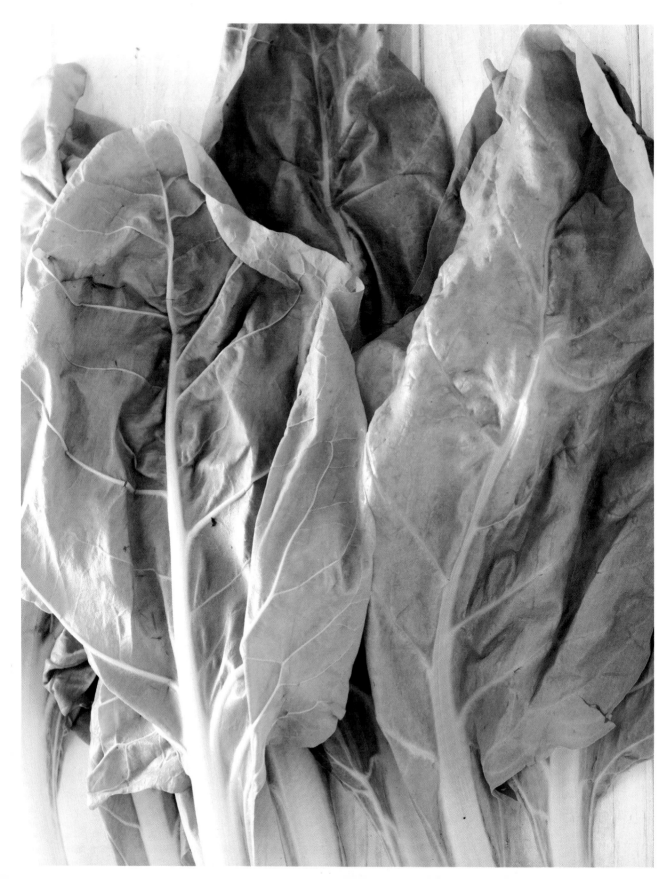

RESOURCES

Bob's Red Mill
www.bobsredmill.com
Toll-free (USA): (800) 349-2173
Telephone: (503) 607-6455
You can find many gluten-free and low
FODMAP grains and products through
this mail-order resource, including Dédé's
favorite, Gluten-Free 1 to 1 Baking Flour.
Also look for Bob's Red Mill products in
well-stocked supermarkets.

Boyajian Incorporated
www.boyajianinc.com
customerservice@boyajianinc.com
Toll-free (USA): (800) 965-0665
Telephone: (781) 828-9966
For Alaska and Hawaii, please call to order.
Boyajian makes many flavored oils, sweet
(lemon and orange, for instance) as well
as savory (garlic, various herbs). Its Garlic
Oil is based on olive oil and comes in three
sizes, from 8 ounces (240 ml) to 25.4 ounces
(752 ml).

Casa de Santé
https://casadesante.com
A variety of spice blends, including BBQ
Rub, Indian Spicy Hot, Italian Tuscan
Herb, Lemon Herb, Mexican Mix, artisan
savory granola, and low FODMAP stock,
many items are certified low FODMAP by
FODMAP Friendly.

Cuisinart
www.cuisinart.com
Toll-free (USA): (800) 211-9604
The recipes were tested using a Prep 11
Plus 11-cup food processor, which comes in
handy when grating large amounts of cheese
or carrots, such as for carrot cake.

Cuisipro
www.cuisipro.com
Toll-free (USA): (866) 849-4715
This company makes very high-quality,
properly calibrated stainless-steel measuring
cups and spoons as well as excellent graters
of all sizes.

FODY Food Co.
www.fodyfoods.com
Certified low FODMAP food products. A variety of convenience products from salsa and marinara to trail mix and bars for on the go, all certified low FODMAP by Monash University.

King Arthur Flour
The Baker's Catalogue
www.kingarthurflour.com
Toll free (USA): (800) 827-6836
King Arthur offers high-quality measuring cups (including ones in odd sizes) as well as scales, baking pans, and other high-quality baking ingredients and implements.

KitchenAid
www.kitchenaid.com
Toll-free (USA): (800) 541-6390 (small appliance information)
Look no further for quality stand mixers in a variety of sizes. These recipes were tested with a 5-quart size.

La Tourangelle
www.latourangelle.com
Toll-free (USA): (866) NUT-OILS
Telephone (USA): (510) 970-9960
This company makes a true garlic-infused oil with sunflower seed oil as the base, and all the ingredients are organic. Perfect for sautéing and high-heat cooking and comes packed in a well-designed lightproof can with easy-pour spout.

Lodge Cast Iron
www.lodgemfg.com
Telephone (USA): (423) 837-7181
Grill pans, cast-iron pans, and enameled cast-iron Dutch ovens from a Tennessee company founded in 1896. Their preseasoned cast-iron pans are inexpensive, a joy to use, and will last literally more than a lifetime.

O Roasted Garlic Olive Oil
www.ooliveoil.com
Toll-free (USA): (888) 827-7148
Telephone (USA): (707) 766-1755
This company makes excellent oils and vinegars. Garlic is roasted with vegetable oil and nothing else. The resulting garlic-flavored oil is used to flavor the olive oil.

Penzeys Spices
www.penzeys.com
customerservice@penzeys.com
Toll-free (USA): (800) 741-7787
Look to this company for its comprehensive selection of herbs and spices (and other items, such as poppy seeds) and excellent customer service. Freshness with spices and herbs is key in our low FODMAP kitchen for maximum flavor.

Savory Choice
www.savorychoice.com
Chicken and beef stock made with low FODMAP ingredients. Comes in a concentrate that dissolves easily in water to make just the amount you need. We like the reduced-sodium versions.

Vitamix
www.vitamix.com
service@vitamix.com
Toll-free (USA): (800) 848-2649
International: +1 (440) 235-4840
High-performance blenders. Dédé uses a 5200 model in the test kitchen. These are

expensive machines, but they are built to last and the company offers refurbished models at a discount.

Williams-Sonoma
www.williams-sonoma.com
Toll-free (USA): (800) 541-2233
Famous for its mail-order catalog, the company also has stores nationwide. You will find well-made, accurate measuring cups and spoons and digital scales as well as many other high-quality kitchen tools.

Zeroll
www.zeroll.com
sales@zeroll.com
Toll-free (USA): (800) 872-5000
Be sure to check out its Universal EZ Disher, which is a scoop with a springlike action (although there are no springs to break). Available in various sizes, they are perfect for making uniform meatballs (page 249) and cookies and for getting muffin and cupcake batter into pans. And as portion control is so important, we find them handy when cooking low FODMAP. We recommend the #40 for a few recipes in the book, which makes a portion about the size of a golf ball. They also make an incomparable ice-cream scoop.

NUTRITION AND HEALTH WEBSITES AND ADDITIONAL RESOURCES

FODMAPS

For a Digestive Peace of Mind
www.katescarlata.com
Kate Scarlata RDN, LDN, FODMAP and Gut Health expert educational blog and website

Kate Scarlata Low FODMAP Grocery Guide app
https://itunes.apple.com/us/app/fodmap-grocery-guide/id1220227921?mt=8

FODMAP Everyday
FODMAPeveryday.com
Dédé's FODMAP educational and lifestyle brand and website

IBS-Free at Last
www.ibsfree.net
Patsy Catsos, MS, RDN LD, expert website

Monash University
www.med.monash.edu/cecs/gastro/fodmap/
Monash University low FODMAP diet app
www.med.monash.edu/cecs/gastro/fodmap/iphone-app.html

My Nutrition GI Health
www.myginutrition.com/index.html

FUNCTIONAL GUT DISORDERS

International Foundation for Functional Gastrointestinal Disorders
www.iffgd.org

ALLERGIES

The Food Allergy and Anaphylaxis Network
www.foodallergy.org

American Academy of Allergy Asthma and Immunology (AAAAI)
www.aaaai.org

CELIAC DISEASE

Gluten Intolerance Group
www.gluten.net

Celiac Disease Foundation
www.celiac.org

Beth Israel Deaconess Medical Center,
Celiac Center
www.celiacnow.org

INFLAMMATORY BOWEL DISEASE

Crohn's and Colitis Foundation
of America
www.ccfa.org

US Probiotic Guide
http://usprobioticguide.com
This site provides details about probiotic
brands and indications for use. It is also
available in app form for your mobile device.

NOTES

Chapter 1

1. "Functional GI Disorders," http://iffgd.org/gi-disorders/functional-gi-disorders.html, accessed June 30, 2016.
2. "Statistics," www.aboutibs.org/facts-about-ibs/statistics.html, accessed July 18, 2016.
3. "IBS in Men," www.aboutibs.org/what-is-ibs/ibs-in-men-2.html, accessed July 18, 2016.
4. R. H. de Roest, B. R. Dobbs, B. A. Chapman, B. Batman, L. A. O'Brien, J. A. Leeper, C. R. Hebblethwaite, and R. B. Gearry, "The Low FODMAP Diet Improves Gastrointestinal Symptoms in Patients with Irritable Bowel Syndrome: A Prospective Study," *International Journal of Clinical Practice* 67, no. 9 (2013): 895–903; E. P. Halmos, V. A. Power, S. J. Shepherd, P. R. Gibson, and J. G. Muir, "A Diet Low in FODMAPs Reduces Symptoms of Irritable Bowel Syndrome," *Gastroenterology* 146, no. 1 (2014): 67–75.
5. H. B. El-Serag, S. Sweet, C. C. Winchester, J. and Dent, "Update on the Epidemiology of Gastro-oesophageal Reflux Disease: A Systematic Review," Gut 63, no. 6 (2014): 871–880.
6. T. Piche, D. B. des Varnnes, S. Sacher-Huvelin, J. J. Holst, J. C. Cuber, and J. P. Galmiche, "Colonic Fermentation Influences Lower Esophageal Sphincter Function in Gastroesophageal Reflux Disease, *Gastroenterology* 124, no. 4 (2003): 894–902.
7. R. B. Gearry, P. M. Irving, J. S. Barrett, D. M. Nathan, S. J. Shepherd, and P. R. Gibson PR, "Reduction of Dietary Poorly Absorbed Short-Chain Carbohydrates (FODMAPs) Improves Abdominal Symptoms in Patients with Inflammatory Bowel Disease—A Pilot Study," *Journal of Crohn's and Colitis* 3, no. 1 (2009): 8–14.
8. B. Chassaing, O. Koren, J. Goodrich, A. Poole, S. Srinivasan, R. E. Ley, and A. T. Gewirtz, "Dietary Emulsifiers Impact the Mouse Gut Microbiota Promoting Colitis and Metabolic Syndrome," *Nature* 519, no. 7541 (2015): 92–96.

9. Celiac Disease Facts and Figures," www.uchospitals.edu/pdf/uch_007937.pdf, accessed June 30, 2016.

10. J. R. Biesiekierski, S. L. Peters, E. D. Newnham, O. Rosella, J. G. Muir, and P. R. Gibson, "No Effects of Gluten in Patients with Self Reported Non-Celiac Gluten Sensitivity After Dietary Restriction of Fermentable, Poorly Absorbed, Short-Chain Carbohydrates," Gastroenterology 145 (2013): 320–328.

11. D. Piacentino, S. Rossi, L. Piretta, D. Badiali, N. Pallotta, and E. S. Corazziari, "Low FODMAP Diet in Irritable Bowel Syndrome Offers Benefit Not Only in Terms of Gastrointestinal Symptoms, but Also in Terms of Psychopathology in the Medium and Long Term," *European Psychology* 33 (2016): suppl. 395.

12. Halmos et al., "A Diet Low in FODMAPs."

Chapter 2

1. K. McIntosh, D. E. Reed, T. Schneider, F. Dang, A. H. Keshteli, G. De Palma, K. Madsen, P. Bercik, and S. Vanner, "FODMAPs Alter Symptoms and the Metabolome of Patients with IBS: A Randomized Controlled Trial," *Gut* (2016), ePub March 14, 2016.

2. www.who.int/foodsafety/fs_management/en/probiotic_guidelines.pdf, accessed June 5, 2017.

Chapter 3

1. http://www.nationalacademies.org/hmd/~/media/Files/Activity%20Files/Nutrition/DRIs/DRI_Macronutrients.pdf, accessed July 25, 2016; S. Eswaran, J. Muir, and W. D. Chey, "Fiber and Functional Gastrointestinal Disorders," *American Journal of Gastroenterology* 108, no. 5 (2013): 718–727.

ACKNOWLEDGMENTS

KATE SCARLATA

I want to thank my family, my husband, Russ; daughter, Chelsea; and sons, Kevin and Brennan, for putting up with my long hours of work on this manuscript and for their constant love and support. A big thanks to Sara Caton, my office manager and running buddy, who helps keep me organized, smiling, and healthier. If not for the generous help of the Monash University low FOD-MAP research team, I would not be the FODMAP expert I am today. Not only do I value their innovative research, I appreciate their willingness to answer my countless questions. I am particularly thankful for Dr. Jane Muir, on whom I relied heavily as I learned about this novel nutritional approach. Thank you to my colleagues, Bill Chey, MD; Mark Pimentel, MD; Gerry Mullin, MD; Allison Siebecker, ND; and Patsy Catsos, MS, RDN, who have been indispensable collaborators with me. And last but not least, a big thanks to literary agent, Marilyn Allen, who has been a great support and advocate throughout the publishing process.

DÉDÉ WILSON

I want to thank my husband, Damon Herring, who absolutely knew and believed that my recipe development career would continue, even after we recognized that I had to change my entire relationship with food. I am truly appreciative of my daughter Ravenna; her partner, Alvin; and my son Forrester, all of whom have been treading the low FODMAP waters with me, and feeling better for it. My son Freeman took on the task of catering our wedding with an entire low FODMAP menu and did it in style. We are all in the food business and these experiences proved to me that eating low FODMAP could be integrated in one's life in a real, meaningful, and delectable way and gave me the creative spark that resulted in this book. Thank you to my agent, Marilyn Allen, who assured us from the start that our book would find a great home. I am grateful to my connection with Jane Muir, Marina Iacovou, Elizabeth Ly and the entire Monash University FODMAP Initiative team. Your work is bringing a new lease on life to millions of people and I am humbled and excited to be part of this journey. I am also extremely excited about my new relationship with the folks from FODY Foods: Steven J. Singer, Sean Surkis, and Delaney Brown, who are working hard to make sure all of us have great low FODMAP food to eat! And to Robin Jaffin, my business partner at FODMAPeveryday.com—you are the best collaborator one could hope for. Our complementarity continues to astound me and I have immense gratitude for your presence in my life.

INDEX